W9-BMZ-407

## Eating Your Vitamins

### Vitamin A

*Preformed*
Beef liver
Fatty fish (mackerel)
Milk
Egg yolks
Cheese

### Beta Carotene

Peaches
Sweet potatoes
Carrots
Spinach
Acorn squash

### B Vitamins:

### Thiamin

Wheat germ
Ham
Beef liver
Peanuts
Green peas

### Riboflavin

Beef liver
Milk
Yogurt
Avocados
Collard greens

### Niacin

Chicken
Salmon
Beef
Peanut butter
Potatoes

### Pyridoxine

Bananas
Avocados
Beef
Chicken
Fish

### Folic Acid

Beef liver
Spinach
Orange juice
Romaine lettuce
Beets

### Cobalamin

Beef liver
Clams
Tuna
Yogurt
Milk

### Biotin

Beef liver
Almonds
Peanut butter
Eggs
Oat bran

### Pantothenic Acid

Beef liver
Eggs
Avocados
Mushrooms
Milk

### Vitamin C

Oranges
Brussels sprouts
Strawberries
Broccoli
Collard greens

### Vitamin D

Canned sardines
Mackerel
Herring
Shrimp
Fortified milk

### Vitamin E

Wheat germ oil
Safflower oil
Sunflower oil
Spinach
Wheat germ

### Vitamin K

Turnip greens
Broccoli
Cabbage
Spinach
Beef liver

alpha
books

# Eating Your Minerals

## Calcium
Yogurt
Canned sardines
Milk
Cheese
Tofu

## Magnesium
Peanuts
Bananas
Avocados
Milk
Collard greens

## Phosphorus
Beef liver
Yogurt
Chicken
Milk
Eggs

## Potassium
Avocados
Bananas
Potatoes
Milk
Beans

## Chromium
Corn kernels
Beef
Apples
Sweet potatoes
Eggs

## Copper
Oysters
Lobster
Beef liver
Avocados
Potatoes

## Iodine
Iodized table salt
Milk
Eggs
Cheese
Nuts

## Iron
Beef liver
Blackstrap molasses
Raisins
Beans
Spinach

## Manganese
Tea
Raisins
Spinach
Carrots
Broccoli

## Selenium
Organ meats
Seafood
Lean beef
Chicken
Brazil nuts

## Zinc
Oysters
Dark-meat turkey
Lean meats
Beans
Almonds

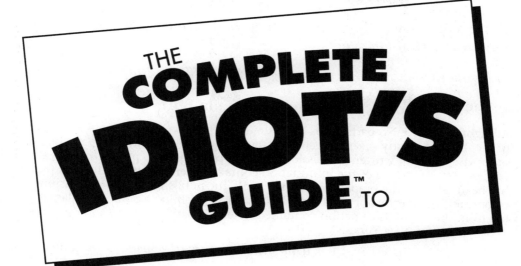

# THE COMPLETE IDIOT'S GUIDE™ TO

# Vitamins and Minerals

*by Dr. Alan H. Pressman*
*with Sheila Buff*

## alpha books

A Division of Macmillan General Reference
A Simon and Schuster Macmillan Company
1633 Broadway, New York, NY 10019-6705

*To my son Corey and my daughter Meghan because they are my life.*
*—Alan H. Pressman*

*In loving memory of Grace Darling Griffin.—Sheila Buff*

## © 1997 by Alan H. Pressman and Sheila Buff

THE COMPLETE IDIOT'S GUIDE name and design are trademarks of Macmillan, Inc.

International Standard Book Number: 0-02-862116-6
Library of Congress Catalog Card Number: 97-80861

99  98      4  3

Interpretation of the printing code: the rightmost number of the first series of numbers is the year of the book's printing; the rightmost number of the second series of numbers is the number of the book's printing. For example, a printing code of 97-1 shows that the first printing occurred in 1997.

**Executive Editor**
*Gary M. Krebs*

**Managing Editor**
*Robert Shuman*

**Senior Editor**
*Nancy Mikhail*

**Development Editor**
*Joan Paterson*

**Production Editor**
*Linda Seifert*

**Technical Editor**
*Carl Germano, RD, CNS, LDN*

**Copy Editor**
*Patricia A. Solberg*

**Editorial Assistant**
*Maureen Horn*

**Illustrator**
*Judd Winick*

**Designer**
*Glenn Larsen*

**Cover Designer**
*Kevin Spears*

**Indexer**
*Joelynn Gifford*

**Production Team**
*Kim Cofer*
*Kristy Nash*
*Nicole M. R. Ritch*

# Contents at a Glance

**Part 1: The Vital Keys to Good Health**                                  **1**

  1  The Alphabet Soup of Nutrition                              3
      *What all those letters mean—and why you need them all.*

  2  Choosing What's Right for You                             15
      *Read this before you go to the vitamin store!*

**Part 2: The A to K of Vitamins**                                          **27**

  3  Vitamin A and Carotenes: Double-Barreled Health
     Protection                                                29
      *Why Bugs Bunny has such great eyesight.*

  4  Meet the B Family                                         45
      *Family togetherness means better health.*

  5  Thiamin: The Basic B                                      57
      *The grandaddy of the B family.*

  6  B Energetic: Riboflavin                                   65
      *Burn off energy with this bouncing B.*

  7  Niacin: Cholesterol B Gone                                73
      *The B that boots out cholesterol.*

  8  Pyridoxine: Have a Healthy Heart                          85
      *Keep your heart beating beautifully with this B.*

  9  Folic Acid: Healthy Babies, Healthy Hearts               95
      *The breakthrough B that's good for young and old.*

 10  Cobalamin: The B for Healthy Blood                       107
      *Are you sure you've got enough?*

 11  Pantothenic Acid: It's Everywhere                        115
      *The B you can't run low on.*

 12  The Unofficial B Vitamins                                121
      *Biotin, choline, inositol, and PABA: When is a B not a B?*

 13  Vitamin C: The Champion                                  129
      *If there's a miracle vitamin or a cure for the common cold,*
      *this is it.*

 14  Vitamin D: Look on the Sunny Side                        149
      *Life's a beach when it comes to this vitamin.*

 15  Vitamin E: E for Excellent                               157
      *Tops on the vitamin report card.*

 16  Vitamin K: The Band-Aid in Your Blood                    169
      *Getting you through life's rough spots.*

**Part 3: Minerals: The Elements of Good Health**     **175**

17   Calcium: Drink Your Milk!     177
      *It's not just for kids—grownups need strong bones, too.*

18   Magnesium: Magnificent for Your Heart     195
      *Also magnificent for migraines, blood pressure, asthma, and
      more.*

19   Zinc: Immune System Booster     207
      *Think zinc for colds, wound healing, and prostate problems.*

20   Electrolytes: Keeping Your Body in Balance     215
      *The electrifying news about potassium, sodium, and chloride.*

21   The Trace Minerals: A Little Goes a Long Way     225
      *Did you know you need molybdenum?*

**Part 4: Exploring Other Supplements**     **243**

22   Amino Acids: The Building Blocks of Life     245
      *How you make 50,000 proteins from just 22 amino acids.*

23   Essential Fatty Acids: When Is Fat Good?     259
      *When it's fishy or flaxy.*

24   Super Antioxidants     271
      *Win the free radical battle with these power supplements.*

25   Flavonoids for Humanoids     277
      *If it's orange, eat it—then have a cup of tea, some blueberries,
      and a few garlic cloves.*

26   Coenzyme $Q_{10}$: Cellular Spark Plug     289
      *Natural energy for heart patients.*

27   Help from Natural Hormones     295
      *Melatonin, genistein, DHEA—what's this stuff really all
      about?*

28   Fiber: Moving Things Along     303
      *High fiber means high health.*

A   Quick Reference Chart of Ailments and Suggested
      Supplements     317

B   Resources     319

C   Glossary     325

    Index     337

# Contents

**Part 1: The Vital Keys to Good Health**    **1**

**1 The Alphabet Soup of Nutrition**    **3**

Vitamins: Why They're Vital ................................................ 4
     Fat-Soluble Vitamins................................................ 4
     Water-Soluble Vitamins............................................. 4
How Much Do You Need?...................................................... 5
     The Measure of Good Health ....................................... 6
Beyond the Basics ........................................................ 6
Minerals: Essential Elements of Health .................................. 7
     Minerals ......................................................... 7
     Trace Minerals .................................................... 8
Do You Need Vitamin and Mineral Supplements? ........................... 9
On the Edge: Marginal Deficiencies ..................................... 10
The Antioxidant Revolution .............................................. 12
Radicals on the Loose ................................................... 12
Fighting Back with Antioxidants ........................................ 12
The Least You Need to Know .............................................. 13

**2 Choosing What's Right for You**    **15**

Who Decides This Stuff, Anyway? ......................................... 16
What Are Your Needs? .................................................... 17
     Tests for Vitamin and Mineral Deficiencies ..................... 18
Nutritionally Oriented Health Care ..................................... 19
Vitamins and Minerals for Everyone ..................................... 19
Special Needs of Older Adults .......................................... 20
Vitamins for Kids and Teens ............................................ 21
Vitamins for Vegetarians ............................................... 22
Supplements and Common Health Problems ................................. 22
     High Cholesterol ................................................ 22
     High Blood Pressure.............................................. 23
     Diabetes ........................................................ 24
Getting the Most from Vitamin and Mineral
   Supplements .......................................................... 24
     Taking Your Vitamins............................................. 26
The Least You Need to Know .............................................. 26

## Part 2: The A to K of Vitamins

**27**

### 3 Vitamin A and Carotenes: Double-Barreled Health Protection

**29**

Why You Need Vitamin A ............................................................ 30
Why You Need Carotenes Even More ...................................... 30
The RDA for Vitamin A .............................................................. 32
    Measuring Vitamin A ............................................................ 32
    Vitamin A Cautions .............................................................. 34
    Beta Carotene Cautions ....................................................... 35
    Carotenes and CARET ......................................................... 35
Are You Deficient? ..................................................................... 35
Eating Your A's .......................................................................... 37
Getting the Most from Vitamin A and Carotenes ................. 39
Which Type Should I Take? ...................................................... 40
Bugs Bunny Had Great Eyesight ............................................. 41
    Preventing Night Blindness ................................................ 41
    Preventing Cataracts ........................................................... 41
    Preserving Eyesight .............................................................. 41
A as in Aging Skin ..................................................................... 42
To Beta or Not to Beta ............................................................... 42
Carotenes and Cardiac Cases ................................................... 43
Boosting Your Immunity with Vitamin A ............................. 43
The Least You Need to Know ................................................... 44

### 4 Meet the B Family

**45**

One Big Happy Family .............................................................. 46
    What the Little Numbers Mean .......................................... 47
    The Unofficial B's ................................................................. 47
RDAs for B Vitamins ................................................................. 48
Are You Deficient? ..................................................................... 50
Eating Your B's .......................................................................... 51
Getting the Most from B Vitamins .......................................... 52
The Three B's for Heart Health ................................................ 53
Aging and the B Vitamins ........................................................ 53
Don't Worry, B Happy .............................................................. 54
Boosting Your Immune System ............................................... 54
The Least You Need to Know ................................................... 55

### 5 Thiamin: The Basic B

**57**

Why You Need Thiamin ............................................................ 58
The RDA for Thiamin ................................................................ 58

Are You Deficient? ................................................................ 59
Eating Your Thiamin ............................................................ 60
Getting the Most from Thiamin ........................................... 62
Protecting Your Heart .......................................................... 62
Thiamin and Diabetes .......................................................... 63
Thiamin and Canker Sores ................................................... 63
The Least You Need to Know ............................................... 63

**6  B Energetic: Riboflavin                                    65**

Why You Need Riboflavin ..................................................... 66
The RDA for Riboflavin ........................................................ 66
Are You Deficient? ................................................................ 67
Eating Your Riboflavin ......................................................... 68
Getting the Most from Riboflavin ........................................ 69
Producing Energy ................................................................. 70
Faster, Higher, Stronger ...................................................... 70
Preventing Migraines ........................................................... 70
Riboflavin and Your Eyes ..................................................... 71
The Least You Need to Know ............................................... 72

**7  Niacin: Cholesterol B Gone                               73**

Why You Need Niacin ........................................................... 74
The RDA for Niacin .............................................................. 74
Are You Deficient? ................................................................ 76
Eating Your Niacin ............................................................... 77
Getting the Most from Niacin .............................................. 79
Producing Energy ................................................................. 79
Lowering High Cholesterol .................................................. 80
    Boy, Was My Face Red ..................................................... 81
Niacin and Diabetes ............................................................. 82
Other Problems Helped by Niacin ....................................... 82
The Least You Need to Know ............................................... 83

**8  Pyridoxine: Have a Healthy Heart                        85**

Why You Need Pyridoxine ..................................................... 86
The RDA for Pyridoxine ........................................................ 86
Are You Deficient? ................................................................ 87
Eating Your Pyridoxine ........................................................ 88
Getting the Most from Pyridoxine ....................................... 89
Help for Heart Disease ......................................................... 90
Immune Booster ................................................................... 91
Helping Asthmatics .............................................................. 91
Preventing Diabetic Complications ..................................... 92

Relief for Carpal Tunnel Syndrome.......................... 92
Pyridoxine for PMS.................................................. 93
Other Problems and Pyridoxine .............................. 93
The Least You Need to Know .................................. 94

## 9 Folic Acid: Healthy Babies, Healthy Hearts        95

Why You Need Folic Acid ...................................... 96
The RDA for Folic Acid .......................................... 96
Are You Deficient?.................................................. 97
Eating Your Folic Acid .......................................... 99
Getting the Most from Folic Acid ........................ 101
Folic Acid for Healthy Babies .............................. 102
Folic Acid Forestalls Heart Disease ...................... 103
Preventing Cancer with Folic Acid...................... 104
   Folic Acid Helps Prevent Colon Cancer ...................... 104
   Preventing Cervical Cancer .......................... 104
Folic Acid and Depression .................................... 104
The Least You Need to Know ................................ 105

## 10 Cobalamin: The B for Healthy Blood        107

Why You Need Cobalamin .................................... 108
The RDA for Cobalamin ........................................ 108
Are You Deficient?................................................ 109
Who's at Risk?...................................................... 110
Eating Your Cobalamin ........................................ 112
Getting the Most from Cobalamin ........................ 113
The Least You Need to Know ................................ 114

## 11 Pantothenic Acid: It's Everywhere        115

Why You Need Pantothenic Acid .......................... 116
Safe and Adequate Intake .................................... 116
Are You Deficient?................................................ 117
Eating Your Pantothenic Acid .............................. 117
Getting the Most from Pantothenic Acid .............. 118
Helping High Cholesterol .................................... 118
Pantothenic Acid for Pentathletes ........................ 118
Quack, Quack, QUACK! ........................................ 119
The Least You Need to Know ................................ 119

## 12 The Unofficial B Vitamins        121

When Is a B Not a B?............................................ 121
Biotin: The B from Your Body .............................. 122

Getting Your Biotin ............................................................ 122
Are You Deficient? ............................................................. 123
Eating Your Biotin .............................................................. 123
Biotin for Your Hair and Nails ......................................... 124
Choline: Brain Food ................................................................ 124
Eating Your Choline ........................................................... 125
Choline for Your Liver ...................................................... 125
Help for Alzheimer's Disease? ......................................... 125
Choosing a Choline Supplement ..................................... 125
Inositol: Choline's Close Cousin .......................................... 126
PABA: Protecting Your Skin .................................................. 126
The Least You Need to Know ................................................. 127

**13  Vitamin C: The Champion                               129**

Why You Need Vitamin C ...................................................... 130
The RDA for Vitamin C .......................................................... 130
Are You Deficient? ................................................................. 132
Eating Your C's ...................................................................... 134
Getting the Most from Vitamin C ........................................ 138
Which Type Should I Take? ................................................... 139
Front-Line Antioxidant ......................................................... 141
Preventing Cardiovascular Disease ..................................... 141
Lowering Cholesterol Levels ............................................ 142
Lowering Blood Pressure .................................................. 142
Enhancing Your Immune System ........................................ 142
Curing the Common Cold .................................................. 143
Healing Wounds and Recovering from Surgery ................. 143
Fighting Allergies and Asthma ............................................ 144
Fighting Asthma Attacks ................................................... 144
Diabetes and Vitamin C ........................................................ 145
Cancer and Vitamin C ........................................................... 145
Preventing Cancer .............................................................. 145
Curing Cancer .................................................................... 146
Treating Cancer ................................................................. 146
Making Babies with Vitamin C ............................................ 146
C-ing Is Believing ................................................................. 147
Other Health Problems Helped by Vitamin C .................... 147
The Least You Need to Know ................................................. 148

**14  Vitamin D: Look on the Sunny Side                     149**

Why You Need Vitamin D ...................................................... 149
The Sunshine Vitamin ........................................................... 150
The RDA for Vitamin D .......................................................... 151

Are You D-ficient? ............................................................ 151
Eating Your D's ............................................................... 153
Getting the Most from Vitamin D ................................... 154
Vitamin D and Cancer .................................................... 155
Other Health Problems Helped by Vitamin D ................. 155
    Helping Psoriasis ......................................................... 156
    Helping Your Hearing ................................................. 156
The Least You Need to Know ........................................... 156

**15 Vitamin E: E for Excellent**             **157**

Why You Need Vitamin E ................................................ 157
The Alpha, Beta, and Gamma of E .................................. 158
The RDA for Vitamin E .................................................... 159
Are You Deficient? .......................................................... 160
Eating Your E's ............................................................... 160
Getting the Most from Vitamin E .................................... 161
    Natural or Synthetic? ................................................... 162
    I'm All Mixed Up ........................................................ 162
    Wet or Dry? ................................................................ 162
    What About Selenium? ................................................ 163
E-vading Heart Disease ................................................... 163
Is It Really that E-Z? ....................................................... 164
E-luding Cancer .............................................................. 165
Excellent for the Elderly ................................................. 165
Other Health Problems Helped by Vitamin E ................. 166
The Least You Need to Know ........................................... 167

**16 Vitamin K: The Band-Aid in Your Blood**     **169**

Why You Need Vitamin K ................................................ 170
The RDA for Vitamin K .................................................... 170
Are You Deficient? .......................................................... 171
Eating Your K's ............................................................... 172
Getting the Most from Vitamin K .................................... 173
Vitamin K and Clotting ................................................... 174
Vitamin K and Osteoporosis ........................................... 174
K Kills Cancer Cells ........................................................ 174
The Least You Need to Know ........................................... 174

**Part 3: Minerals: The Elements of Good Health**    **175**

**17 Calcium: Drink Your Milk!**                 **177**

Why You Need Calcium .................................................. 178
Boning Up on Calcium ................................................... 178

The DRI for Calcium ............................................................ 179
Are You Deficient? ............................................................... 180
Calcium-Robbing Drugs ...................................................... 181
    Cortisone and Other Steroid Drugs ............................... 181
    Thyroid Drugs ................................................................ 182
    Drugs for High Cholesterol ........................................... 182
    Aluminum Antacids ........................................................ 182
    Alcohol and Tobacco ...................................................... 182
Other Prescription Drugs and Calcium .............................. 182
Eating Your Calcium ........................................................... 183
Picking the Right Calcium Supplement ............................. 185
    Calcium Supplements to Avoid ..................................... 187
Getting the Most from Calcium ......................................... 188
    The Dynamic Duo: Calcium and Vitamin D ................. 189
The Function of Phosphorus ............................................... 189
Avoiding Osteoporosis ........................................................ 190
Not for Women Only .......................................................... 192
Calcium and High Blood Pressure ..................................... 192
Calcium and Colon Cancer ................................................. 193
Calcium and Kidney Stones ................................................ 193
Calcium and Heart Disease ................................................. 193
The Least You Need to Know .............................................. 193

**18 Magnesium: Magnificent for Your Heart          195**

Why You Need Magnesium .................................................. 196
The DRI for Magnesium ...................................................... 196
Are You Deficient? ............................................................... 197
Eating Your Magnesium ...................................................... 198
Getting the Most from Magnesium .................................... 200
Magnesium and Your Heart ................................................ 201
Magnesium Manages Blood Pressure ................................. 202
Help for Asthma ................................................................. 203
Magnesium and Diabetes .................................................... 203
Magnesium for Healthy Bones ........................................... 203
Magnesium and Migraines .................................................. 204
Other Problems Helped by Magnesium ............................. 204
The Least You Need to Know .............................................. 205

**19 Zinc: Immune System Booster          207**

Why You Need Zinc ............................................................ 208
The RDA for Zinc ............................................................... 208
Are You Deficient? ............................................................... 208
Eating Your Zinc ................................................................. 209
Getting the Most from Zinc ............................................... 211

Fighting Off Colds ............................................................ 211
Zinc Club for Men ............................................................ 212
Healthy Skin, Nails, and Hair ........................................ 213
Zinc for Healing ............................................................... 213
Think Zinc for Other Problems ..................................... 213
The Least You Need to Know ......................................... 214

## 20 Electrolytes: Keeping Your Body in Balance      215

What's an Electrolyte? ..................................................... 216
Why You Need Electrolytes ............................................. 216
The RDAs for Electrolytes .............................................. 217
Are You Deficient? ........................................................... 217
Potassium Pitfalls............................................................. 218
    Other Prescription Drugs .......................................... 219
Eating Your Electrolytes ................................................. 219
Getting the Most from Electrolytes ............................... 220
Shaking Up Salt ............................................................... 221
Electrifying News on High Blood Pressure ................... 222
Preventing Strokes with Potassium .............................. 223
The Least You Need to Know ......................................... 223

## 21 The Trace Minerals: A Little Goes a Long Way      225

What's a Trace Mineral? .................................................. 226
Why You Need Trace Minerals ....................................... 227
RDAs and Safe and Adequate Intakes ........................... 227
Are You Deficient? ........................................................... 227
Eating Your Trace Minerals ............................................ 227
Getting the Most from Trace Minerals .......................... 228
Singling Out Sulfur ......................................................... 228
Iron: Basic for Blood ....................................................... 229
    The RDA for Iron ....................................................... 230
    Eating Your Iron ........................................................ 230
    Getting the Most from Iron ...................................... 232
Iodine: Important for the Thyroid ................................ 232
    The RDA for Iodine .................................................... 233
Chromium: Boon for Diabetics? .................................... 234
Selenium: An Essential Element .................................... 235
Copper: Crucial for Your Circulation ........................... 236
Fluoride: Fighting Tooth Decay .................................... 237
Manganese: Mystery Metal............................................. 238
Molybdenum: Making Enzymes ..................................... 239
Other Trace Minerals ...................................................... 240
Minerals You Should Miss .............................................. 241
The Least You Need to Know ......................................... 242

## Part 4:  Exploring Other Supplements                          243

### 22  Amino Acids: The Building Blocks of Life                 245

Why You Need Amino Acids ............................................. 246
50,000 Proteins from Just 22 Aminos ........................... 247
The RDA for Amino Acids ................................................ 248
Eating Your Aminos ......................................................... 250
Amino Alert! ...................................................................... 251
Arginine for Immunity ..................................................... 252
Carnitine for Cardiac Cases ........................................... 252
Cysteine for Pollution Protection ................................. 253
Glutamine for the Gut ..................................................... 254
Lysine: Help for Herpes? ................................................ 254
Methionine and Taurine .................................................. 255
Tryptophan for Natural Sleep ....................................... 255
Phenylalanine, Tyrosine, and Migraines ...................... 256
Glucosamine: Real Help for Arthritis .......................... 257
The Least You Need to Know ........................................... 258

### 23  Essential Fatty Acids: When Is Fat Good?               259

What's So Essential about Fat? ....................................... 260
Good Fat versus Bad Fat .................................................. 260
The Good Fats .................................................................... 261
Omega-3 and Omega-6 .................................................... 261
   Why You Need Omega-6 ............................................... 262
   Why You Need Omega-3 ............................................... 262
   Getting the Most from Essential Fatty Acids ............. 263
   Fish Oil Supplements .................................................... 263
Nothing Fishy About It: Omega-3 Helps Your Heart ....... 265
Fish Oil and Fat Levels .................................................... 266
Helping High Blood Pressure ......................................... 267
Fish Oil and Diabetes ...................................................... 267
Calming Crohn's Disease ................................................ 267
Helping Rheumatoid Arthritis ....................................... 267
Fish Oil Fights Cancer ..................................................... 267
GLA: The Promise of Evening Primrose Oil ................ 268
Other Good Fats ................................................................ 268
   The Weight Loss Pill ..................................................... 268
   Helping Senility ............................................................. 268
   Building Brain Cells ...................................................... 269
The Least You Need to Know ........................................... 269

## 24 Super Antioxidants                                271

The Crucial Role of Glutathione ...................................... 271
Are You Deficient? ........................................................... 272
Boosting Your Glutathione Level ..................................... 273
Supplements to Boost Glutathione .................................. 274
Lipoic Acid: The Vitamin That's Not a Vitamin .............. 275
  Helping Diabetic Neuropathy .................................... 276
The Least You Need to Know ........................................... 276

## 25 Flavonoids for Humanoids                           277

What Are Flavonoids? ...................................................... 278
Carotenoids: Orange You Glad You Know ....................... 279
The Carotenes ................................................................. 280
  Alpha Carotene .......................................................... 280
  Beta-Cryptoxanthin .................................................... 280
  Lycopene .................................................................... 280
The Xanthophylls ............................................................ 281
  Lutein and Zeaxanthin ................................................ 282
  Capsanthin .................................................................. 282
Have a Nice Cup of Tea ................................................... 282
Quercetin: The Flavonoid from Onions ........................... 283
Garlic: It's Good for You ................................................. 284
Anthocyanins for Healthy Eyes ....................................... 285
Resveratrol: Red Wine Rescuer ....................................... 285
Unexpected Health from Unlikely Plants ......................... 286
Ginkgo Biloba and Your Brain ......................................... 287
The Least You Need to Know ........................................... 288

## 26 Coenzyme $Q_{10}$: Cellular Spark Plug            289

Co Q What? ..................................................................... 290
$CoQ_{10}$ for Cardiac Cases .......................................... 290
Lowering Your Blood Pressure ........................................ 291
Cholesterol and $CoQ_{10}$ ............................................ 292
Other Benefits of Coenzyme $Q_{10}$ ............................. 292
Getting Your Coenzyme $Q_{10}$ .................................... 293
The Least You Need to Know ........................................... 294

## 27 Help from Natural Hormones                        295

What's a Hormone? .......................................................... 296
Melatonin: From A to Zzzz .............................................. 296
  Melatonin for a Good Night's Rest .............................. 296
  Relieving Jet Lag ........................................................ 297
  Maximizing Your Melatonin ........................................ 297

It's Soy Good for You .......................................................... 297
Eating Your Soy ................................................................. 299
Wild about Yams ............................................................... 300
DHEA: Eternal Youth? ...................................................... 301
The Least You Need to Know ............................................ 302

**28 Fiber: Moving Things Along                                   303**

Why Fiber Is Fabulous ...................................................... 304
How Much Fiber Is Enough? ............................................. 304
Insoluble and Soluble Fiber ............................................. 304
   Insoluble Fiber .......................................................... 304
   Soluble Fiber ............................................................. 304
Eating More Fiber ............................................................. 305
Which Type of Fiber? ........................................................ 307
Fiber Supplements ............................................................ 308
Water, Water Everywhere .................................................. 310
It's Official: Oatmeal Lowers Cholesterol ........................ 310
Oatmeal for Breakfast ....................................................... 311
Help for Bowel Problems .................................................. 312
Beneficial Bacteria ........................................................... 313
Fiber Fights Cancer .......................................................... 315
Fiber for Diabetes ............................................................. 315
The Least You Need to Know ............................................ 315

**A Quick Reference Chart for Health Problems                    317**

**B Resources                                                     319**

Finding Nutritionally Oriented Health Care .................... 319
Nutrition and the Elderly ................................................. 320
Testing Labs ..................................................................... 320
Supplement Manufacturers .............................................. 321
Supplement Information and Regulation ......................... 321
   General Information ................................................... 321
   Federal Regulations and Industry Associations ............. 322
Help for Medical Problems ............................................... 322

**C Glossary                                                      325**

**Index                                                           337**

# Foreword

You don't have to be an idiot to understand how simple, easy, and beneficial this book is to your overall well-being. Dr. Alan Pressman has included all of the information you need to help you decide which vitamins, minerals, and supplements you need for good health. We live in an age where there is a need to merge hard science with everyday practical use with reader-friendly techniques. This book serves that purpose.

Knowing that you're getting the right amount of nutrients is important whether you're 18 or 80. This book gives you the knowledge you need to look and feel better—it's just a matter of looking in the index and going to the right page. There you'll see a synthesized, easy-to-follow understanding to all of your health questions.

Gary Null, Ph.D.

Host of the nationally syndicated "Gary Null Show" which airs daily on WBAI in New York City, and is carried weekly to 32 stations nationwide. In addition, Mr. Null is author of over 50 books on health and nutrition including *The Woman's Encyclopedia of Natural Healing* and *The New Vegetarian Cookbook*.

# Introduction

## Live Better with Vitamins

Every year Americans spend more than $4 billion on vitamins, minerals, and other supplements. Why? They're seeking better health, perhaps a longer and more vigorous life, or maybe help for a painful health problem. Are they finding it? Yes! Can you? Yes! If you understand how important vitamins and minerals are and what they can—and can't—do, you too can achieve better health.

## Why Are They So Important?

You need thirteen different vitamins and at least ten minerals to stay alive. Vitamins and minerals are essential to your health—you have to have them to stay alive and to be healthy. Vitamins and minerals are also needed to make the thousands of enzymes, hormones, and other chemical messengers your body uses to grow, repair itself, make energy, remove wastes, defend you against infection, and generally keep you running smoothly. You also need them to keep your bones strong, your eyes sharp, and your brain alert. And, most important of all, you need them to help protect you against cancer and heart disease.

The *only* way you can get all those vitamins and minerals into your body is to eat them. That's why we'll talk about your diet over and over again in this book—the foods you eat are your best way to get the nutrients you need. But even if you could eat right all the time—and most people can't—you might still benefit from some extra vitamins and minerals.

## Do You Really Need Vitamin Pills?

The short answer is yes—the long answers are found in each chapter of this book. Try as we might, most of us just can't eat a good, nutritious diet at every meal every day. We need the help vitamin and mineral supplements can give. And sometimes we need a vitamin or mineral boost to help deal with health problems. Finally, some vitamins, like Vitamin E, are most valuable in large doses—doses far greater (though very safe) than the amounts you could ever get only from your food.

Supplements are an easy, safe, and inexpensive way to make sure you're getting the vitamins and minerals your body has to have for optimum health. Taking supplements can improve your health now and ensure it for the future. As there are too many herbal remedies to discuss in this book, we had to omit any discussion of them.

# How to Use This Book

We've divided this book into four parts. In Part 1, "The Vital Keys to Good Health," we explain the basics of vitamins and minerals: Why you need them, how much you need, and the best ways to get them. In Part 2, "The A to K of Vitamins," we discuss each vitamin in detail, explaining how it works in your body, specific health problems it can help, and how to get the amounts you need. In Part 3, "Minerals: The Elements of Good Health," we do the same for minerals. In Part 4, "Exploring Other Supplements," we discuss many other nutritional supplements, like essential fatty acids, flavonoids, and natural hormones. This part gives you the information you need to understand which supplements have real value, what conditions they can help, and how best to use them. We end the book with a quick-reference chart for finding which supplements are helpful for particular health problems, a list of resources for finding more information, and a glossary.

To get the most from this book, we urge you to read through the first two chapters carefully. These give you the background you need to understand the overall importance of vitamins and minerals to your health.

Throughout this book, we give you plenty of charts, including many that list good food sources for the various vitamins, minerals, and other supplements. Look for Thumbs Up/ Thumbs Down boxes to get more details on the best ways to take your vitamins and minerals. We also give a lot of useful information and tips in sidebars.

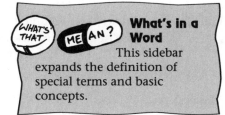

**What's in a Word**

This sidebar expands the definition of special terms and basic concepts.

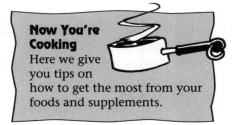

**Now You're Cooking**

Here we give you tips on how to get the most from your foods and supplements.

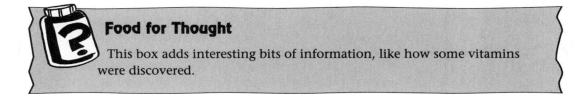

**Food for Thought**

This box adds interesting bits of information, like how some vitamins were discovered.

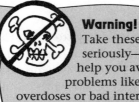

**Warning!** Take these boxes seriously—they help you avoid problems like overdoses or bad interactions with other drugs or supplements.

**Quack, Quack** We also have a special sidebar reserved for exploding some of the sillier ideas about supplements. These boxes help you avoid supplements that don't work.

# Acknowledgments

We'd like to thank all the people who have, over the years, shared their knowledge and enthusiasm with us. Special thanks to Carl Germano, Director of Product Development at Solgar Vitamin and Herb Company, and to his assistant Joanne DeCandia RD, Assistant Director of Technical Services. Thanks also to Jerry Hickey of Hickey Chemists, Martin Kohl for research assistance, Gary Krebs for getting this project started, and Deborah Quilter for her expertise in repetitive strain injuries. Extra special thanks to our hardworking editors at Macmillan: Nancy Mikhail, Joan Paterson, and Linda Seifert.

# Trademarks

# Part 1
# The Vital Keys to Good Health

*You've been hearing a lot about all the great things vitamins and minerals can do for your health, and you've decided to try them. Good decision. Now what?*

*What you need now is information—the knowledge that will let you unlock the door to good health. The knowledge you need isn't a secret and it's not hard to understand. In fact, after you've learned the basics of vitamins, minerals, and other supplements, you'll easily be able to decide what's right for you.*

*Your own good health, both for now and the future, is in your hands. Let's get started.*

# Chapter 1

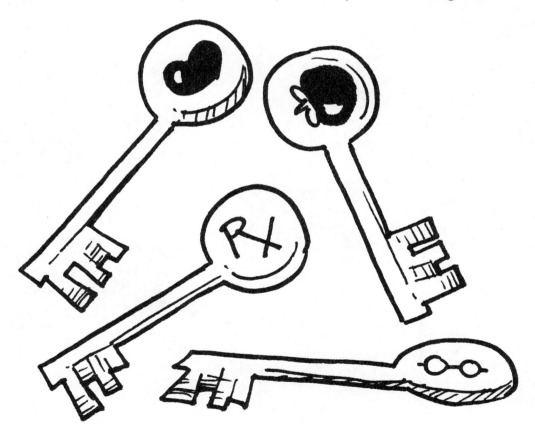

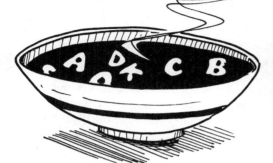

# The Alphabet Soup of Nutrition

## In This Chapter

➤ Why you need vitamins and minerals

➤ How much do you need?

➤ Vitamins, minerals, and your diet

➤ How vitamins and minerals protect you from damaging free radicals

Walk into any health-food store or drugstore and you're faced with shelf after shelf crammed with vitamins, minerals, and supplements of all sorts. What is all this stuff? How can you choose? What's best for *you?*

To decide wisely for your health, you need to understand what each vitamin does—and why you need them *all.* You need to understand what minerals do for you—and why you need them *all.* You need to understand how the vitamins and minerals in your food affect you—and how everything else in your food affects you as well. You need to under-stand which of those other supplements are valuable to your health—and which aren't.

Although all those bottles on the shelves may seem confusing and a little scary, they're really not. Once you understand the easy basics of vitamins and minerals, you'll be able to pick the supplements that will help *your* health.

# Vitamins: Why They're Vital

A *vitamin* is an organic (carbon-containing) chemical compound your body must have in very small amounts for normal growth, metabolism (creating energy in your cells), and health. You need vitamins to make *enzymes* and *hormones*—important substances your body uses to make all the many chemical reactions you need to live. You *must* get your vitamins from your food or from supplements—you can't make them in your body.

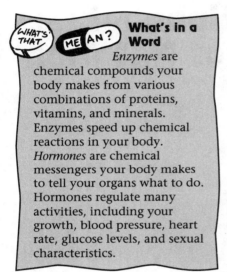

**What's in a Word**

*Enzymes* are chemical compounds your body makes from various combinations of proteins, vitamins, and minerals. Enzymes speed up chemical reactions in your body. *Hormones* are chemical messengers your body makes to tell your organs what to do. Hormones regulate many activities, including your growth, blood pressure, heart rate, glucose levels, and sexual characteristics.

There are 13 vitamins in all, and you need every single one of them, no exceptions. Vitamins aren't food or a substitute for food. They have no calories and give you no energy directly—but your body needs vitamins, especially the B vitamins, to convert food to energy. We'll look at each vitamin in detail in the later chapters of this book, but for now we'll divide them into two groups: *fat-soluble* and *water-soluble*.

## Fat-Soluble Vitamins

Fat-soluble vitamins are stored in your body, mostly in your fatty tissues and in your liver. Vitamins A, E, D and K are fat-soluble—that is, they dissolve in fat but not water. Because you can store these vitamins, you don't have to get a supply of them every day. On the other hand, getting too much of these vitamins means they could build up in your body and cause problems.

## Water-Soluble Vitamins

Water-soluble vitamins can't really be stored in your body for very long. That's because these vitamins dissolve in water, so any extra is carried out of your body. Vitamin C and all the B vitamins are water-soluble. Because you can't store these vitamins, you need to get a fresh supply every day. You can't really overdose on water-soluble vitamins. Unless you take truly massive doses, the extra just washes harmlessly out.

**Food for Thought**

For centuries, we've known that there's a relationship between your diet and certain kinds of diseases. It was only in the early 1900s that research really got going on exactly what it was in food that prevented certain diseases. By 1912, researchers had decided that the vital substances, whatever they were, had to be amines—chemicals that contain nitrogen, hydrogen, and carbon. The Polish biochemist Casimir Funk coined the word "vitamine," from vital and amine. As it turns out, not all vitamins are amines, so to avoid confusion the word was changed to vitamin in 1920.

# How Much Do You Need?

How much you need of each vitamin is a question that has a lot of different answers, depending on who you are and who you ask. For now, we're going to tell you what the doctors and scientists at the Food and Nutrition Board of the Institute of Medicine think is enough to meet your basic needs for each vitamin, assuming you're an average healthy adult man or woman. The Institute of Medicine is the group that brings you the Recommended Dietary Allowances, better known as RDAs. (We'll talk a lot more about RDAs and other ways of looking at your vitamin and mineral needs in the next chapter.) Check out the chart to see the RDAs for vitamins. These are the *minimum* amounts you should be getting every day, preferably from your food (and from vitamin pills if you need to).

| Adult RDAs for Vitamins | | |
| --- | --- | --- |
| Vitamin | RDA for Men | RDA for Women |
| *Fat-Soluble* | | |
| Vitamin A | 1,000 RE or 5,000 IU | 800 RE or 4,000 IU |
| Vitamin D | 5 mcg or 200 IU | 5 mcg or 200 IU |
| Vitamin E | 10 mg or 15 IU | 8 mg or 12 IU |
| Vitamin K | 80 mcg | 65 mcg |
| *Water-Soluble* | | |
| Vitamin C | 60 mg | 60 mg |
| B Vitamins: | | |
| Thiamin | 1.5 mg | 1.1 mg |
| Riboflavin | 1.7 mg | 1.3 mg |
| Niacin | 19 mg | 15 mg |
| Pyridoxine | 2.0 mg | 1.6 mg |
| Folic acid | 200 mcg | 180 mcg |
| Cobalamin | 2.0 mcg | 2.0 mcg |

If you were counting, you noticed that the chart only listed 11 vitamins, even though we said you need 13. Two B vitamins, biotin and pantothenic acid, aren't listed. That's because even though you need to have them, they don't have RDAs. Why not? Because you get these vitamins so easily from your food, even if you have incredibly bad eating habits, no one is ever really deficient in them. And if no one's ever deficient, there's no point in bothering to set an RDA.

**Food for Thought**

The Food and Nutrition Board of the Institute of Medicine first established Recommended Dietary Allowances (RDAs) for vitamins and minerals in 1941. The RDAs are revised and changed as needed about once every five to ten years. The parent organization of the Institute of Medicine is the National Academy of Science, a private, nonprofit, self-perpetuating society of distinguished scholars. Founded by Congressional charter in 1863, the NAS has a mandate to advise the federal government on scientific and technical matters.

## The Measure of Good Health

The other thing you may have noticed about the vitamins chart is the way we gave the RDAs in funny measurement units: mg and mcg. Usually the amounts of vitamins (and minerals and other supplements) are given using the metric system. (We'll explain the difference between an RE and an IU in Chapter 3 on Vitamin A.)

Most of us stubbornly refuse to use metric measurement unless we really have to, but when it comes to vitamins, minerals, and supplements, you have to. Here's how to understand the measurements:

**One gram (g) contains 1,000 milligrams (mg).** A gram is roughly equivalent to one-quarter teaspoon, or 0.035 of an ounce. There are about 4,000 mg in a teaspoon.

**One milligram contains 1,000 micrograms (mcg).** That means a microgram is 1/1,000 of a milligram, or 1/1,000,000 (yes, one millionth) of a gram. That's less than the amount that would fit on the head of a pin.

**Quack, Quack**

The only thing a vitamin can cure is a deficiency disease caused by a shortage of that vitamin. In other words, Vitamin C cures scurvy. It doesn't cure the common cold, although it can help shorten how long you're sick. Megadoses of vitamins can help prevent or treat health problems such as heart disease and diabetes, but they don't cure them.

## Beyond the Basics

Throughout this book, we'll use the RDA as the rock-bottom, bare minimum amount you need to get every day for a particular vitamin or mineral. That's because the RDAs are only the amounts needed to prevent disease in ordinary healthy people. They are, in our opinion and the opinion of many other nutritionists, doctors, and researchers, the *least* you should get. (In fairness, we should say that the Institute of Medicine is looking carefully at the current RDAs and will probably revise some of them upward over the next few years.) In many cases, we believe the RDAs are far from the amount you need to reach optimal good health or to prevent many serious health problems, like heart disease. As you'll discover in the chapters to come, there are many, many good reasons for taking more—sometimes much more—than the RDA. There are also sometimes many good reasons to stick to the RDA and *not* take any extra—and we'll cover those issues as well.

# Minerals: Essential Elements of Health

A *mineral* is an inorganic chemical element, such as calcium or potassium, that your body must have in very small amounts for normal growth, metabolism, and health and to make many enzymes and hormones. Like vitamins, you must get your minerals from your food.

We use the word mineral in a broad sense to mean all the many inorganic substances you need every day, but we should really be a little more exact. Nutritionally speaking, a mineral is an inorganic substance that you need every day in amounts over 100 mg. If you need less than 100 mg a day, we call the mineral a *trace mineral* or *trace element*. Even though the amounts you need for a trace mineral are very small—sometimes no more than 50 mcg—they're just as important to your health as the major minerals.

## Minerals

The minerals you need every day include calcium, chloride, magnesium, phosphorus, potassium, sodium, and sulfur. We deal with these all in separate chapters (potassium, sodium, and chloride are combined in Chapter 20 on electrolytes). Take a look at the chart to see the RDAs for the major minerals.

| Adult RDAs for Minerals | |
| --- | --- |
| **Mineral** | **RDA for adults** |
| Calcium | 1000 mg |
| Chloride | 750 mg |
| Magnesium | 350 mg |
| Phosphorus | 700 mg |
| Potassium | 2,000 mg |
| Sodium | 500 mg |

One mineral is missing from the chart: sulfur. You need over 100 mg of sulfur a day, but this mineral is so common in foods that nobody is ever deficient. Like biotin and pantothenic acid in the vitamins, there's no real need to set an RDA for sulfur, so nobody has.

**Food for Thought**

Your body has about 60 *trillion* cells in it. Every moment of every day, thousands of different chemical reactions are happening inside *each* cell. To make each one of those reactions happen, your body makes a specific enzyme just for that particular purpose and no other. When the reaction is over, still other enzymes break down the specific enzyme and recycle it. To make all those enzymes and keep your body running smoothly, you need plenty of vitamins, minerals, and trace minerals.

## Trace Minerals

How many trace elements you need to get and in what amounts is open to a lot of discussion (see Chapter 21). We know for sure that you need very small amounts of boron, chromium, cobalt, copper, iodine, iron, manganese, molybdenum, nickel, selenium, silicon, tin, vanadium, and zinc. What about the tiny, tiny amounts of other minerals, like aluminum and lithium, that are found in your body? We don't really know why you have them or how much you need.

A lot of the trace minerals don't have RDAs—we just don't know enough to set any. Your need for boron, for example, was only discovered in the mid-1980s, and researchers are still trying to figure what the RDA should be. Instead, some of these minerals have Safe and Adequate Intakes (SAIs). These are best guesses as to how much you probably need. They're often given as a fairly broad range. For example, the SAI for chromium seems to be anywhere from 50 to 200 mcg. The chart lists the RDAs and SAIs for the trace minerals that have them—we've left off the ones that don't.

### Adult RDAs or SAIs for Trace Minerals

| Trace Mineral | RDA | SAI |
|---|---|---|
| Chromium | | 50–200 mcg |
| Copper | | 1.5–3.0 mg |
| Iodine | 150 mcg | |
| Iron | 10–15 mg | |
| Manganese | | 2.5–5.0 mg |
| Molybdenum | | 75–250 mcg |
| Selenium | 55–70 mcg | |
| Zinc | 12–15 mg | |

What's missing from the chart? Boron, cobalt, nickel, silicon, tin, and vanadium. You easily get these trace minerals from your food. Very few people will ever be deficient in them.

# Do You Need Vitamin and Mineral Supplements?

The average person can get the RDAs for vitamins and minerals simply by eating a reasonable diet containing plenty of whole grains and fresh fruits and vegetables. Yeah, right. First of all, who's that mythical average person? Not anyone we know. The RDAs assume you're an adult under age 60 who's in good health, has perfect digestion, isn't overweight, leads a totally stress-free life, doesn't ever have any sort of medical problem, and never needs to take any sort of medicine. The RDAs also assume that you really manage to eat a good diet every day.

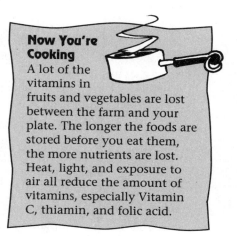

**Now You're Cooking**

A lot of the vitamins in fruits and vegetables are lost between the farm and your plate. The longer the foods are stored before you eat them, the more nutrients are lost. Heat, light, and exposure to air all reduce the amount of vitamins, especially Vitamin C, thiamin, and folic acid.

Let's get real here: Even on a good day, you can't always manage a completely healthful diet. Who has the time or energy to do all that shopping and food preparation? On any given day, half of us eat at least one meal away from home anyway. You just can't always eat healthfully, even when you try.

The fact is, most of us don't try all that hard, and most of us don't meet all the RDAs from our diet. Just look at the results of the 1994 Department of Agriculture's Continuing Survey of Food Intakes by Individuals (CSFII):

➤ Most adult women don't meet the RDAs for iron, zinc, Vitamin $B_6$ (pyridoxine), calcium, magnesium, and Vitamin E.

➤ Most adult men don't meet the RDA for zinc and magnesium.

➤ Young children drink 16 percent less milk than they did in the late 1970s, but they drink 23 percent more carbonated soft drinks.

➤ Americans eat very few dark-green leafy vegetables and deep yellow vegetables. Fewer than one out of five people eats five fresh fruits and vegetables a day—and about one person in five doesn't eat any.

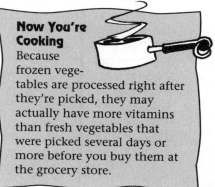

**Now You're Cooking**

Because frozen vegetables are processed right after they're picked, they may actually have more vitamins than fresh vegetables that were picked several days or more before you buy them at the grocery store.

If it's that hard to meet the RDAs through diet, what about reaching the higher amounts of vitamins and minerals many health professionals now recommend? You could just try harder to eat better or differently. For example, women between the ages of

25 and 50 should get at least 1,000 mg of calcium every day to keep their bones strong. That's the calcium in three glasses of milk a day. You could easily drink that much milk, but would you? Do you even like milk? What if you hate the stuff or have trouble digesting it?

One of the biggest problems with the RDAs is that they assume you're in good health and eat about 2,000 calories a day. What if you don't eat that much? Many people over age 70, for example, only take in about 1,500 calories a day. And in our weight-conscious society, at any given time one in six Americans are dieting—usually in a way that doesn't provide good nutrition. There's no way these people are getting the vitamins and minerals they need from their food.

We'd be the first to tell you that vitamin and mineral supplements aren't a substitute for healthy eating. They're also not a magic shield against the effects of bad health habits, like smoking or not getting much exercise. But we know that you can't always eat like you should—and that sometimes you need more of a vitamin or mineral than you can reasonably get just from your food.

That's why vitamin and mineral supplements are so important. Taking a daily multivitamin and mineral supplement is sensible insurance—it makes sure you get everything you need. You may also need extra of one or more vitamins or minerals—more than you could get from your diet. Here too supplements make sure you're getting enough.

Generally speaking, vitamin and mineral supplements are safe even in large doses. More isn't always better, though, and some supplements can be harmful in big doses. Use your common sense. Read what we have to say about the vitamins and minerals, talk it over with your doctor, and then decide which supplements are best for you.

# On the Edge: Marginal Deficiencies

If you don't get a particular vitamin for a long time, you develop a *deficiency*. If the deficiency goes on long enough, you get a deficiency disease. The classic example of a deficiency disease is scurvy, caused by a lack of Vitamin C (we'll explain more about this in Chapter 13). Long before you start having any of the signs of a deficiency disease—and long before the deficiency shows up in the usual medical tests—you could be *marginally deficient* in a vitamin or mineral. Here's a very good example: Many older adults are marginally deficient in cobalamin (Vitamin $B_{12}$). The main symptom of classic cobalamin deficiency is anemia, which a doctor can easily diagnose with a simple blood test. Long before anemia sets in, though, marginal cobalamin deficiency leads to depression, confused thinking, and other mental symptoms that look a lot like senility. So, is your Uncle George ga-ga from old age, or is he just low on B vitamins from the over-processed, overcooked food he gets at the nursing home? The chances are good that poor diet is playing a bigger role in his mental condition than you—or his doctor—might realize. The chances are also good that a supplement containing all the B vitamins could do a lot to restore Uncle George to his old self.

What about you? You might be marginally deficient if:

➤ You rarely eat fresh fruits and vegetables. These are the best natural sources of vitamins and minerals.

➤ You've been going through a long period of high stress or overwork. You're probably not eating right, plus you're using up a lot vitamins and minerals to make extra stress hormones. Think of yourself as a battery running down.

➤ You're sick with something—bronchitis, say—or you're recovering from surgery. At a time when you probably don't feel much like eating, you need lots of extra vitamins and minerals to help you heal faster.

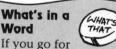

**What's in a Word**
If you go for a long period without getting enough of a vitamin or mineral, you become *deficient*. A *marginal* or *subclinical deficiency* is an early stage. Your body's supply of a vitamin or mineral is gradually drained and your body's normal workings are gradually impaired. If a marginal deficiency goes on long enough, you will get a deficiency disease.

➤ You have a chronic disease such as asthma or diabetes. Low levels of a vitamin or mineral might be causing the problem or making it worse. Many people with asthma are low on magnesium, for example; many diabetics are very low on Vitamin C. Chronic diseases change how well your body absorbs and uses vitamins and minerals, so your needs change as well.

➤ You're pregnant or nursing. You need extra vitamins and minerals because you're passing some of yours on to your baby.

➤ You're seriously depressed. When you're depressed, you don't eat well. That can make the depression worse, because marginal deficiencies of many vitamins and minerals *cause* depression.

➤ You smoke. Smoking sharply increases your need for vitamins, especially Vitamin C.

➤ You drink a lot of alcohol. Heavy drinkers are often marginally deficient in almost all the vitamins and minerals, especially B vitamins.

How do you know you have a marginal deficiency? Deficiencies can be hard to pin down. You might just be feeling a little below par, or more tired than usual. That's easy to blame on all sorts of things, so you might not think a vitamin or mineral deficiency is the problem. Even if you go to your doctor with other deficiency symptoms, like irritability, anxiety, or insomnia, you're more likely to come home with a prescription for Valium® than for a vitamin supplement. If you feel your health isn't what it could be—if you get frequent minor illnesses, for example, or bad colds you just can't seem to shake, ask yourself if you're getting enough of the vitamins and minerals you need.

# The Antioxidant Revolution

You need vitamins and minerals to make all those thousands of enzymes, hormones, and other chemicals your body needs to work right. But vitamins and minerals have another crucial role in your body: They act as powerful *antioxidants* that capture *free radicals* in your body. It's only in the past few decades that we've begun to understand how damaging free radicals can be and how important it is to have plenty of antioxidants in your body to neutralize them.

# Radicals on the Loose

WHAT'S THAT ME AN?

**What's in a Word**

*Free radicals* are unstable oxygen atoms created by your body's natural processes and by the effects of toxins such as cigarette smoke. Free radicals, especially the types called singlet oxygen and hydroxyl, are very reactive and cause a lot of damage to your cells, but they're not all bad. You use free radicals as part of your immune system to defend against invading bacteria.

When you drive your car, you burn gasoline by combining it with oxygen in the pistons of the engine. Your car zips along on the released energy, but it also gives off exhaust fumes as a byproduct. Something very similar happens in the cells of your body. When oxygen combines with glucose in your cells, for example, you make energy—and you also make free radicals, your body's version of exhaust fumes. Free radicals are oxygen atoms that are missing one electron from the pair the atom should have. When an atom is missing an electron from a pair, it becomes unstable and very reactive. That's because a free radical desperately wants to find another electron to fill in the gap, so it grabs an electron from the next atom it gets near. But when a free radical seizes an electron from another atom, the second atom then becomes a free radical, because now it's the one missing an electron. One free radical starts a cascade of new free radicals in your body. The free radicals blunder around, grabbing electrons from your cells—and doing a lot of damage to them at the same time.

# Fighting Back with Antioxidants

Antioxidants are your body's natural defense against free radicals. Antioxidants are enzymes that patrol your cells looking for free radicals. When they find one, they grab hold of it and neutralize it without being damaged themselves. The antioxidant enzymes stop the invasion and remove the free radical from circulation.

WHAT'S THAT ME AN?

**What's in a Word**

*Antioxidant* enzymes protect your body by capturing free radicals and, in a complex series of steps, escort them out of your body before they do any additional damage.

You have to have plenty of vitamins and minerals, especially Vitamin A, beta carotene, Vitamin C, Vitamin E and selenium, in your body to make the antioxidant enzymes that do the neutralizing. If you're short on the right vitamins and minerals, you can't make enough of the antioxidant enzymes. That lets the free radicals get the upper hand and do extra damage to your cells before they get quenched.

Oxidation isn't the only thing that can cause free radicals in your cells. The ultraviolet light in sunshine can do it—that's why people who spend too much time in the sun are more likely to get skin cancer and cataracts. Toxins of all sorts—tobacco smoke, the natural chemicals found in our food, the poisonous wastes of your own metabolism, and man-made toxins like air pollution and pesticides—trigger free radicals as well.

On average, every cell in your body comes under attack from a free radical once every ten seconds. Your best protection is to keep your antioxidant levels high. How? That's what we're going to explain in just about every chapter for the rest of this book.

**Warning!**
If free radicals damage the DNA in your cells often enough, they can cause the genetic changes that trigger cancer. If free radicals oxidize cholesterol in your blood, they can cause the artery-clogging plaque that leads to heart disease.

# The Least You Need to Know

➤ Vitamins (organic substances) and minerals (inorganic substances) are necessary for life and good health.

➤ Vitamins A, D, E, and K are fat-soluble: They are stored in your body's fatty tissues.

➤ The B vitamins and Vitamin C are water-soluble: Your body can't store them, so you need some every day.

➤ Vitamins and minerals are needed to make the thousands of different enzymes your body needs to live.

➤ Free radicals are unstable oxygen atoms made in your body as part of normal metabolism. They are very reactive and can damage your cells.

➤ Antioxidant enzymes capture and neutralize free radicals.

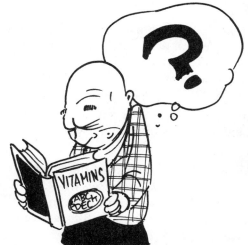

# Chapter 2

# Choosing What's Right for You

**In This Chapter**

➤ Interpreting the Recommended Dietary Allowance (RDA)

➤ Deciding which vitamins and minerals you need—and how much

➤ Vitamins and minerals for kids, adults, older adults, and vegetarians

➤ How vitamins and minerals can help common health problems

➤ Best buys in vitamin and mineral supplements

➤ Getting the most from your supplements

Your next-door neighbor tells you that a friend of her mother's feels a thousand times better since she started taking this new vitamin pill. Should you take the same pill? Of course not! You need real information, not third-hand stories, to make a good choice about which supplements are right for *you*.

It's not hard to make good choices. All you need is some reliable information based on real research, not anecdotes you hear by the supplements counter at your local health-food store. That's what we're here for. In this chapter we'll give you the basics you need to select the vitamins and minerals that are best for you, choose products you can rely on, and get the most out of them.

# Who Decides This Stuff, Anyway?

Two major players set the national standards for your daily vitamins and minerals: the nonprofit, independent Institute of Medicine and the federal Food and Drug Administration (FDA). The FDA is an agency within the Public Health Service, which in turn is part of the Department of Health and Human Services. One big part of the FDA's job is to make sure foods are safe and are labeled truthfully with useful information.

The two organizations use some similar abbreviations to explain their recommendations, which has created a lot of confusion among consumers. Here's what all those initials mean:

➤ **RDA.** As we explained in Chapter 1, the Food and Nutrition Board of the Institute of Medicine, an arm of the nonprofit American Academy of Sciences, sets the Recommended Dietary Allowances. RDAs set the national guidelines for the minimum amounts you need to get every day. They're the basis for all the scientific research on nutrition—and for the information we give in this book.

➤ **USRDA.** These are the "other" RDAs, set by the FDA. US stands for United States, of course, but this time RDA stands for Recommended Daily Allowance. The USRDAs are really just somewhat simplified versions of the Institute of Medicine's RDAs. This standard is being phased out in favor of a new one called RDI.

➤ **DRI.** Starting in 1997, the Institute of Medicine has begun issuing a new standard, the Daily Reference Intake. For each vitamin and mineral, the DRI is sort of an average based on four measurements: the estimated average requirement; the RDA; the adequate intake; and the tolerable upper intake level. The new DRIs will gradually replace the old RDAs.

➤ **RDI.** Get used to this one, because it will eventually replace USRDA on all food and supplement labels. RDI stands for Reference Daily Intake. The amounts are still pretty much the same as the old USRDAs, which are pretty much the same as the RDAs, which are now becoming part of the DRIs. With us so far?

➤ **DRV.** Now it starts to get complicated. DRV stands for Daily Recommended Values. The FDA created this new standard to cover energy-producing nutrients, which aren't covered in the RDIs. The DRVs are the amounts of fats, carbohydrates, fiber, protein, cholesterol, sodium, and potassium you should get every day. As you can see from the chart, the DRVs are percentages based on a diet that contains 2,000 calories.

➤ **DV.** In its wisdom, the FDA has combined the RDIs and DRVs into one, easy-to-understand standard called the Daily Value (DV). This is the basis for the detailed labels you now see on food packages. The labels include the DRVs and selected RDIs for some vitamins and minerals, usually Vitamin A, Vitamin C, calcium, and iron, but sometimes others (depending on whether the food is a good source of those nutrients or not). The label gives both the total amount of each nutrient per serving and what percentage of your recommended daily intake that amount is.

| Daily Recommended Values for Adults | |
|---|---|
| **Nutrient** | **Portion of Daily Diet** |
| Total fats | 30%, 65 g, or 600 calories |
| Saturated fat | 10%, 20 g, or 200 calories |
| Cholesterol | 300 mg |
| Carbohydrates | 60%, 300 grams, or 1,200 calories |
| Protein | 10%, 50 g, or 200 calories |
| Fiber | 25 grams |
| Sodium | 2,400 mg |
| Potassium | 3,500 mg |

*Notes: Based on a daily diet of 2,000 calories. If you eat fewer or more calories, the percentages remain the same. Saturated fat should be no more than 10% of total fat. Children under age 4 and pregnant and nursing women need more protein.*

Other agencies and organizations also get into the standards act. The nonprofit American Heart Association, for example, says your daily cholesterol intake should be no more than 300 mg a day—the same as the DRV. The federal National Institutes of Health recommends 1,000 mg of calcium for women aged 25 to 50 and 1,500 mg for women over age 65. Both amounts are higher than the current RDI—and the RDIs don't really consider the different needs of older adults. These recommendations don't have the force of law the way the ones from the FDA do, but they carry a lot of weight in the medical community.

**Now You're Cooking**

The American Heart Association's Food Certification Program began in 1994 to help consumers easily select foods in the grocery store that are part of balanced, heart-healthy diet. These foods are generally low in fat, saturated fat, and cholesterol. Foods that have been certified can carry the AHA's red heart-check logo.

No matter how you look at it—RDA, RDI, DV— there's still one big problem. In the opinion of many health professionals, the amounts for vitamins and minerals are too low. More and more research tells us that larger doses of some vitamins and minerals not only keep you healthier now, they can also help diseases from getting started and can help control them once they do.

# What Are Your Needs?

Everybody's different, which is one reason minimum averages like the RDAs aren't always helpful. In many cases, you might want to take supplements to get more than the RDAs. But how can you decide what's best for you?

We can't tell you exactly how much to take of anything. What we can do is explain, in the chapters on the individual vitamins and minerals, why you might want more of each and how much more is safe. The amounts you decide to take will depend on your personal health, family medical history, age, sex, and other factors. We also explain why it's safe to take supplements of some vitamins and minerals and why sometimes you should stick to the RDA.

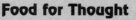

### Food for Thought

According to Harvard Medical School's ongoing Physician's Health Study, people who take a daily multivitamin have a 25 percent lower risk of developing a cataract.

You won't see instant changes in your health as soon as you start taking more vitamins and minerals. The improvements come slowly, over a period of a few weeks or even months. You may notice that you just feel better overall—more energetic and more optimistic. Nagging problems, like a lingering cold or minor skin rash, may finally clear up. If you have a chronic disease such as diabetes, you may find that your symptoms are easier to deal with and some side effects and complications improve.

What may be most important about supplements, though, are the things that *won't* happen. By taking extra vitamins and minerals now as part of a healthy diet, you may be preventing future problems, like osteoporosis, cancer, heart disease, stroke, and senility.

## Tests for Vitamin and Mineral Deficiencies

Today many doctors routinely check your blood for some vitamin and mineral deficiencies, especially iron and Vitamin $B_{12}$ (cobalamin). There are blood and urine tests for most vitamins and minerals, but some are complicated or inconvenient, to say nothing of the costs. Generally there's no real reason to do them, unless you have a medical problem that affects your ability to absorb nutrients. Today many nutritionally oriented health practitioners think that your blood antioxidant level is a better test of your vitamin and mineral levels and overall health. That's because you need vitamins and minerals to make antioxidant enzymes. If you're low on the enzymes, you're also low on their building blocks. If you're interested in antioxidant testing, discuss it with your doctor or nutritionist.

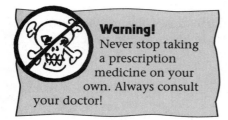

### Warning!
Never stop taking a prescription medicine on your own. Always consult your doctor!

# Nutritionally Oriented Health Care

Nutritionally oriented doctors often describe their approach as *functional medicine* or sometimes *orthomolecular medicine*. They believe that fixing the underlying biochemical imbalance that is causing an illness is just as important as treating the symptoms. Vitamins, minerals, and other nutrients, along with lifestyle changes, are important parts of functional medicine.

Prestigious institutions like the Harvard Medical School are now seriously studying the value of alternative treatments. Many doctors today have come to realize how important diet and vitamins and minerals are to the health of their patients. Sadly, many more haven't. If your doctor is among the unenlightened, you may want to consult a nutritionally oriented doctor, nutritionist, or other health care professional. We list several national professional organizations in Appendix B "Resources" at the back of this book. These groups can help you find a qualified professional in your area.

Whenever you visit any health-care professional, be sure to bring along a list of everything you take—including *all* prescription and nonprescription drugs and *all* vitamins, minerals, and other supplements. Otherwise, you might end up with an accidental bad reaction to a drug.

# Vitamins and Minerals for Everyone

We feel almost everyone can benefit from vitamins and minerals beyond the RDAs. To help you decide how much more, we've done a very conservative chart showing the safe ranges for healthy adults. Remember, more isn't always better. When in doubt, less is always best. Don't exceed the maximum safe dose!

**What's in a Word**

The great Linus Pauling, two-time winner of the Nobel Prize, coined the term *orthomolecular* medicine. The prefix *ortho-* means "right" or "correct." Many doctors today prefer the term *functional* medicine, meaning that they work to restore your body to its proper functioning.

**Quack, Quack**

One in three Americans will seek an "alternative" therapy for a serious illness. They're easy targets for unscrupulous companies and unlicensed "natural medicine" practitioners peddling phony treatments and formulas that "cure" ailments like arthritis or Alzheimer's disease. If the advertising pitch includes words like *special, instant relief, secret, miracle, rediscovered,* or *ancient,* beware! The only thing miraculous about these products is how quickly your money vanishes.

| Safe Dosage Ranges for Vitamins and Minerals for Healthy Adults | |
|---|---|
| **Vitamins** | **Safe Daily Dosage Range** |
| Vitamin A | 5,000–25,000 IU |
| B Vitamins: | |
| Thiamin | 2–100 mg |
| Riboflavin | 50–100 mg |
| Niacin | 20–100 mg |
| Pyridoxine | 3–50 mg |
| Folic acid | 800 mcg–2 mg |
| Cobalamin | 500–1,000 mcg |
| Pantothenic acid | 4–7 mg |
| Biotin | 30–100 mcg |
| Vitamin C | 500–2,000 mg |
| Vitamin D | 400–600 IU |
| Vitamin E | 200–400 IU |
| **Minerals** | **Safe Daily Dosage Range** |
| Calcium | 1,000–1,500 mg |
| Copper | 1.5–3.0 mg |
| Chromium | 50–200 mcg |
| Iron | 15–30 mg |
| Magnesium | 300–500 mg |
| Manganese | 2.5–5.0 mg |
| Molybdenum | 75–250 mcg |
| Potassium | 2,000–3,500 mg |
| Selenium | 70–200 mcg |
| Zinc | 15–50 mg |

# Special Needs of Older Adults

As you get older, your nutritional needs change. By the time you're 65, for instance, you just don't absorb Vitamin D and some B vitamins as well as you used to. If you're an older woman, you need more calcium and less iron. And by the time you're 65 you may well be taking at least one prescription drug to treat some sort of chronic condition. In fact, nearly half of all people over age 75 take three or more prescription drugs every day. As you'll learn in the chapters of this book, some common prescription drugs can seriously affect your vitamin and mineral levels—and some vitamins and minerals could keep the drugs from working right.

Many older people just don't eat right or eat enough. Many older women eat only 1,250 to 1,500 calories a day, while many older men eat only about 1,600 to 1,900 calories daily. Even worse, studies show that 30 percent of the elderly regularly skip at least one meal a day. If you're not taking in enough good, nutritious calories, you're not taking in enough vitamins and minerals from your food.

If you're over age 65, discuss your vitamin and mineral needs with your doctor. Look carefully at your diet and be sure you're getting of all the B vitamins, but especially thiamin (Vitamin $B_1$), riboflavin (Vitamin $B_{12}$), pyridoxine (Vitamin $B_6$), and cobalamin (Vitamin $B_{12}$). Because your ability to absorb the B's drops with age, talk to your doctor about taking a complete B vitamins supplement. You also need to be sure you're getting enough Vitamin E, Vitamin C, iron, calcium, magnesium, and zinc. Supplements could help here as well.

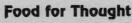

## Food for Thought

A 1997 international study showed that women who took multivitamin supplements throughout their pregnancy had children who were 40 percent less likely to get brain tumors. Vitamins A, C, E, and folic acid seemed to be the most important for providing the protection. If you're planning a family or are already pregnant, talk to your doctor about which vitamins and minerals to take.

# Vitamins for Kids and Teens

Kids and teenagers grow fast. To fuel that growth, they need good nutrition, including plenty of vitamins and minerals. Unfortunately, kids today don't always get what they need. One out of every ten toddlers is low on iron, for example, and teenage girls need extra. Many teens, male and female, are low on zinc.

How can you be sure your kids are getting their vitamins? The standard answer is to make sure they eat a variety of foods, including lots of fresh fruits and vegetables. That's easy for the nutritionists to say. Anyone who's ever been a parent knows that it's a *lot* harder to do. It's tough enough to get a six-year-old to eat vegetables—just try getting a sixteen-year-old to eat them!

Vitamin and mineral supplements can be very helpful here. Give children under age two vitamin and minerals supplements only if your doctor

**Warning!**
Keep all supplements and drugs of any sort safely away from small children. The amount of iron in just three or four adult iron supplements, for example, could cause serious poisoning in a young child.

recommends them. Many doctors do suggest an iron supplement or a formula containing iron for babies under 24 months, especially if you are breastfeeding. For young children over age two, liquid multi supplements are convenient—all you have to do is add a squirt to their morning milk or juice. Older kids like chewable tablets and you might even be able to get your teenagers to swallow a daily supplement. There are a lot of different brands from which to choose. We suggest looking for one that has the RDA for your child's age group and is made without artificial colorings and preservatives. As a rule, there's no real reason to give a child or teen supplements of individual vitamins and minerals—stick to a good multi instead.

# Vitamins for Vegetarians

> **WHAT'S THAT MEAN? What's in a Word**
> *Vegetarians* are people who don't eat meat. Most vegetarians will eat eggs and dairy foods, and some will eat fish. *Vegans* are people who don't eat any animal foods at all.

Because they don't eat meat—and sometimes don't eat any animal foods at all—*vegetarians* and *vegans* need to be sure they're getting enough vitamins and minerals from their food. This is fairly easy to do with a little planning and a good understanding of what's in their foods. Even so, vegetarians and vegans may end up on the low side for some nutrients, especially the B vitamins, calcium, and iron. To be on the safe side, we recommend a good daily multi supplement, especially for kids who don't eat animal foods.

# Supplements and Common Health Problems

We're going to talk a lot in this book about how vitamins, minerals, and other supplements can help high cholesterol, high blood pressure, and diabetes. Rather than explain these very common health problems over and over, we're going to deal with them here instead.

# High Cholesterol

> **WHAT'S THAT MEAN? What's in a Word**
> *Low-density lipoprotein (LDL)*—a form of cholesterol—is often called "bad" cholesterol because excess amounts in your blood can lead to health problems, including heart disease. *High-density lipoprotein (HDL)*—another form of cholesterol—is often called "good" cholesterol because it can help remove LDL cholesterol from your blood.

We worry so much about our cholesterol these days that we sometimes forget that you need cholesterol to live. Cholesterol is a waxy fat your body needs to make your cell membranes and many hormones, among other important roles. Most of your cholesterol you make in your liver, but also you get some from eating animal foods. Just like oil and water, cholesterol and blood don't mix. To get the cholesterol to where it has to go, your liver coats it with a layer of protein. The protein keeps the cholesterol together so that it doesn't just float around in your blood. The technical name for the cholesterol-protein package is *lipoprotein*.

There are several different kinds of lipoproteins, but the two most important are *low-density lipoprotein (LDL)* and *high-density lipoprotein (HDL).* Most of the cholesterol in your blood is carried as LDL cholesterol; only about a third to a quarter is carried as HDL cholesterol. But too much LDL cholesterol in the blood can lead to *atherosclerosis*—"clogging" of the arteries—which can lead to heart disease, stroke, and other problems. That's why LDL cholesterol is often called "bad" cholesterol. HDL cholesterol actually helps remove cholesterol from the blood—that's why it's often called "good" cholesterol. Ideally, you want to have a relatively low LDL level and a relatively high HDL level.

What's a good level and how do you know? To measure your blood cholesterol levels, your doctor sends a sample of your blood to a laboratory, where the amounts of LDL and HDL in it are measured. (To make sure the results are accurate, don't eat for twelve hours before the test.) The results come back as milligrams per deciliter, abbreviated as mg/dL (a deciliter is one-tenth of a liter). Usually there are two numbers: your total cholesterol (LDL plus HDL) and your LDL stated separately. In general, if your total cholesterol is below 200 mg/dL, you don't have to worry. If it's above 200 mg/dL but below 240 mg/dL, you have borderline high cholesterol. If it's above 240 mg/dL, you have high cholesterol.

If your cholesterol is borderline high or high, lowering it by even 10 percent could prevent a heart attack or stroke. Eating less fat, getting more exercise, and quitting smoking are the most important steps, along with cholesterol-lowering drugs if your doctor recommends them. In addition, throughout this book we'll talk about how vitamins, minerals, and other supplements, along with diet and lifestyle changes, can help.

> **What's in a Word**
> *Atherosclerosis* happens when fatty deposits called *plaques* build up inside one your arteries, often an artery that nourishes your heart or leads to your brain. Many researchers today believe that plaque forms when LDL cholesterol is oxidized by free radicals. Keeping your antioxidant levels high may help prevent atherosclerosis.

> **Now You're Cooking**
> Some foods that are advertised as having no cholesterol are still loaded with fat—it's just that the fat comes from plant oils. Take potato chips, for instance. One ounce (and who can eat just an ounce?) of regular chips has nearly 10 grams of fat and 150 calories, but no cholesterol.

## High Blood Pressure

Every time your heart beats (about 60 to 70 times a minute when you're resting), it pumps blood out through large blood vessels called arteries. Blood pressure is the force of that blood as it pushes against the walls of the arteries. Your blood pressure is at its highest when your heart beats and pushes the blood out—doctors call this the *systolic* pressure. When the heart is at rest between beats, your blood pressure falls. This is called *diastolic* pressure. Blood pressure is always given as two numbers: first the systolic and then the diastolic pressure.

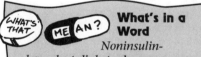

### What's in a Word

*Hypertension*, or high blood pressure, is a disease with many causes, no symptoms at first, and no cure. Early detection and treatment could save your life. Your doctor looks at two numbers when checking your blood pressure. The *systolic* pressure is the pressure against your arteries when your heart pumps out blood. The *diastolic* pressure is the pressure when your heart is at rest between beats. If your pressure is 140/90 or more, you have hypertension.

### What's in a Word

*Noninsulin-dependent diabetes* happens when cells, for unknown reasons, become resistant to insulin, a hormone made in the pancreas. Insulin carries glucose (sugar) into cells, where it is then burned for fuel. When your cells are resistant to insulin, glucose builds up in your blood while your cells literally starve. This form of diabetes usually begins after age 40 and is most common after age 55.

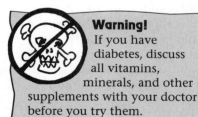

### Warning!

If you have diabetes, discuss all vitamins, minerals, and other supplements with your doctor before you try them.

Normal blood pressure ranges from below 130 to 140 systolic and below 85 to 90 diastolic. If your blood pressure is less than 140/90, then, it's normal. High blood pressure, or *hypertension*, is anything above 140/90. High blood pressure gets more serious as the numbers get higher. Your risk of heart attack, stroke, and kidney disease go up along with your blood pressure.

If your blood pressure is high, there are many lifestyle steps you can take to lower it, like losing weight, getting more exercise, avoiding salt, giving up cigarettes, and drinking less alcohol. If that doesn't help, or if your blood pressure stays high, your doctor may prescribe drugs to bring it down. As you'll learn in the rest of this book, vitamins, minerals, and other supplements, along with diet and lifestyle changes, can help.

## Diabetes

The recommendations in this book are for the 13 to 14 million Americans who have *noninsulin-dependent diabetes*. People with this disease have trouble getting glucose, your body's main fuel, from their blood into their cells, where it can be turned into energy. Diabetes can lead to serious complications. It's the single biggest cause of kidney disease, for example; it's also a leading cause of blindness. Diabetics have double the risk of the general population for heart attack and stroke.

Noninsulin-dependent diabetes can be controlled by losing weight, watching your diet carefully, getting more exercise, and taking the medicine your doctor prescribes. As we'll discuss throughout this book, many of the problems diabetics get, including a painful condition called diabetic neuropathy, can be helped by vitamin, minerals, and supplements.

## Getting the Most from Vitamin and Mineral Supplements

We hope by now we've made a pretty good case for taking extra vitamins and minerals every day. The best way to do that is with a good multivitamin/mineral supplement. According to the Dietary Supplement Health and Education Act (DSHEA) of 1994, a dietary supplement is a product that contains one or more dietary ingredients, such as vitamins, minerals, herbs, amino acids or other ingredients used to supplement the diet.

How can you choose the right one out of all the many, many brands available? Here's what to look for:

➤ A reliable manufacturer who follows good manufacturing practices (GMPs). These are set out by the National Nutritional Foods Association (a trade organization for the supplements industry), the United States Pharmacopeia (USP) Standards (the same standards used for making prescription drugs), FDA guidelines, and the guidelines set out in the Dietary Supplement Health and Education Act (DSHEA) of 1994. If you're in doubt, call the manufacturer and ask.

➤ A formula that contains all the vitamins except Vitamin K. Be sure the supplement contains all the B vitamins, including cobalamin (Vitamin $B_{12}$).

➤ A formula that contains mixed carotenoids along with Vitamin A. (See Chapter 3 on Vitamin A and Chapter 25 on flavonoids to learn why.)

➤ A formula that contains *chelated* forms of calcium, magnesium, potassium, selenium, and zinc, along with boron, chromium, manganese, and molybdenum. Because a tablet that had the RDAs for calcium and the other minerals would be too large to swallow, it's OK if the formula doesn't have the full amounts. Just be sure you're getting some calcium from your diet as well.

➤ A formula that contains iron, if you want to take extra of this mineral, or is iron-free if you don't. (See Chapter 21 on trace minerals to decide.)

➤ A formula that contains the minerals in forms you can easily absorb. We go into that in more detail in each mineral chapter, but here's an easy rule of thumb: The calcium should be in the form of calcium citrate or an amino acid chelate. If it's not, choose a different brand.

What about picking individual supplements, like calcium or Vitamin C? Check out what we have to say about each vitamin or mineral in the rest of this book, then pick the kind best for you. The same rules for quality apply.

> **What's in a Word**
> *Chelated* minerals have been treated to alter their electrical charge, usually by binding them chemically a harmless salt such as gluconate, citrate, picolinate, aspartate, or another -ate substance. That's why the label often reads "zinc picolinate" or "magnesium citrate" rather than just plain zinc or magnesium. You absorb minerals better if they've been chelated.

> **Quack, Quack**
> Colloidal minerals are the latest hot product to hit the supplement market. Stay away. Colloidal supplements are basically clay, which naturally contains a wide range of minerals, dissolved in water. They're expensive, they're unregulated, and you can't be sure of what you're getting.

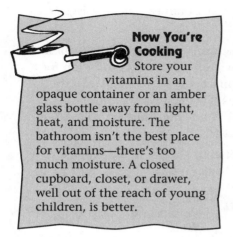

**Now You're Cooking**

Store your vitamins in an opaque container or an amber glass bottle away from light, heat, and moisture. The bathroom isn't the best place for vitamins—there's too much moisture. A closed cupboard, closet, or drawer, well out of the reach of young children, is better.

Not too many manufacturers, in our opinion, meet the requirements for producing quality supplements. The leader for quality, research, and integrity is Solgar. Other leading manufacturers include Twin Labs and Enzymatic Therapy. To find a retailer near you, call the companies (we list them in Appendix B "Resources"). We suggest you avoid "no-name" or "store-brand" supplements—you can't be sure of the quality.

## Taking Your Vitamins

Many people like the convenience of taking a one-a-day supplement—a pill you can pop first thing in the morning and not have to think about again. One-a-days have some drawbacks, though. First, many one-a-days just don't have enough in them. To keep them small enough to swallow easily, they don't have the RDAs for calcium, magnesium, or potassium. Most don't have the RDA for selenium, either. Another problem is that the water-soluble B vitamins and Vitamin C will be washed from your body fairly quickly if you take them all at once.

It's much more effective to take your vitamins and minerals in divided doses throughout the day. That way, you can easily get the full RDAs for calcium and other minerals without having to swallow big pills, and your levels of the water-soluble vitamins remain high throughout the day. You'll get the most from your supplements if you make a habit of taking them with meals.

Check the freshness and potency guarantee date on supplements before you buy them. Pass on products that are near or past their expiration. To keep supplements fresh after you open them, buy only as much as you normally use in a month and put the lids back on tightly.

## The Least You Need to Know

➤ The minimum daily amounts for vitamins, minerals, and other nutrients such as fiber are set by the independent National Research Council and the federal Food and Drug Agency (FDA).

➤ Many doctors, nutritionists, and researchers today believe these amounts are far too low.

➤ You can safely take more than the RDA for almost all vitamins and minerals.

➤ Everyone's needs are different. Kids, older adults, and vegetarians have special nutritional needs.

➤ Almost everyone can benefit from taking a daily multivitamin/mineral supplement.

➤ Choose high-quality supplements and take them regularly.

# Part 2
# The A to K of Vitamins

*We could write this part of the book using just six letters: A, B, C, D, E, and K. These are the vitamins you absolutely, positively must have in very small amounts to live. No one vitamin is any more important than any other.*

*After you get beyond your basic needs, though, some vitamins may be more useful to you than others. But which ones? And how much? Here is where you need an understanding of how vitamins work and the effects they have on you.*

*Remember when you were a kid and had alphabet soup for lunch? You'd poke around in the bowl until you came up with the letters of your name. That's a little what the alphabet soup of vitamins is like—you can arrange those six letters to spell good health for yourself.*

# Chapter 3

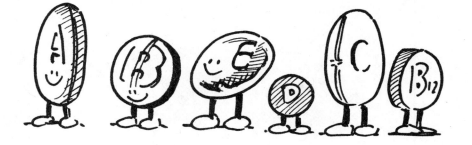

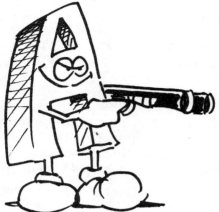

# Vitamin A and Carotenes: Double-Barreled Health Protection

## In This Chapter

➤ Why you need Vitamin A and carotenes

➤ Foods that are high in Vitamin A and carotenes

➤ Choosing the right supplements

➤ How Vitamin A helps protect your vision and boost your immune system

➤ How carotenes help protect you against the free radicals that can cause cancer and heart disease

Vitamin A was the first vitamin to be discovered, back in 1913. Twenty-four centuries ago in ancient Greece, the importance of Vitamin A was already well known. Back then, Hippocrates, the father of modern medicine, told patients with failing eyesight to eat beef liver. When they did, they were able to see much better, especially at night. Hippocrates didn't know why liver helped so much, but today we know that animal liver is a rich source of Vitamin A—and we know that our eyes need plenty of Vitamin A to work properly in the dark.

Today we know a lot more than Hippocrates about the importance of Vitamin A for a wide range of body functions—from keeping your skin smooth to warding off cancer. We also know that Vitamin A is only half the story. Health researchers are very excited about carotenes, the natural plant forms of Vitamin A. Your body converts some of the carotenes in plant foods into the Vitamin A you need and uses the leftovers to help you fight off the free radicals that can cause cancer, heart disease, and other problems.

# Why You Need Vitamin A

When Vitamin A was first discovered, it was called the "anti-infective agent." Lab animals fed a diet low in animal foods, vegetables, and fruits soon got eye infections—infections that cleared up as soon as these foods were put back into their diet. The mysterious "agent" in the foods turned out to be a fat-soluble substance that was dubbed Vitamin A.

> **What's in a Word**
>
> Your *epithelial tissues* cover the internal and external surfaces of your body. Because your skin covers all of your outside, for example, it's one giant external epithelial tissue. Epithelial tissue also lines your nose and your eyes. Your entire digestive tract, from start to finish, is lined with epithelial tissue. So are your lungs and your urinary and reproductive tracts.

To fend off infections and illnesses, Vitamin A helps you put up strong front-line barriers to infection. How? By helping your body's *epithelial tissues*—the cells that make up your skin and line your eyes, mouth, nose, throat, lungs, digestive tract, and urinary tract—grow and repair themselves. These tissues line your body's external and internal surfaces and keep out trespassers. Without enough Vitamin A, these cells become stiff, dry, and much more likely to let their guard down. When that happens, germs can easily pass through them and into your body.

Even if your body has plenty of Vitamin A, those nasty germs still sometimes get through your outer defenses. When that happens, Vitamin A helps your immune system come riding to the rescue.

Vitamin A is essential for healthy eyes—an important subject we'll talk a lot about later in this chapter.

Children and teens need plenty of Vitamin A to help them grow properly and build strong bones and teeth. Your need for Vitamin A doesn't stop then, though. Even after you're full grown, your body constantly replaces old, worn-out cells with new ones. You need Vitamin A to produce healthy replacement cells and to keep your bones and teeth strong.

# Why You Need Carotenes Even More

Now that you know why you need Vitamin A, we're going to confuse you by explaining why you need carotenes even more. Bear with us as we journey back into vitamin history again to explain why.

After Vitamin A was first discovered, researchers believed that the only way to get your A's was by eating animal foods such as eggs or liver that naturally contain *retinoids,* or *preformed* Vitamin A. Your body can use this Vitamin A as is just as soon as you eat it.

In 1928, researchers discovered the other way to get your A's: by eating plant foods that contain *carotenes*—the orange, red, and yellow substances that give plant foods their colors. The most abundant of the carotenes in plant foods is *beta carotene.* Your body easily converts beta carotene to Vitamin A in your small intestine, where special enzymes split one molecule of beta carotene in half to make two molecules of Vitamin A.

If you don't happen to need any Vitamin A just then, you don't convert the beta carotene. Instead, a lot of it circulates in your blood and enters into your cells; the rest gets stored in your fatty tissues. Whenever you need some extra A's, your liver quickly converts the stored beta carotene.

Carotenes are just one small group of plant substances in the much larger *carotenoid* family. In this chapter we'll focus on the two main carotenes that are converted to Vitamin A: *alpha carotene* (sometimes written α-carotene) and *beta carotene* (sometimes written β-carotene). (A few other carotenes have some Vitamin A activity, but it's so minor we don't really need to discuss them.)

Why is it better to convert your A's from the carotenes in plant foods rather than getting them straight from animal foods or supplements? There are some very good reasons:

➤ The *antioxidant power* of carotenes. About 40 percent of the carotenes you eat are converted to Vitamin A in your liver and small intestine as you need it. The rest act as powerful antioxidants. Beta carotene is especially good at quenching singlet oxygen. (Remember that destructive little molecule from Chapter 1?) Alpha carotene is an

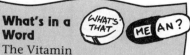

**What's in a Word**

**The Vitamin**
A found in animal foods such as egg yolks is *preformed*—your body can use it immediately. Actually, there are three kinds of preformed Vitamin A: *retinol, retinaldehyde,* and *retinoic acid.* These names refer to your retina, the light-sensitive layer of cells at the back of your eye. One of the first signs of Vitamin A deficiency is trouble seeing at night, because your retina needs Vitamin A to function properly.

**What's in a Word**

*Carotenes* are natural pigments in red, orange, and yellow plant foods (like cantaloupes, carrots, and tomatoes). Carotenes are also found in potatoes and dark green leafy vegetables. The name comes from carrots. Because your body has to change the carotenes into Vitamin A before you can use them, carotenes are sometimes called *precursor* (meaning something that precedes or goes before) *Vitamin A* or *provitamin A* (where *pro-* means "before").

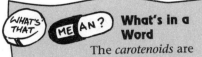

**What's in a Word**

The *carotenoids* are a large family of red, orange, and yellow plant substances found in many fruits and vegetables. Your body can convert two related carotenoids, *alpha carotene* and *beta carotene*, into Vitamin A. The two carotenes are similar, but beta carotene is much more abundant in foods and accounts for most of the Vitamin A you make from plant foods.

even better antioxidant—it may be ten times as effective for mopping up free radicals.

➤ The *safety* of carotenes. Large doses of supplemental Vitamin A can be toxic—and some people show overdose symptoms even at lower doses. Your body converts carotenes to Vitamin A only as needed, however, so it's almost impossible to overdose. Also, beta carotene is nontoxic—even if you store so much in your fatty tissues that you turn yellow, it's harmless.

➤ The *health benefits* of fruits and vegetables. Carotenes are found in almost every fruit and vegetable. Five servings a day will give you all the Vitamin A you need, along with plenty of other vitamins, minerals, antioxidants, and fiber. What you won't get are calories and the cholesterol found in animal sources of preformed Vitamin A such as beef liver (and let's not even discuss the yucky taste).

# The RDA for Vitamin A

If you eat a typical diet, you'll get some of your Vitamin A the preformed way from milk, eggs, and meat. You'll get the rest in the form of carotenes (mostly beta) from the fruits and vegetables you eat. That means the RDA for Vitamin A assumes that you get some of your A's from animal foods and some from plant foods. But that leads to a problem. How can you measure how much Vitamin A you're actually making from the beta carotene you eat in plant foods?

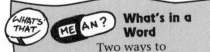

**What's in a Word**

Two ways to measure Vitamin A are currently in use: *International Units (IU)* and *Retinol Equivalents (RE)*. One IU equals 0.3 micrograms of Vitamin A in the form of retinol or 0.6 micrograms of beta carotene. One RE equals one microgram of retinol or 6 micrograms of beta carotene. IUs continue to be used as a standard measurement on vitamin labels, but researchers today prefer the more accurate Retinol Equivalent.

## Measuring Vitamin A

Up until 1980, the RDA for Vitamin A was given in *International Units (IU)*. One IU was defined as 0.3 micrograms of retinol (the most common type of preformed Vitamin A) or 0.6 micrograms of beta carotene. After 1980, the measurement unit for Vitamin A was changed. International Units didn't take into account the difference in absorption between preformed Vitamin A and beta carotene. About 80 percent of the preformed Vitamin A you take in gets absorbed into your body, but only about 40 percent of the beta carotene does, so you need more beta carotene to make the same amount of Vitamin A. After much deliberation (the idea was first proposed in 1967), the measurement unit was changed to give a more accurate idea of how much Vitamin A is really in a food or supplement. The new unit is called a *Retinol Equivalent (RE)*. One microgram of preformed

Vitamin A in the form of retinol equals one Retinol Equivalent. You need 6 micrograms of beta carotene to make one Retinol Equivalent; you need 12 micrograms of alpha carotene to make one RE.

Are you with us so far? There's one more complicating fact: Most vitamin manufacturers still list the Vitamin A and beta carotene content on the label in International Units. To convert from IUs to REs, divide by five (in other words, 4,000 IUs is equal to 800 REs). To help you figure out what's in your vitamins, we list the amounts in the RDA charts in both REs and IUs.

## The RDA for Vitamin A

| Age | RE | IU |
| --- | --- | --- |
| **Infants** | | |
| 0–1 year | 375 | 1,875 |
| **Children** | | |
| 1–3 years | 400 | 2,000 |
| 4–6 | 500 | 2,500 |
| 7–10 | 700 | 3,500 |
| **Adults** | | |
| Men 11+ | 1,000 | 5,000 |
| Women 11+ | 800 | 4,000 |
| Pregnant women | 800 | 4,000 |
| Nursing women | 1,300 | 6,500 |

Vitamin A is an essential nutrient, so it's got an established RDA. Beta carotene, although it's certainly important, isn't considered essential, so it doesn't have an RDA. How can you decide how much to take? The U.S. Department of Agriculture and the National Cancer Institute suggest a daily dose of 6 mg, but many nutritionists feel this is too low. Some think you should take as much as 30 mg a day. A good compromise might be 15 mg a day—roughly the equivalent of 25,000 IU (5,000 RE) of Vitamin A. That's about five times the RDA for Vitamin A, but without the toxic side effects.

Studies show that most people get the RDA for Vitamin A every day, but only a few get anywhere near the suggested 6 mg of beta carotene. Most people eat only about 1.5 mg of beta carotene daily. On an average day, only about 20 percent of the population eats any fruits and vegetables rich in beta carotene.

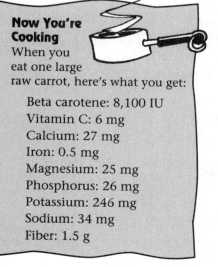

**Now You're Cooking**
When you eat one large raw carrot, here's what you get:

Beta carotene: 8,100 IU
Vitamin C: 6 mg
Calcium: 27 mg
Iron: 0.5 mg
Magnesium: 25 mg
Phosphorus: 26 mg
Potassium: 246 mg
Sodium: 34 mg
Fiber: 1.5 g

# Vitamin A Cautions

Taking supplements that contain the RDA for Vitamin A is generally safe for everyone, but use caution. Vitamin A in large doses can be toxic, causing a condition called *hypervitaminosis A*. Symptoms of A overload include blurred vision, bone pain, headaches, diarrhea, loss of appetite, skin scaling and peeling, and muscular weakness. Vitamin A toxicity doesn't usually occur until you've been taking really large doses (more than 25,000 IU daily) for a long time, but don't take any chances—stick to the RDA.

 **Warning!** Excess Vitamin A during pregnancy can cause birth defects! If you are a woman of childbearing age, talk to your doctor about taking beta carotene supplements instead of Vitamin A.

Babies and children can reach toxic Vitamin A levels at much smaller doses. Most multivitamin supplements contain only the RDA, but some contain 10,000 IU (2,000 RE) or even more. Read labels carefully and talk to your doctor before giving vitamins to babies and children. Fortunately, most symptoms of Vitamin A toxicity gradually go away without lasting damage when you stop taking it.

 **Warning!** Vitamin A can cause serious problems for people with kidney disease. If you have kidney disease, talk to your doctor about taking Vitamin A or beta carotene supplements.

Be very careful about Vitamin A supplements if you are or might become pregnant. Too much Vitamin A (over 5,000 IU or 1,000 RE) can cause birth defects, especially if taken in the first seven weeks of pregnancy—when you might not even realize you're pregnant. Today many doctors suggest that women of childbearing age take beta carotene instead of Vitamin A supplements.

---

### Symptoms of Vitamin A Toxicity

| *Children* | *Adults* |
|---|---|
| Appetite loss | Appetite loss |
| Bone pain | Blurred vision |
| Bulging fontanelle (the soft spot on an infant's skull) | Diarrhea |
| Irritability | Drowsiness |
| Lethargy | Hair loss |
| Stunted growth | Headaches |
| | Irritability |
| | Lethargy |
| | Muscle weakness |
| | Skin scaling and peeling |
| | Vomiting |

## Beta Carotene Cautions

There's an easy way to avoid any possible problems from taking Vitamin A supplements—take beta carotene supplements instead. You'll safely get all the Vitamin A you need, along with the bonus of powerful antioxidant protection. It's almost impossible to take too much beta carotene. If you do, the only side effect is that you might turn yellow. Extra beta carotene builds up in the fat under your skin, giving your fat an orange-yellow color that shows through your skin—technically, *hypercarotenodermia*. You may look a little odd, but the color is harmless and goes away in a few weeks when you cut back your dosage.

## Carotenes and CARET

Recently a major study that was supposed to prove the positive effects of beta carotene against lung cancer turned out to suggest just the opposite. The Beta Carotene and Retinol Efficacy Trial (better known as CARET) studied the effects of beta carotene and Vitamin A supplements on people who had been or still were heavy smokers. The researchers expected that the people who took the supplements would have lower rates of lung cancer. In fact, they ended up with higher rates. The researchers were so upset by the results that they stopped the study nearly two years early.

Does all this mean that excitement about beta carotene is just so much hype? Not at all—numerous other studies show over and over that people with high beta carotene levels are generally healthier. For now, the one thing the CARET study suggests for sure is that people who smoke shouldn't take beta carotene supplements.

## Are You Deficient?

Generally speaking, a real Vitamin A deficiency is rare in the Western world, because so many common foods, including milk and breakfast cereals, are fortified with it.

### Food for Thought

Although Vitamin A deficiency is rare in Westernized countries, it's all too common in the less developed world. According to UNICEF, Vitamin A supplements could prevent millions of cases of blindness and one to three million child deaths each year in countries such as Bangladesh, Malawi, Haiti, and Brazil. The cost? Just two cents a capsule. Your donations to UNICEF help prevent this tragedy.

Almost everyone gets the RDA or pretty close to it, but some people are at high risk of a Vitamin A deficiency. If you fall into any of these categories, you may need more Vitamin A than you're actually getting:

➤ You have liver disease, cystic fibrosis, or chronic diarrhea. These problems can reduce the amount of Vitamin A you absorb or store.

➤ You abuse alcohol. Alcohol reduces the Vitamin A and beta carotene stored in your liver. On the other hand, animal studies suggest that beta carotene combined with alcohol is a one-two punch that could do a lot of damage to your liver.

➤ You smoke. People who smoke cigarettes have low beta carotene levels.

➤ You take birth control pills. The Pill raises the amount of Vitamin A in your blood but reduces the amount you store in your liver. (This doesn't happen with beta carotene.)

➤ You're sick or have a chronic infection. Being sick makes you produce extra free radicals, which lowers your Vitamin A level.

➤ You're under a great deal of stress—physical or psychological. Overwork, fatigue, and exercising too much all create free radicals, which lower your Vitamin A level. Also, when you're too busy or tired to eat right you don't get enough beta carotene.

➤ You're pregnant or breastfeeding. You're passing a lot of your Vitamin A on to your baby. You need some extra for yourself—but talk to your doctor first. Too much Vitamin A during pregnancy can cause birth defects.

➤ You take a bile-sequestering drug such as Cholybar®, Colestid®, or Questran® to lower your cholesterol. These drugs can keep you from absorbing fat-soluble vitamins such as Vitamin A correctly. If you take these drugs, your doctor will probably recommend vitamin supplements and tell you to take them at a different time than the medicine. Discuss any other supplements with your doctor before you try them.

➤ You take the drug methotrexate (Folex®, Methotrate®, Mexate®, Rheumatrex®) to treat arthritis, psoriasis, or cancer. This drug affects your intestines, making it harder to absorb Vitamin A and beta carotene. Discuss supplements with your doctor before you try them.

After several weeks without much Vitamin A in your diet, you'd start to have some signs of deficiency. One of the earliest is night blindness and other eye problems (we'll talk about these later on). Another sign of Vitamin A deficiency is a condition called *follicular hyperkeratosis*. When this happens, your epithelial tissues, especially your skin, start to make too much of a hard protein called keratin. You start to get little deposits of keratin that look like goose bumps around your hair follicles and make your skin feel rough and dry. Vitamin A deficiency can also cause reproductive problems for both men and women. A shortage of Vitamin A can also make you more likely to get respiratory infections, sore throats, sinus infections, and ear infections.

# Eating Your A's

The RDA assumes that you'll be getting most of your Vitamin A from animal sources such as eggs, liver, poultry, milk, and dairy products. That's a pretty good assumption, because most people don't eat that many fruits and vegetables and don't get much beta carotene from their diet. Animal foods that are high in Vitamin A, however, also tend to be high in calories and cholesterol.

## Food for Thought

The richest food source of Vitamin A is polar bear liver, which has 13,000 to 18,000 IU per *gram*—more than enough to give you Vitamin A poisoning if you ate even a small amount. That's not very likely—the only people who've actually gotten Vitamin A toxicity this way are Arctic explorers who have been trapped on the ice with nothing else to eat. And Antarctic explorers don't have to worry—there are no polar bears at the South Pole.

Nutritionists today strongly recommend getting your A's the beta carotene way, through five daily servings of fresh fruits and vegetables. One medium carrot contains over 8,000 IU of beta carotene—with no toxic side effects, no fat, and only 35 calories. Plus, you'll be getting the antioxidant protection carotenes provide. How many of these foods do you regularly eat?

## The Vitamin A in Food

| Food | Amount | Vitamin A in RE |
| --- | --- | --- |
| American cheese | 1 ounce | 82 |
| Beef liver | 3 ounces | 9,000 |
| Butter | 1 teaspoon | 35 |
| Cheddar cheese | 1 ounce | 86 |
| Chicken leg, with skin | 1 | 45 |
| Chicken liver | 3 1/2 ounces | 4,913 |
| Egg | 1 large | 97 |
| Ice cream, vanilla | 1 cup | 133 |
| Milk, skim | 1 cup | 149 |
| Salmon | 3 ounces | 11 |
| Sole | 3 ounces | 10 |
| Swiss cheese | 1 ounce | 72 |
| Swordfish | 3 ounces | 35 |
| Yogurt, low fat | 8 ounces | 36 |

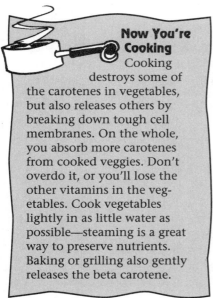

**Now You're Cooking** Cooking destroys some of the carotenes in vegetables, but also releases others by breaking down tough cell membranes. On the whole, you absorb more carotenes from cooked veggies. Don't overdo it, or you'll lose the other vitamins in the vegetables. Cook vegetables lightly in as little water as possible—steaming is a great way to preserve nutrients. Baking or grilling also gently releases the beta carotene.

The old saying "Have a lot of color on your plate" is the best advice for eating your carotenes. Remember, carotenes are the substances that give foods such as carrots, tomatoes, sweet potatoes, and apricots their vivid color. Actually, carotenes are found in practically all vegetables and fruits, including dark green leafy vegetables such as spinach and broccoli. The carotenes are there—you just can't see the bright reddish colors because they're disguised by the green.

Traditional food tables from standard sources treat beta carotene and Vitamin A as if they were interchangeable. The beta carotene contents of plant foods varies quite a bit, even within the same food. Farmers grow different carrot varieties, for example, depending on which kind does best on their land. Any listing of beta carotene content is approximate. In general, though, the listings are accurate enough to give you a good idea of how much beta carotene is in the foods you eat. Check the beta carotene content in your favorite fruits and veggies.

### The Beta Carotene in Food

| Food | Amount | Beta Carotene in IU |
|---|---|---|
| Apple | 1 | 120 |
| Apricots, fresh | 3 | 2,890 |
| Asparagus, cooked | 1 cup | 1,220 |
| Banana | 1 | 230 |
| Beet greens | 1/2 cup | 3,700 |
| Broccoli, cooked | 1/2 cup | 1,940 |
| Brussels sprouts | 1/2 cup | 405 |
| Cabbage | 1/2 cup | 90 |
| Cantaloupe | 1 cup | 2,720 |
| Carrot, raw | 1 medium | 8,100 |
| Cauliflower | 1 cup | 80 |
| Collard greens, cooked | 1/2 cup | 7,410 |
| Corn kernels | 1/2 cup | 330 |
| Grapefruit | 1/2 medium | 80 |
| Green beans, cooked | 1/2 cup | 340 |
| Kale, cooked | 1/2 cup | 4,560 |
| Orange | 1 medium | 400 |

| Food | Amount | Beta Carotene in IU |
|---|---|---|
| Peach | 1 large | 2,030 |
| Peas | 1/2 cup | 430 |
| Pepper, green | 1/2 cup | 210 |
| Pepper, sweet red | 1/2 cup | 2,225 |
| Prunes, stewed | 1/2 cup | 1,065 |
| Spinach, cooked | 1/2 cup | 7,290 |
| Squash, winter | 1/2 cup | 6,560 |
| Sweet potato, cooked | 1 medium | 9,230 |
| Tomato | 1 medium | 1,110 |
| Tomato juice | 6 ounces | 1,460 |
| Turnip greens, cooked | 1/2 cup | 4,570 |
| Watermelon, cubed | 1 cup | 940 |
| Zucchini | 1/2 cup | 270 |

# Getting the Most from Vitamin A and Carotenes

Vitamin A and beta carotene are fat-soluble, which means you store them in your liver and in the fatty tissues of your body. To avoid any chance of a toxic buildup, we suggest you stick to the Vitamin A in your daily multivitamin supplement and skip any additional A supplements.

## Food for Thought

Americans eat more carrots than they used to. According to the Department of Agriculture, in 1970, per capita consumption of carrots was 6.0 pounds. In 1995, per capita consumption was up to 10.1 pounds. To grow all those carrots, farmers planted over 106,000 acres, mostly in the top carrot-growing states of California, Washington, and Michigan. The total value of the carrot crop in 1994 was $310 million.

But if you're having one of those frantic days where eating right is way down on your priority list, taking a mixed carotenoid supplement can help make up for that skipped breakfast, fast-food lunch, and takeout dinner. These supplements contain beta carotene, lycopene, lutein, and other carotenoids. (We'll talk about these more when we get to Chapter 25 on flavonoids.)

To get the most out of your Vitamin A and beta carotene, be sure to also get at least the RDA for Vitamin E, zinc, and selenium. You need Vitamin E to help Vitamin A work more effectively; you also need extra Vitamin E if you take large doses (more than 15 g daily) of beta carotene supplements (see Chapter 15 for more information about Vitamin E). You need zinc to help transport Vitamin A around your body and you need selenium to help beta carotene work more effectively (for more on the important trace minerals see Chapter 21).

| Thumbs Up/Thumbs Down | |
|---|---|
| **Vitamin A and beta carotene work better if you also take:** | **Vitamin A and beta carotene are blocked by:** |
| All other vitamins and minerals | Alcohol |
| Vitamin E | Birth control pills |
| Selenium | Bile-sequestering cholesterol drugs |
| Zinc | Cigarette smoke |
| | Methotrexate, a drug used to treat arthritis, psoriasis, or cancer |

# Which Type Should I Take?

Vitamin A supplements usually come in soft gel caps in retinol or retinyl palmitate form—either is fine, but retinyl palmitate is best for people with intestinal problems. An old-fashioned way to get your A's is by taking cod liver oil. Aside from the fact that it's truly horrible tasting—even the cherry-flavored kind is awful—cod liver oil isn't a good choice. It's high in calories and often causes digestive upsets. Don't overdo on the Vitamin A supplements—more than 5,000 IU (1,000 RE) a day can be harmful. To avoid possible problems, we suggest taking mixed carotenes instead—you'll get your A's along with extra antioxidant protection.

For many years, the only beta carotene supplements you could buy were made synthetically and were oil-based. Today you have the option of buying water-based supplements made either from a type of algae called *Dunaliella* or

**Quack, Quack**

Some manufacturers offer micellized or emulsified Vitamin A, which means that the Vitamin A is broken up into very tiny droplets. The manufacturers claim that this improves absorption. In fact, you absorb about 80 to 90 percent of plain old Vitamin A. If you buy the micellized or emulsified brands, you'll be spending a lot more, but you won't really be absorbing much more.

from palm oil. Water-based carotenes do seem to be absorbed better. In general, oil-based supplements come in gel caps while the water-based ones come in solid form. No matter which form you buy, look for a product that is bright orange-red in color and store it away from light.

Most nutritionists today recommend mixed carotenoid supplements instead of just beta carotene. To be sure you're getting a good product, choose mixed carotenoids that contain beta carotene along with at least 20 percent alpha carotene and also xanthophylls and lycopene.

# Bugs Bunny Had Great Eyesight

Elmer Fudd never catches that pesky wabbit because Bugs always sees him coming. Why does Bugs have such great eyesight? It's all those carrots. What's good for Bugs is good for you too. Vitamin A and beta carotene are essential for your eyesight. Here are three reasons why:

## Preventing Night Blindness

Vitamin A helps you see well in the dark. Your retina (the layer of light-sensitive cells at the back of your eye) contains large amounts of Vitamin A, especially in the tiny structures called rods that are used for night vision. If you don't get enough Vitamin A, you develop night blindness—you can't see well in the dark or in dim light. We all lose a little of our night vision as we grow older, but Vitamin A can help slow or even prevent the loss. If you've noticed that you don't see as well at night as you used to, see your eye doctor to rule out other eye problems. If your eyes are OK otherwise, extra Vitamin A or beta carotene might help. Discuss the right amount with your doctor before you try it.

## Preventing Cataracts

A cataract forms when the lens of your eye becomes cloudy, reducing or even blocking completely the amount of light that enters your eye. At one time cataracts were a leading cause of blindness, but today simple outpatient surgery can fix the problem. But wouldn't it be better if a cataract never developed in the first place? There's solid evidence that a diet rich in carotenoids, especially beta carotene, helps prevent cataracts by mopping up free radicals before they can damage the lens.

## Preserving Eyesight

Vitamin A helps prevent age-related macular degeneration (AMD). Your macula is a tiny cluster of very sensitive cells in the center of your retina. It's essential for sharp vision. As you grow older, your macula may start to degenerate, causing vision loss and eventual blindness. AMD is the leading cause of blindness in people over 65, and about 30 percent of Americans over 75 suffer from it. What about the other 70 percent? It's likely they eat more foods that are high in beta carotene. According to one study, eating just one serving a day of a food high in beta carotene could reduce your chances of AMD by 40 percent.

Helpful as beta carotene is for preventing AMD, other carotenoids such as lutein and zeaxanthin are even better—we'll talk about them more in Chapter 25 on flavonoids.

# A as in Aging Skin

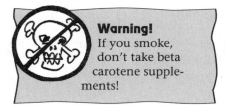

**Warning!** Millions of grateful teenagers treat their severe acne with prescription drugs such as Accutane® (isotretinoin) and Retin-A® (tretinoin) derived from Vitamin A. Another drug, Tegison® (etretinate), helps severe psoriasis. Taking large doses of Vitamin A will not have the same effect as taking these drugs! Large doses of Vitamin A are toxic!

**Warning!** If you smoke, don't take beta carotene supplements!

The cells of your skin grow very rapidly—your outer skin turns over completely in just about four weeks. All rapidly growing cells, including those in your skin, need plenty of Vitamin A. An early symptom of Vitamin A deficiency is skin that is rough, dry, and scaly. To help keep your skin smooth and supple, make sure to get the RDA for Vitamin A. This is especially important as you get older and your risk of skin cancer rises. One recent study shows that taking Vitamin A could cut your chances of getting basal cell carcinoma, the most common type of skin cancer, by 70 percent.

## To Beta or Not to Beta...

... that is the cancer question. There's been a lot of controversy recently about beta carotene and cancer. Does it prevent cancer or not? Yes—or maybe not. Let's try and sort out the issues here.

Study after study shows that if you have a high beta carotene level because you eat a lot of foods that contain carotenoids, you're less likely to get cancer. In one important study, for example, 8,000 men were followed for five years. The ones who had the lowest intake of beta carotene had the highest risk of lung cancer. Almost all researchers today agree that beta carotene *foods* play a major role in preventing cancer, especially cancer of the lung, stomach, and cervix. The real question is, do beta carotene *supplements* prevent cancer? Here's where the evidence is growing that they don't.

Three recent studies come down hard against beta carotene supplements: the CARET study we talked about earlier, the Alpha-tocopherol, Beta-carotene Cancer Prevention Study Group (the ABC study), and the Physicians' Health Study. Like the CARET study, the ABC study found that people taking beta carotene supplements had an *increased* risk of lung cancer. The Physicians' Health Study found that beta carotene supplements had no protective effect against cancer or heart disease.

So what do these studies prove? Only that beta carotene supplements may have a bad effect on people who are already at high risk for lung cancer. The people in the CARET and ABC studies all smoked cigarettes and drank alcohol. Among the people in the Physicians' Health Study, about 11 percent were smokers. In the bigger picture, the studies suggest two things. First, beta carotene supplements alone can't overcome a lifetime of smoking, drinking, and eating a diet low in the valuable nutrients found in fruits and vegetables. Second, people who eat foods high in beta carotene are also eating lots of other carotenoids—and *you need a range of carotenoids, not just beta carotene, to help ward off cancer.*

Researchers have focused on beta carotene because it's easy to measure in your blood, but perhaps now it's time to look further. In the meantime, get your beta carotene from your food whenever possible. If you want to take supplements, take mixed carotenoids, not beta carotene alone.

## Carotenes and Cardiac Cases

As with cancer, so with heart disease. People who eat foods high in beta carotene definitely have fewer heart attacks and strokes. In one major study of women nurses, for example, the ones who ate the most beta carotene foods had 22 percent fewer heart attacks than those who ate the least. The biggest beta carotene eaters did even better when it came to strokes—they had 40 percent fewer.

Once again, though, just taking beta carotene supplements doesn't necessarily give you the same protection. In the Physicians' Health Study, for example, people who took beta carotene supplements didn't really have any less heart disease than people who didn't. The message? You need *all* the carotenoids, not just beta carotene. The best way to get them all is to eat plenty of fruits and vegetables. If you want to take supplements, take mixed carotenoids.

## Boosting Your Immunity with Vitamin A

The anti-infective powers of Vitamin A have been known ever since the vitamin was discovered. Today Vitamin A is being used to help boost immunity in some cases—and some very exciting research suggests more uses in the future. Here's the current rundown:

➤ **Treating measles and respiratory infections.** Extra Vitamin A has been shown to help children get over the measles faster and with fewer complications. It also seems to help babies with respiratory infections. Talk to your doctor before you give Vitamin A supplements to babies or children.

➤ **Treating viral infections.** If you're low on Vitamin A you're more susceptible to illness, especially viral infections. If you're sick with a virus, extra Vitamin A in the form of beta carotene could help you fight it off.

➤ **Preventing complications from cancer treatment.** Chemotherapy and radiation therapy really lower your immunity. Very large doses of Vitamin A can help raise it again, but the amounts needed are too toxic to be used for long. In animal tests, large doses of beta carotene boost the immune system without the toxic danger. It's still too soon to tell if this will work in humans.

> ➤ **Boosting immune cells**. Large doses of beta carotene may help increase the number of infection-fighting cells in your immune system. This could be very beneficial for AIDS patients and anyone whose immune system is depressed.

Research continues on the benefits of Vitamin A and beta carotene for your immune system. We believe that the future will bring solid evidence that these nutrients can help not only immunity but many other health problems as well.

## The Least You Need to Know

> ➤ You need Vitamin A for healthy eyes, cell growth, and a strong immune system.

> ➤ Your body converts the beta carotene found in many fruits and vegetables into Vitamin A as needed.

> ➤ Beta carotene is also a powerful antioxidant that can help protect you against cancer and heart disease.

> ➤ The adult RDA for Vitamin A is between 800 and 1,000 RE (4,000 to 5,000 IU). There is no RDA for beta carotene, but 15 mg is often recommended.

> ➤ Vitamin A can be toxic in large amounts—don't exceed the RDA. Beta carotene is safe even in very large doses.

> ➤ Foods high in Vitamin A include eggs, milk, liver, and meat.

> ➤ Foods high in beta carotene include orange, yellow, and red fruits and vegetables such as cantaloupes, tomatoes, carrots, and butternut squash. Potatoes and dark green leafy vegetables are also high in beta carotene.

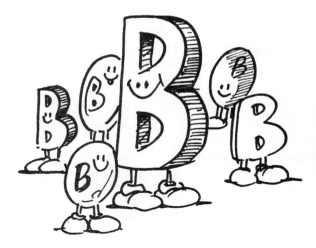

# Meet the B Family

## In This Chapter

➤ Why you need the entire B family of vitamins

➤ Foods that are high in B vitamins

➤ Choosing the right supplements

➤ How the B family protects your heart, gives you energy, boosts your immune system, and keeps you mentally alert

What big brood of vitamins is basic for keeping your brains, your blood, and a broad bunch of body functions in balance? Are you baffled? It's the B complex—that bunch of vitamins with the little numbers underneath and the weird names.

The B family members pull together to keep you healthy. You need each and every one of them—two doses of $B_6$ don't equal one of $B_{12}$. The range of jobs the B's do is pretty amazing. You need all the B's to help your cells grow and reproduce properly. You also need them all to send messages back and forth from your brain along your nerves. Another big chore done by most of the B's is helping you produce energy by breaking down the foods you eat into fuel your body can use. And we're just starting to realize that three different B's—folic acid, cobalamin, and pyridoxine—work together to do another very important job: keeping your heart healthy. On their own, each B vitamin also has special jobs to do, like keeping your red blood cells healthy and preventing birth defects.

# One Big Happy Family

The vitamins in the B family are all closely related. You could think of them as eight siblings and four cousins. We'll discuss all the siblings in later chapters, but for now, here are the main branches of the family tree:

➤ **Thiamin, or Vitamin $B_1$.** You need thiamin to keep all your body's cells, but especially your nerves, working right. Thiamin is important for mental functions, especially memory. You also need it to convert food to energy.

➤ **Riboflavin, or Vitamin $B_2$.** Riboflavin is really important for releasing energy from food. It's also vital for normal growth and development, normal red blood cells, and for making many of your body's hormones.

➤ **Niacin, or Vitamin $B_3$.** More than 50 body processes, from releasing energy from food to making hormones to detoxifying chemicals, depend on niacin.

➤ **Pantothenic acid, or Vitamin $B_5$.** This vitamin works closely with several of the other B's in the breakdown of fats, proteins, and carbohydrates into energy. You also need it to make Vitamin D, some hormones, and red blood cells.

➤ **Pyridoxine, or Vitamin $B_6$.** The main job of pyridoxine is shuffling around your amino acids to make the 5,000-plus proteins your body needs to run properly. It's also involved in making more than 60 different enzymes.

➤ **Biotin, or Vitamin $B_7$.** Biotin is needed for a lot of body processes that break down fats, proteins, and carbohydrates into fuel you can use. Biotin is sometimes called Vitamin H.

➤ **Folic acid, or Vitamin $B_9$.** The main job for folic acid is helping your cells grow and divide properly—it's important for preventing birth defects. You also need it for making the natural chemicals that control your mood, your appetite, and how well you sleep. And folic acid is vital for keeping your arteries open and lowering your chances of a heart attack or stroke.

➤ **Cobalamin, or Vitamin $B_{12}$.** You need cobalamin to process the carbohydrates, proteins, and fats in your food into energy. It also forms the protective covering of your nerve cells and keeps your red blood cells healthy, and helps prevent heart disease.

When you have plenty of all the B's in your body, they work together to keep your body running efficiently, producing the energy and the many complicated chemicals your body needs to function normally. But just as no one but Aunt Rose can make her famous potato salad, and just as it wouldn't be a family barbecue without it, each member of the B family has its own essential role to play. You need them all—if you're low on any one B vitamin, the others can't do their jobs.

# What the Little Numbers Mean

Why do most of the B vitamins have those little numbers underneath? And what happened to $B_4$, $B_8$, $B_{10}$ and $B_{11}$? The first B vitamin to be discovered was called "water-soluble B." That meant only that it was the second vitamin ever identified (the first was fat-soluble A). Riboflavin was discovered next, so water-soluble B became $B_1$ and riboflavin became $B_2$. The system began to get confusing in 1926, when researchers realized that Vitamin $B_1$ was actually two vitamins, thiamin and niacin. Thiamin kept the $B_1$ name. $B_2$ was already taken, so niacin got $B_3$. As vitamin research continued, scientists found a number of substances they thought at first were new B vitamins. Some turned out to be the same as B's that had already been discovered, while others turned out not to be vitamins at all. These phantom B's are the missing numbers. To avoid confusion, scientists now prefer to use the B vitamin names instead of the numbers.

| The B's at a Glance | |
|---|---|
| **B Vitamin** | **Function** |
| Thiamin (Vitamin $B_1$) | Helps regulate nerve growth, mental functions, and memory. Helps convert food to energy. |
| Riboflavin (Vitamin $B_2$) | Releases energy, aids in growth and development, needed for normal red blood cells and hormones. |
| Niacin (Vitamin $B_3$) | Needed for over 50 body processes. Releases energy, makes hormones, removes toxins, helps keep cholesterol normal. |
| Pantothenic acid (Vitamin $B_5$) | Releases energy from food. Necessary to make Vitamin D, hormones, and red blood cells. |
| Pyridoxine (Vitamin $B_6$) | Needed to make proteins, hormones, enzymes. Helps prevent heart disease. |
| Biotin (Vitamin $B_7$) | Releases energy from food. |
| Folic acid (Vitamin $B_9$) | Cell growth and division. Prevents birth defects and heart disease. |
| Cobalamin (Vitamin $B_{12}$) | Releases energy from food. Necessary for healthy red blood cells. Helps prevent heart disease. |

# The Unofficial B's

The four cousins of the main B family are sometimes called the "unofficial" B vitamins, because they're important for your health but don't have RDAs. They don't have RDAs because technically they're not vitamins—you make them in your body from other substances. We'll talk more about choline, inositol, and PABA in Chapter 12. We'll also talk a lot about lipoic acid in Chapter 23 on super antioxidants. For now, these are the twigs that come off the main B branch:

➤ **Choline.** Your brain uses choline to help store memories. It's also sometimes helpful for treating depression and may be useful for treating hepatitis.

➤ **Inositol.** You need inositol to make healthy cell membranes and messenger chemicals. It's also sometimes helpful for relieving nerve damage from diabetes.

➤ **PABA.** The initials stand for Para-aminobenzoic acid. This powerful antioxidant protects your skin from sun damage and is found in many sunscreen lotions and creams.

➤ **Lipoic acid.** A helper for the B vitamins, lipoic acid works closely with thiamin, riboflavin, niacin, and pantothenic acid to convert carbohydrates, fats, and proteins in your food into energy. Lipoic acid is also a powerful antioxidant and helps recycle Vitamin C and Vitamin E.

# RDAs for B Vitamins

The RDAs for the B vitamins are a little controversial these days. That's because several of the RDAs were lowered in the 1989 recommendations. At the same time, however, increasing evidence shows that you really need considerably larger doses to get the benefits of some B's, such as folic acid. Also, many doctors are starting to realize that their older patients show subtle signs of B vitamin deficiencies, even though they're getting the RDA. When new RDAs for B vitamins are released in the spring of 1998, it is likely that the amounts for folic acid and possibly some of the other B's will be raised.

Because one of the major roles of the B vitamins is converting food to energy, the RDAs are based on the number of calories you take in every day. The amount varies from vitamin to vitamin within the family. For thiamin, it's 0.5 mg per 1,000 calories; for niacin, it's 6.6 mg per 1,000 calories.

Another major role for the B's is cell growth and division. Growing children and teens need plenty of B's, and their needs go up as they enter their young adult years. Women who are pregnant or breastfeeding also need extra B's because they are passing a lot of their vitamins on to their babies.

Because none of the unofficial B's are essential to your diet (you can make them in your body from other things), there's no need to have RDAs for them. Almost everybody gets enough of the building blocks to make all they need.

We'll discuss the RDAs further when we get to each B in the upcoming chapters. In the meantime, check out the charts to see the RDAs for the six major B vitamins and the Safe and Adequate Intakes for biotin and pantothenic acid.

## RDAs for the B Vitamins

| Age/Sex | Thiamin | Ribo-flavin | Niacin | Pyri-doxine | Folic Acid | Cobal-amin |
|---|---|---|---|---|---|---|
| *Infants* | | | | | | |
| 0–0.5 year | 0.3 mg | 0.4 mg | 5.0 mg | 0.3 mg | 25 mcg | 0.3 mcg |
| 0.5–1 year | 0.4 mg | 0.5 mg | 6.0 mg | 0.6 mg | 35 mcg | 0.5 mcg |
| *Children* | | | | | | |
| 1–3 years | 0.7 mg | 0.8 mg | 9.0 mg | 1.0 mg | 50 mcg | 0.7 mcg |
| 4–6 | 0.9 mg | 1.1 mg | 12.0 mg | 1.1 mg | 75 mcg | 1.0 mcg |
| 7–10 | 1.0 mg | 1.2 mg | 13.0 mg | 1.4 mg | 100 mcg | 1.4 mcg |
| *Adolescents and Young Adults* | | | | | | |
| Males, 11–14 years | 1.3 mg | 1.5 mg | 17.0 mg | 1.7 mg | 150 mcg | 2.0 mcg |
| Males, 15–18 | 1.5 mg | 1.8 mg | 20.0 mg | 2.0 mg | 200 mcg | 2.0 mcg |
| Females, 11–18 | 1.1 mg | 1.3 mg | 15.0 mg | 1.4 mg | 150 mcg | 2.0 mcg |
| *Adults* | | | | | | |
| Men, 19–50 years | 1.5 mg | 1.7 mg | 19.0 mg | 2.0 mg | 200 mcg | 2.0 mcg |
| Men, 50+ | 1.2 mg | 1.4 mg | 15.0 mg | 2.0 mg | 200 mcg | 2.0 mcg |
| Women 19–50 | 1.1 mg | 1.3 mg | 15.0 mg | 1.6 mg | 180 mcg | 2.0 mcg |
| Women, 50+ | 1.0 mg | 1.2 mg | 13.0 mg | 1.6 mg | 180 mcg | 2.0 mcg |
| Pregnant women | 1.5 mg | 1.6 mg | 17.0 mg | 2.2 mg | 400 mcg | 2.2 mcg |
| Nursing women | 1.6 mg | 1.8 mg | 20.0 mg | 2.1 mg | 280 mcg | 2.1 mcg |

Two B vitamins, pantothenic acid and biotin, work closely with the other B's to help convert your food into energy. Pantothenic acid is also needed for making Vitamin D and normal red blood cells. Because pantothenic acid and biotin are found so widely in foods, nobody is ever deficient. For that reason, these vitamins don't have RDAs—instead, researchers have figured out Safe and Adequate Intakes.

| Safe and Adequate Intakes for Biotin and Pantothenic Acid | | |
|---|---|---|
| Age/Sex | Biotin | Pantothenic Acid |
| *Infants* | | |
| 0–0.5 year | 10 mcg | 2 mg |
| 0.5–1 year | 15 mcg | 3 mg |
| *Children* | | |
| 1–3 years | 20 mcg | 3 mg |
| 4–6 | 25 mcg | 3–4 mg |
| 7–10 | 30 mcg | 4–5 mg |
| *Adolescents and Young Adults* | | |
| Males, 11–14 years | 30–100 mcg | 4–7 mg |
| Males, 15–18 | 30–100 mcg | 4–7 mg |
| Females, 11–18 | 30–100 mcg | 4–7 mg |
| *Adults* | | |
| Men, 19–50 years | 30–100 mcg | 4–7 mg |
| Men, 50+ | 30–100 mcg | 4–7 mg |
| Women 19–50 | 30–100 mcg | 4–7 mg |
| Women, 50+ | 30–100 mcg | 4–7 mg |
| Pregnant women | 30–100 mcg | 4–7 mg |
| Nursing women | 30–100 mcg | 4–7 mg |

# Are You Deficient?

The B vitamins are found in many different foods; they're also added to a lot of foods such as bread and breakfast cereals. Almost everybody gets enough to cover the RDA and then some. If your diet is poor or you have a digestive problem, though, you might be deficient in B's. Some people are especially at risk:

➤ **Alcohol abusers.** Alcohol blocks your ability to absorb B vitamins and also makes you excrete them faster. Alcoholics are most likely to be deficient in thiamin, riboflavin, pyridoxine, and folic acid.

➤ **The elderly.** You absorb less of some of the B's as you age. Also, elderly people who live alone or in nursing homes often don't eat properly and don't get enough B's from their food.

➤ **Smokers.** Tobacco smoke decreases your absorption of B vitamins across the board.

➤ **People with chronic digestive problems.** These people may not be absorbing enough B vitamins through their intestines.

➤ **People on strict diets.** Vegetarians and vegans (vegetarians who don't eat any animal foods such as milk or eggs) may not get enough B vitamins. Vegetarian children and people following macrobiotic diets are especially at risk.

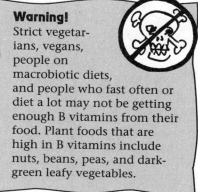

**Warning!**
Strict vegetarians, vegans, people on macrobiotic diets, and people who fast often or diet a lot may not be getting enough B vitamins from their food. Plant foods that are high in B vitamins include nuts, beans, peas, and dark-green leafy vegetables.

The B vitamins all pull together to do the larger jobs of producing energy, making body chemicals such as hormones, and controlling how your cells grow and divide. When it comes to releasing energy, for example, niacin, riboflavin, folic acid, pantothenic acid, and biotin all work together. A shortage of any one of these B's can throw off the entire process. And because the B's are found in many of the same foods, if you're deficient in one you're likely to be deficient in the others too.

Because the B's work together so often, sometimes a shortage of one covers up a shortage of another. A good example is folic acid, which can mask a shortage of cobalamin. Other vitamin shortages also affect your B levels. If you're low on Vitamin C, you're probably also low on folic acid—and vice versa.

# Eating Your B's

Some or all of the B vitamins are found in just about every food you're likely to eat: milk, meat, fish, oranges, peanut butter, bread, breakfast cereal, eggs, yogurt, and a lot more. Here's a rundown of the best foods for each B:

➤ Thiamin: Pork, liver, fish, oranges, peas, peanut butter, wheat germ, beans, and whole grains.

➤ Riboflavin: Milk, dairy products, meat, beans, nuts, green leafy vegetables, avocados.

➤ Niacin: Meat, chicken, fish, beans, peas, peanut butter, milk, diary products, nuts.

➤ Pantothenic acid: Liver, meat, fish, chicken, whole grains, beans.

➤ Pyridoxine: Meat, fish, chicken, peanuts, beans, peas, bananas, avocados, potatoes.

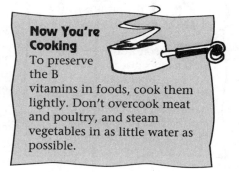

**Now You're Cooking**
To preserve the B vitamins in foods, cook them lightly. Don't overcook meat and poultry, and steam vegetables in as little water as possible.

➤ Biotin: Liver, oatmeal, eggs, peanut butter, milk, salmon, clams, bananas.

➤ Folic acid: Dark-green leafy vegetables, liver, orange juice, beans, avocados, beets.

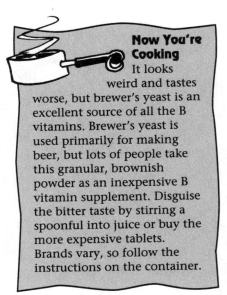

**Now You're Cooking**
It looks weird and tastes worse, but brewer's yeast is an excellent source of all the B vitamins. Brewer's yeast is used primarily for making beer, but lots of people take this granular, brownish powder as an inexpensive B vitamin supplement. Disguise the bitter taste by stirring a spoonful into juice or buy the more expensive tablets. Brands vary, so follow the instructions on the container.

➤ Cobalamin: Meat, chicken, fish, milk, yogurt, cheese, eggs.

Light can actually destroy some of the B's, especially riboflavin. To preserve the B's, store foods out of the light. Pyridoxine is easily destroyed by freezing. Use fresh meats and vegetables whenever you can.

# Getting the Most from B Vitamins

The B vitamins are all water-soluble, which means that you need daily doses to keep your levels high. It also means that your body excretes what you don't absorb. For most of the B's, there are no toxic effects even with very large doses—but there are two important exceptions.

1. **Niacin.** Large doses of niacin (over 1,000 mg) in the form of nicotinic acid can give you a niacin "flush." The sensation is sort of like blushing badly: your face turns red and feels hot or tingly. The flush goes away fairly soon with no lasting harm. Super-large doses of niacin (over three grams a day) could cause liver problems. Three grams is thousands of times more than the RDA—few people would have any reason at all for taking so much.

2. **Pyridoxine.** The one B vitamin that might do real damage in megadoses is pyridoxine. If you take more than 2,000 mg a day for a long time you might get a tingling sensation in your neck and feet, lose coordination, and have permanent nerve damage. In a few cases, people who took 200 mg a day for a number of years also had these symptoms. The RDA for pyridoxine is only about 2 mg a day, though, so you're not likely to have problems unless you take at least a hundred times more than that.

**Warning!**
B vitamins can interfere with medicines for some conditions such as Parkinson's disease and epilepsy. If you take medicine for these or any other chronic condition, discuss B supplements with your doctor before you try them.

Any good multivitamin supplement contains all the extra B vitamins you need. Pick one that has at least 400 mcg of folic acid (we'll tell you why in Chapter 10). You can also buy each B in separate supplements or in assorted combinations. In general, you don't need to bother with these unless your doctor recommends them. If you have a cobalamin deficiency, your doctor will probably recommend shots every two weeks (see Chapter 9 to learn why).

Choline is found in most good multivitamins, but the amount is usually only 10 or 20 percent of the RDA.

To get more choline than that, you'll need to take a separate supplement—but there's rarely any reason to. To get extra lipoic acid or inositol, you'll have to buy separate supplements. Lipoic acid supplements can be helpful for diabetics (see Chapter 24 on antioxidants for more information). Inositol supplements don't do anything for you—skip them.

The best use for PABA is in sunscreen products. It's available as a supplement, but we don't recommend it. As we'll explain in Chapter 12, PABA pills won't do anything positive for you and they could be harmful.

## The Three B's for Heart Health

B vitamins can help keep your heart beating beautifully. A major study in the prestigious *New England Journal of Medicine* in 1995 showed that people with high blood levels of a substance called homocysteine were much more likely to have clogged arteries, which means they were more likely to have a heart attack. Folic acid, pyridoxine, and cobalamin break down homocysteine. The higher your levels of these three B's, the lower your homocysteine level and the healthier your heart. How much healthier? The people with the highest B levels cut their risk of a heart attack *in half*.

**Food for Thought**

Preventing heart disease is a really good example of how the B family pulls together. Folic acid, pyridoxine, and cobalamin are all needed to break down homocysteine, a normal waste product in your body, and convert it to a harmless amino acid called methionine. Too little of any of these three B's, and you can't remove homocysteine quickly. The result could be damage to your arteries and your heart.

Two-thirds of the people with dangerously high homocysteine had inadequate levels of the three vital B's. Could there be a better example of how important vitamins are to your health? We'll talk about this in more detail in Chapter 10 on folic acid, because folic acid seems to be the most important of the three B's that help your heart.

## Aging and the B Vitamins

You may have noticed that your elderly grandmother has started to get a little forgetful and confused, even depressed. Well, you think, that's normal for someone who's in her 80s. But is it? Not necessarily. There are lots of medical problems that can make an elderly person seem senile, but bad nutrition can also play a big role—especially for someone who falls into the risk categories we talked about in Chapter 1.

Studies show that many elderly people are low in B vitamins, particularly cobalamin. Part of the reason is that you just don't absorb as many B's from your food as you grow older. Because some of the B's aren't absorbed all that well in the first place, older people can easily start to be deficient. Then the deficiency makes them a little depressed, so they eat less and get even fewer B's, which makes them more depressed or so forgetful that they eat even less, which makes them so forgetful, confused, and depressed that they end up in a nursing home. The food there might not help—institutional food often has most of its vitamins processed or cooked away.

**Warning!**
Low levels of B vitamins are common among the elderly. That's because we naturally absorb fewer B vitamins as we age. The problem is made worse if you don't eat a healthy diet or don't eat large enough portions. If you're over age 60, discuss taking a complete B vitamins supplement with your doctor.

Studies show that a large number of elderly people have overall B vitamin shortages that affect their health and their mental abilities. For example, many elderly people are low on thiamin, folic acid, choline, and cobalamin. The statistics here are disturbing—about a third of the elderly are low on pyridoxine, and thiamin deficiency may affect nearly half of all elderly people sent to hospitals.

B shortages in older people are enough to cause depression, confusion, and memory problems, even though the usual blood tests show normal levels. Instead, the doctor and the family think poor old Grandma has just gotten senile. What she may really need are some extra B's.

## Don't Worry, B Happy

If you're seriously low on any of the B vitamins, depression is one of the earliest symptoms. In fact, studies show that at least one in four of all people hospitalized for depression is deficient in pyridoxine and cobalamin; another study suggests that over three-quarters of all depressed patients have a pyridoxine deficiency. Giving these patients even small doses of pyridoxine improves their depression. Folic acid supplements have been shown to help elderly patients who are depressed.

People who take lithium to control bipolar disorder (manic depression) sometimes benefit from taking additional choline. If you take lithium, read the information in Chapter 12 and discuss choline supplements with your doctor before you try them.

## Boosting Your Immune System

When your body comes under attack from germs, your immune system swings into action. To launch an effective counterattack, your body needs to quickly produce a bunch of complicated proteins and the enzymes that help them work better and faster. And for that, you need all your B vitamins because the B's are all closely involved with moving amino acids around to make proteins, hormones, and enzymes.

Pyridoxine, folic acid, and cobalamin are especially important for your immune system. You need pyridoxine to help regulate and maintain your immune system. Folic acid keeps your front-line defenses—your skin, your lungs, your intestines—against infection strong. And without enough folic acid and cobalamin, you can't produce enough infection-fighting white blood cells.

Although low levels of B vitamins make you more likely to get sick, taking extra B's won't help you get better faster. Your best bet: Keep your B levels high to help avoid illness and infection.

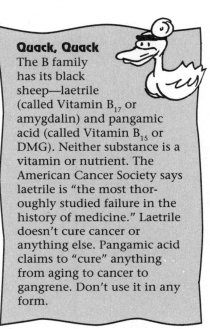

**Quack, Quack**
The B family has its black sheep—laetrile (called Vitamin $B_{17}$ or amygdalin) and pangamic acid (called Vitamin $B_{15}$ or DMG). Neither substance is a vitamin or nutrient. The American Cancer Society says laetrile is "the most thoroughly studied failure in the history of medicine." Laetrile doesn't cure cancer or anything else. Pangamic acid claims to "cure" anything from aging to cancer to gangrene. Don't use it in any form.

## The Least You Need to Know

➤ The B family contains eight vitamins and four related substances that work closely with each other—you need them all.

➤ If you have a shortage of one B vitamin, you probably have a shortage of the others as well.

➤ Foods rich in B vitamins include meat, chicken, fish, milk and dairy products, nuts, beans, peas, and dark-green leafy vegetables.

➤ Most people get all the B's they need from their food. Strict vegetarians, the elderly, and alcohol abusers may not get enough.

➤ High levels of folic acid, pyridoxine, and cobalamin help protect you from heart disease.

➤ The B family helps keep your immune system working at peak efficiency.

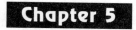

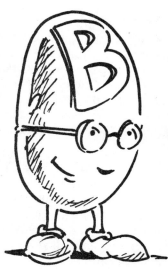

# Chapter 5

# Thiamin: The Basic B

---

## In This Chapter

➤ Why you need thiamin (Vitamin B$_1$)

➤ Foods that are high in thiamin

➤ How thiamin helps gives you energy

➤ Protecting your heart muscles and nerve cells with thiamin

---

Good old thiamin—least glamorous member of the B family. Even though it was the first B vitamin to be discovered, thiamin doesn't do anything spectacular to grab the headlines. It's not a standout or a superstar. Instead, like a good utility infielder or defensive lineman, thiamin works along with the other members of the B team to keep you healthy.

Thiamin's special job on the team is to help you convert carbohydrates in your food into energy your body can use. All you have to do is give yourself a reliable daily supply and your thiamin will chug along, day in and day out, nourishing your brain and nervous system and keeping your heart pumping smoothly.

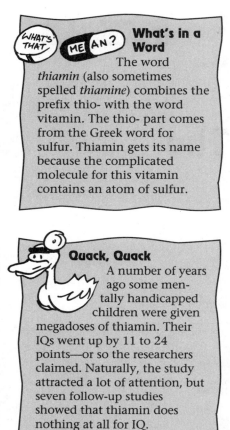

The word *thiamin* (also sometimes spelled *thiamine*) combines the prefix thio- with the word vitamin. The thio- part comes from the Greek word for sulfur. Thiamin gets its name because the complicated molecule for this vitamin contains an atom of sulfur.

**Quack, Quack**

A number of years ago some mentally handicapped children were given megadoses of thiamin. Their IQs went up by 11 to 24 points—or so the researchers claimed. Naturally, the study attracted a lot of attention, but seven follow-up studies showed that thiamin does nothing at all for IQ.

# Why You Need Thiamin

Your body goes through an amazingly complex series of steps to turn the food you eat into energy. All the B vitamins are involved in every one of those steps, alone or working together, but let's focus just on thiamin here. One particular step in the process needs an enzyme called *thiamin pyrophosphate*, or TPP, to work. Without thiamin, you can't make the enzyme—and without the enzyme, the whole process grinds to a halt.

You also need thiamin to keep your brain and nervous system fueled up. Your brain runs on glucose, a type of sugar that's made from the carbohydrates you eat. Thiamin helps your brain and nervous system absorb enough glucose. Without it, they take in only half of what they really need. And when your brain doesn't get enough fuel, you start to get forgetful, depressed, tired, and apathetic.

Thiamin helps keep your heart muscles elastic and working smoothly, which keeps your heart pumping strongly and evenly, with just the right number of beats.

# The RDA for Thiamin

The amount of thiamin you need daily for good health is very small—the RDA for an adult male is only 1.5 mg. That's based on the mythical average man, because the RDA is calculated on the basis of how much you eat. Figure on 0.5 mg of thiamin for every 1,000 calories you eat. If you take in less than 2,000 calories a day, though, make sure you still get at least 1.0 mg of thiamin. Check the following table to make sure you're getting your daily requirement.

| The RDA for Thiamin | |
| --- | --- |
| Age/Sex | Thiamin in mg |
| *Infants* | |
| 0–0.5 year | 0.3 |
| 0.5–1 year | 0.4 |
| *Children* | |
| 1–3 years | 0.7 |
| 4–6 | 0.9 |
| 7–10 | 1.0 |

| Age/Sex | Thiamin in mg |
| --- | --- |
| *Adults* | |
| Men 11–14 years | 1.3 |
| Men 15–50 | 1.5 |
| Men 50+ | 1.2 |
| Women 11–50 | 1.1 |
| Women 50+ | 1.0 |
| Pregnant women | 1.5 |
| Nursing women | 1.6 |

# Are You Deficient?

Starting in the early 1800s, rice mills in Asia began removing the brown outer covering of the rice grains. Polishing, as it was called, produced white rice that cooked quickly and tasted good. People who ate a lot of white rice and little else, however, developed a disease called *beriberi*. Millions of people across Asia lost muscle strength, had leg spasms or paralysis, and became mentally confused.

For a long time, people thought some sort of germ in the white rice was making them sick. It was only in the late 1890s that researchers realized people who ate *brown* rice and not much else didn't get beriberi. Something in the brown rice husk was clearly important to human health, but it wasn't until 1911 that thiamin was isolated.

Today beriberi still occurs in the less developed world, but it is extremely rare in our modern society. You need so little thiamin, and it's so easily found in the typical diet, that few people are seriously deficient.

There's one very big exception to that last statement: people who abuse alcohol. In fact, so many people in the developed world abuse alcohol that thiamin deficiency may be the most common vitamin deficiency of all.

Why does alcohol have such an impact on your thiamin level? There are several related reasons. Alcoholics tend to eat poorly, so their vitamin intake in general is very low. They don't eat enough thiamin, and the alcohol destroys most of what little they do take in. Alcohol also makes them excrete more thiamin. Chronic alcoholics need large amounts of thiamin supplements—anywhere from 10 to 100 mg day.

**What's in a Word**

In Singhalese, a language spoken in Sri Lanka, *beriberi* means "I can't, I can't." That's a pretty good way of describing what happens when you don't get enough thiamin. Muscle weakness, appetite loss, poor coordination, a tingling feeling in the nerves, and severe pain in the calves are among the symptoms. Sometimes a person with beriberi also gets an enlarged heart. The early symptoms of beriberi can start after only ten days without enough thiamin.

Eventually, thiamin deficiency from alcoholism causes a type of nerve damage called *Wernicke-Korsakoff syndrome*. The symptoms can usually be helped by giving up alcohol and eating a good diet, but the syndrome only worsens and leads to death if alcohol abuse continues.

**What's in a Word**

After years of heavy drinking, an alcoholic's thiamin levels can drop so low that *Wernicke-Korsakoff syndrome*—nerve damage from thiamin deficiency—develops. The symptoms include immediate memory loss, jerky eye movements, disorientation, and a staggering gait. The symptoms go away or at least get better if the alcoholic stops drinking and starts eating right. If not, there's permanent damage that leads to psychosis and finally death.

Some other people, especially those with special health problems, may become deficient in thiamin. Mild thiamin deficiency generally causes tiredness, muscle weakness, a pins-and-needles feeling in the legs, depression, and constipation. You could be deficient if:

➤ You're elderly. Many elderly people don't eat well and don't get enough thiamin in their diets, especially if they live in a nursing home. Nearly half of all elderly people sent to hospitals may be deficient in thiamin.

➤ You're pregnant or breastfeeding. You're passing a lot of thiamin on to your baby, so you need about 0.5 mg extra every day.

➤ You diet a lot. If you eat less than 1,500 calories a day, or if you eat only a few different foods, you're probably not getting enough thiamin.

➤ You fast frequently. You need thiamin every day for good health.

➤ You have diabetes. You could be excreting too much thiamin in your urine.

➤ You have kidney disease and are on dialysis. Talk to your doctor about all vitamin supplements before you try them.

➤ You're sick with something, such as a chronic infection, that causes frequent fevers. Fever makes your body run faster, so you need more thiamin.

Most people, even the ones with the health issues listed here, do get enough thiamin. A real deficiency is pretty rare.

# Eating Your Thiamin

What do bagels and brown rice have in common? They're both good sources of thiamin. Actually, thiamin is found in lots of different foods; it's also added to flour, breads, pasta, and breakfast cereals. Because you need less than 2 mg to meet the RDA, most people get enough from their diet. Even someone who eats mostly burgers and fries will get enough thiamin, although just barely.

Wheat germ, sunflower seeds, whole grains, and all kinds of nuts are excellent food sources of thiamin. Beans and peas are also good sources. Some other good sources are oranges, raisins, asparagus, cauliflower, potatoes, milk, and whole wheat bread. Oatmeal, whole wheat, and brown rice are grains that are high in thiamin. Among meats, pork and beef liver are high in thiamin; there's some in all beef and chicken. How many of these thiamin-rich foods do you eat regularly?

## The Thiamin in Food

| Food | Amount | Thiamin in mg |
|---|---|---|
| Asparagus, steamed | 1 cup | 0.12 |
| Bagel | 1 | 0.21 |
| Beans, black | 1/2 cup | 0.21 |
| Beans, kidney | 1/2 cup | 0.14 |
| Beef, lean | 3 ounces | 0.05 |
| Beef liver | 3 ounces | 0.23 |
| Bread, whole wheat | 1 slice | 0.09 |
| Cashews | 3 ounces | 0.18 |
| Chicken, roasted | 3 ounces | 0.06 |
| Corn | 1/2 cup | 0.18 |
| Green peas | 1/2 cup | 0.21 |
| Ham | 3 ounces | 0.82 |
| Milk, nonfat | 1 cup | 0.09 |
| Oatmeal | 1 cup | 0.26 |
| Orange | 1 | 0.13 |
| Peanuts | 3 ounces | 0.36 |
| Pecans | 3 ounces | 0.27 |
| Pork, roasted | 3 ounces | 0.52 |
| Potato | 1 medium | 0.22 |
| Raisins | 1 cup | 0.21 |
| Rice, brown | 1 cup | 0.20 |
| Sunflower seeds | 3 ounces | 1.95 |
| Wheat germ | 1/4 cup | 0.55 |

What you drink with your food affects how much thiamin you get. Alcohol and the tannins found in tea destroy thiamin. To get the most thiamin from your food, skip these beverages during your meal and have them afterward instead.

Sulfites (preservatives sometimes added to prepared foods in restaurants and salad bars) also destroy thiamin in food. Mostly because of customer complaints, a lot of restaurants have stopped adding sulfites to salads and precut fruit, but they're still sometimes used in places where the customers can't complain, like school and company cafeterias and nursing homes. Sulfites are also added to many convenience foods. Read the labels carefully and choose fresh foods whenever possible.

**Now You're Cooking**

To preserve the thiamin (and the other vitamins) in vegetables, cook them lightly in as little water as possible. Don't add baking soda to the cooking water. It helps your green veggies keep their color, but it destroys the thiamin.

Meats preserve their thiamin best if they are cooked only until done—overcooking at high temperatures destroys thiamin. On the other hand, thiamin isn't affected by freezing.

## Getting the Most from Thiamin

Most people don't really need to take a thiamin supplement—the amount in your diet, along with any you take in a daily multivitamin, is fine. Your body doesn't store thiamin, because it's water soluble, so you need to get some every day. There's no known toxicity from taking thiamin supplements—people have taken over 300 mg a day (nearly 200 hundred times the RDA) with no bad effects. There's no reason at all to take that much, but it is safe.

The B vitamins work together to convert the foods you eat into energy you can use. You need all of them. Fortunately, they're all found in many of the same foods, so eating foods high in thiamin will also give you riboflavin, niacin, pyridoxine, biotin, and pantothenic acid.

| Thumbs Up/Thumbs Down | |
|---|---|
| **Thiamin is helped by:** | **Thiamin is hurt by:** |
| All other B vitamins | Alcohol |
| Magnesium | A shortage of other B vitamins |

## Protecting Your Heart

Thiamin helps your heart beat strongly and regularly. It also keeps your heart muscles elastic and lets them bounce back quickly from each beat. If you're low on thiamin, your heart muscles won't be elastic enough, which could lead to abnormal heartbeats.

Although too little thiamin definitely causes heart problems, it's not clear that taking more thiamin than the RDA will help heart problems. Some researchers are looking into using thiamin to treat heart attacks, but it's too soon to say if it will be really valuable. In the meantime, if you have a heart problem, talk to your doctor about thiamin supplements before you try them.

# Thiamin and Diabetes

Because thiamin is involved in glucose production, one symptom of thiamin deficiency is that you don't use glucose normally. That's similar to the problem people with diabetes have, but unfortunately the similarity ends there. A diabetic who is deficient in thiamin—and some are—will use glucose better once the deficiency is fixed, but after that, there won't be any improvement. Diabetics with normal thiamin levels aren't helped by taking thiamin supplements, and thiamin won't help control blood sugar levels.

# Thiamin and Canker Sores

If you're low on thiamin, you're much more likely to get frequent canker sores (aphthous stomatitis)—painful, crater-like sores in your mouth. Interestingly, a recent study showed that taking extra thiamin once the sores have started doesn't help them go away. If you often get canker sores, your best bet is probably prevention. Try getting more thiamin in your diet.

# The Least You Need to Know

➤ Thiamin (Vitamin $B_1$) is a water-soluble vitamin.

➤ Thiamin works closely with all the other B vitamins.

➤ You need thiamin to help convert your food to energy and to keep your brain, nervous system, and heart running well.

➤ The RDA for thiamin is small—adults need only between 1.1 and 1.6 mg a day.

➤ Thiamin is found in many different foods, including meat, whole grains, and nuts, and is usually added to rice, pasta, breads, and breakfast cereals.

➤ Most people get the RDA from their diet and don't need supplements.

# Chapter 6

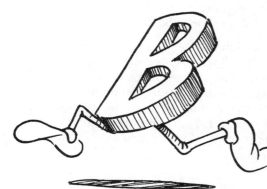

# B Energetic: Riboflavin

### In This Chapter

➤ Why you need riboflavin (Vitamin $B_2$)

➤ Foods that are high in riboflavin

➤ How riboflavin gives you energy

➤ Why athletes need riboflavin

➤ How riboflavin can prevent migraine headaches

Does anybody ever complain about having too much energy? Of course not—most of us go around wishing for more, enough to get through a busy day of work and family with a little bit left over for ourselves. Some sort of subspace energy transference beam would be nice, but until that happens, you'll just have to settle for riboflavin. Your cells need riboflavin to make energy, so you need to be sure you're getting enough of this vital member of the B family.

Riboflavin does lots of other good things for you as well, mostly by working with the other B's to keep your body's systems, like your immune system, running smoothly. Riboflavin works especially closely with niacin and pyridoxine—in fact, without riboflavin, these two B siblings can't do their main jobs at all.

# Why You Need Riboflavin

Riboflavin gives you energy at the most basic level—inside your cells. You need it to make two of the enzymes that are absolutely vital for releasing energy from the fats, carbohydrates, and proteins you eat. To make a complicated story short, riboflavin keeps you alive.

Aside from that little chore, riboflavin also does a bunch of other things in your body, either by itself or along with the other members of the B team (especially pyridoxine and niacin). Riboflavin regulates cell growth and reproduction and helps you make healthy red blood cells. It helps your immune system by keeping the mucous membranes that line your respiratory and digestive systems in good shape. If invading germs still sneak in, riboflavin helps you make antibodies for fighting them off. Your eyes, nerves, skin, nails, and hair all need riboflavin to stay healthy. It might even help your memory—older people with high levels of riboflavin do better on memory tests.

### Food for Thought

Riboflavin was first discovered in milk in 1879. Nobody realized it was a vitamin, mostly because back then nobody knew what a vitamin was. The discoverers just saw it as an interesting yellow-green pigment in the milk. The name riboflavin is a combination of two words: ribose, a type of sugar found in milk, and flavin, from the Latin word *flavus*, which means yellow.

# The RDA for Riboflavin

Important as riboflavin is, you don't really need a lot of it for good health—just under 2 mg a day is enough. Riboflavin is found naturally in many foods, especially meat, milk products, and dark-green leafy vegetables. It's also added to flour, bread, and most breakfast cereals.

The RDA for riboflavin is based on your caloric intake—the more you eat, the more you need. The basic formula is 0.6 mg for every 1,000 calories. Your daily intake should be at least 1.2 mg, even if you eat less than 2,000 calories. Check the table to see how much you need per day.

| The RDA for Riboflavin | |
| --- | --- |
| Age/Sex | Riboflavin in mg |
| *Infants* | |
| 0–0.5 year | 0.4 |
| 0.5–1 year | 0.5 |

| Age/Sex | Riboflavin in mg |
| --- | --- |
| *Children* | |
| 1–3 years | 0.8 |
| 4–6 | 1.1 |
| 7–10 | 1.2 |
| *Adults* | |
| Men 11–14 years | 1.5 |
| Men 15–18 | 1.8 |
| Men 19–50 | 1.7 |
| Men 50+ | 1.4 |
| Women 11–50 years | 1.3 |
| Women 50+ | 1.2 |
| Pregnant women | 1.6 |
| Nursing women | 1.8 |

# Are You Deficient?

Riboflavin is an exception to the water-soluble rule, because you store small amounts of it in your kidneys and liver. Because of that, riboflavin deficiency can take as long as three or four months to show up.

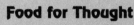

**Food for Thought**

Birth-control pills may increase your need for riboflavin and other B vitamins. If you take the Pill, talk to your doctor about B supplements.

True riboflavin deficiency is quite rare. Most people get plenty of riboflavin in their food. When deficiency symptoms do occur, they're usually related to a shortage of all the B's. You need riboflavin to help niacin and pyridoxine work right. In fact, if you're short on riboflavin you might have deficiency symptoms for one of the other vitamins. Usually, though, riboflavin deficiency shows up as problems with the mucous membranes, skin, eyes, and blood. An early and clear sign is sores and cracks on the lips, especially at the corners. Scaly skin, reddened eyes, and anemia are other deficiency signs.

Some people are at special risk for riboflavin deficiency:

➤ **Athletes.** You need extra riboflavin if you exercise a lot—we'll talk about this more later on in this chapter.

➤ **Diabetics.** You may be excreting a lot of your riboflavin in your urine. Talk to your doctor about vitamin supplements before you try them.

➤ **Pregnant and breastfeeding women.** You're passing a lot of your riboflavin on to your baby, so you need about 0.5 mg more a day.

➤ **Elderly people.** About a third of all elderly people have a riboflavin deficiency, mostly from poor absorption or poor diet.

➤ **People who can't digest milk.** Milk and dairy products such as cottage cheese are important sources of riboflavin. If you can't digest these foods, you might not be getting enough riboflavin.

➤ **People who take tricyclic antidepressants.** Drugs such as amitriptyline (Elavil®) can interfere with riboflavin. If you take a tricyclic antidepressant, talk to your doctor about vitamin supplements before you try them.

Ah, for the good old days, when milk came in clear glass bottles. Nostalgia isn't what it used to be—those glass bottles let in light, which destroys the riboflavin. Because riboflavin is quickly destroyed by light, always store foods such as milk, pasta, grains, and vegetables in opaque containers or a dark place. And when you're eating those healthful sun-dried fruits and vegetables, remember that the sunlight has removed the riboflavin.

# Eating Your Riboflavin

**Now You're Cooking**
Riboflavin does not break down in cooking. Avoid adding baking soda to vegetables, though. It helps the veggies keep their color but it destroys the riboflavin.

Large amounts of riboflavin are found in milk and other dairy foods. Good choices here include cheese, yogurt, and ice cream. Naturally, even this really good justification for indulging in chocolate butternut chip has guilt attached—the higher the fat, the less the riboflavin.

Meat, especially liver, is a good source of riboflavin, as is fish. Vegetable foods that are high in riboflavin include broccoli, spinach, avocados, mushrooms, and asparagus. Most breads, baked goods, and pasta are made with flour that has been enriched with riboflavin and other B vitamins; most breakfast cereals also have riboflavin and other B's added to them.

## The Riboflavin in Food

| Food | Amount | Riboflavin in mg |
| --- | --- | --- |
| Almonds, dry roasted | 1 ounce | 0.22 |
| Asparagus, cooked | 1/2 cup | 0.13 |
| Avocado, California | 1 medium | 0.22 |
| Beef, ground | 3 ounces | 0.20 |

| Food | Amount | Riboflavin in mg |
|---|---|---|
| Beef liver | 3 ounces | 3.60 |
| Bread, whole wheat | 1 slice | 0.05 |
| Broccoli, cooked | 1/2 cup | 0.12 |
| Brie cheese | 1 ounce | 0.15 |
| Cheddar cheese | 1 ounce | 0.11 |
| Chicken breast | 3 ounces | 0.16 |
| Chick peas | 1 cup | 0.10 |
| Cottage cheese, low-fat | 1 cup | 0.42 |
| Egg | 1 large | 0.26 |
| Ice cream, vanilla | 1/2 cup | 0.16 |
| Kidney beans | 1 cup | 0.10 |
| Milk, low-fat | 1 cup | 0.52 |
| Mushrooms, cooked | 1/2 cup | 0.23 |
| Peas | 1/2 cup | 0.12 |
| Pork, roasted | 3 ounces | 0.30 |
| Salmon, canned | 3 ounces | 0.16 |
| Spinach, cooked | 1/2 cup | 0.21 |
| Sweet potato, baked with skin | 1 medium | 0.15 |
| Swiss cheese | 1 ounce | 0.10 |
| Turkey breast | 3 ounces | 0.10 |
| Wheat germ | 1/4 cup | 0.23 |
| Yogurt, low-fat | 8 ounces | 0.49 |

# Getting the Most from Riboflavin

Most people get all the riboflavin they need from their food. Riboflavin is added to so many common foods, like bread and pasta, that even someone with lousy eating habits will probably get enough.

If you're a strict vegetarian or if you exercise a lot (or both), you might need extra riboflavin. You also might need some extra if you fall into the other risk categories we talked about earlier. Most daily multivitamins contain the full RDA for riboflavin. If you think you need more, consider taking a complete B supplement. You need all the B vitamins for your riboflavin to work well—and vice versa.

If you want just extra riboflavin, these supplements come as tablets or capsules. They usually contain either 50 mg or 100 mg—either amount is well over the RDA. You absorb only about 15 percent of the riboflavin from supplements, especially if you take them on an empty stomach. To get the most from your riboflavin, take the supplements with meals.

You can't really overdose on riboflavin, because even very large doses (over 1,000 mg) are safe. There is one side effect from large doses, though: Your urine will turn a bright fluorescent yellow. It may be a little startling, but it's harmless.

# Producing Energy

By itself, riboflavin's most important role is in cell respiration. Just as you breathe in oxygen and exhale the waste product carbon dioxide from your lungs, so does each and every cell in your body. Molecules of oxygen and food enter a cell and are carried into the *mitochondria,* tiny structures within the cell that act like little power plants. Enzymes in the mitochondria release the energy from the oxygen and food. Two of those enzymes, *flavin mononucleotide* and *flavin adenine dinucleotide*, must work together as part of the process. As you can tell from the flavin part of their names, these enzymes contain riboflavin. Not enough riboflavin, not enough enzymes—and therefore not enough energy.

# Faster, Higher, Stronger

The faster you use up energy, the more riboflavin you need. Most people have enough to meet their energy needs, but most people don't really exercise very much. Anyone who exercises even moderately on a regular basis probably needs some extra riboflavin beyond the RDA. Women seem to need the riboflavin boost more than men. You don't need a lot more—the amount in your daily multivitamin supplement will probably be plenty.

Serious athletes who train hard are making their mitochondria work super hard and super fast to provide enough energy. At the same time, they may not be taking in enough riboflavin from their food to make the flavin enzymes they need—especially if they are also watching their weight and avoiding meat and dairy foods. Some athletes and body builders claim that riboflavin supplements help them train harder and longer. They also say riboflavin helps them bounce back faster from training sessions and cuts the time they have to spend resting.

Does this really work? While it's true that exercising hard increases your need for riboflavin, there's no real evidence that taking supplements really improves athletic performance. The supplements don't hurt performance, though, and they are safe to take.

# Preventing Migraines

There's no headache quite so awful as a *migraine*. There's the terrible pain along with nausea, vomiting, and sensitivity to light. Because these headaches are so incapacitating, and because they affect some 11 to 18 million Americans every year, a lot of research goes into them. Despite all the studies, we still don't really know what causes migraines, though there are a lot of good theories (we'll talk about some of the others in Chapter 18 on magnesium and Chapter 27 on natural hormones).

One of the more interesting recent studies showed that high daily doses of riboflavin—400 mg a day—sharply reduced the number and severity of migraine attacks for over half the participants. The researchers think it works because people who get migraines have low cellular energy reserves in their brains. Riboflavin helps the cells use energy better, which seems to help prevent the migraines to begin with and make them less severe when they do happen. And unlike many other drugs used to treat migraines, riboflavin is cheap, safe, and has no side effects. The research is still in the early stages, however, so if you want to try high doses of riboflavin for your migraines, talk to your doctor first.

# Riboflavin and Your Eyes

Whether riboflavin helps your eyes is open to debate. One good example is the cataract question. In theory, people with high levels of riboflavin should have fewer cataracts. Here's how the thinking runs: You need riboflavin to utilize glutathione, one of your body's main antioxidants, most effectively. (We'll talk a lot more about glutathione in Chapter 23 on super antioxidants.) Your eyes need a lot of glutathione to counteract the damaging ultraviolet rays in sunlight, so a shortage of riboflavin leads to a shortage of glutathione, which could lead to cataracts from free radical damage. It's nice in theory, but it's never held up well in studies. Although about a third of the elderly are riboflavin-deficient, their cataract rate isn't any different from the rest of the population.

On the other hand, too much riboflavin could cause cataracts or make them worse if you already have them. The reason is similar: free radical damage. Riboflavin is sensitive to light, so the riboflavin in the cells of your eyes breaks down when light hits it. Free radicals are released in the process, which then damage the lens and cause a cataract. The same free radicals could also damage the macula, the tiny area of super-sensitive cells in your retina, leading to macular degeneration.

Older people who are low on riboflavin should definitely get their levels up, but only by a better diet and riboflavin in small doses—no more than 10 mg a day. If you have cataracts and low riboflavin, raise your level only by eating more riboflavin-rich foods.

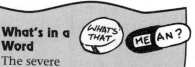

**What's in a Word**

The severe pain of a *migraine* headache is usually felt on just one side of your head. You may also get other unpleasant symptoms, such as nausea, vomiting, sensitivity to light, and cold hands and feet. A typical migraine lasts about six hours. Warning signs, called the *prodrome*, or *aura*, often start an hour or two before the headache strikes. The warning signs are usually visual—many people see flashing lights or zigzag patterns. Sometimes the aura is a strange smell, dizziness, or sudden fatigue. Migraines are fairly common—about 11 to 18 million Americans, 70 percent of them women, get migraines.

Some nutritionists claim that riboflavin helps prevent or reduce eye fatigue. Among the symptoms of riboflavin deficiency are red eyes and dimmed vision, but there's not a lot of evidence to show that taking extra riboflavin helps your eyes.

## The Least You Need to Know

➤ Riboflavin is also called Vitamin $B_2$. Riboflavin works closely with all the other B vitamins, especially niacin and pyridoxine.

➤ You need riboflavin to make energy within your cells, to keep your red blood cells healthy, and to help keep your immune system working well.

➤ The RDA for riboflavin is low—adults need at least 1.2 mg a day.

➤ Riboflavin is found in many different foods, including meat and dairy products, and is usually added to rice, pasta, breads, and breakfast cereals.

➤ Most people get the RDA for riboflavin from their diet and don't need supplements.

# Chapter 7

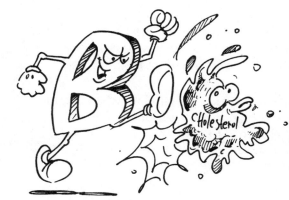

# Niacin: Cholesterol B Gone

## In This Chapter

➤ Why you need niacin (Vitamin B₃)

➤ Foods that are high in niacin

➤ How niacin can help lower your cholesterol

➤ How niacin can help one kind of diabetes

Suddenly it seems that everyone you know is worried about their cholesterol. They're talking about their LDL and HDL levels and cutting back on the fat in their diets. Some are taking two different drugs to lower their cholesterol—maybe you are too.

Are cholesterol drugs the price you have to pay for all those double cheeseburgers with bacon and a big side of fries? Not necessarily. Swap those buckets of fried chicken for green leafy vegetables, give up cigarettes, get more exercise, lose some weight, and watch your cholesterol drop. Add some niacin—but only under your doctor's care—and watch it drop even more.

At the ordinary RDA level, niacin doesn't do anything very dramatic. Except that you do need it for some of the most important functions in your body, like releasing energy in your cells, making hormones, and working with the other members of the B team to keep your body running smoothly.

# Why You Need Niacin

Niacin is essential for more than 50 different processes in your body. What most of these processes boil down to is helping your body produce energy from the foods you eat. Niacin makes enzymes that help your cells turn carbohydrates into energy. As part of the energy end of things, niacin also helps control how much glucose (sugar) is in your blood, which in turn helps give you energy when you need it—when you exercise, for example.

Niacin also acts as an antioxidant within your cells—every little bit helps when it comes to battling free radicals. However, niacin only works as an on-the-spot antioxidant for mopping up the free radicals made when it's being used to release energy. It's nowhere near as powerful as some other vitamins, like Vitamin C, for battling free radicals in general.

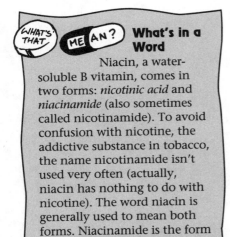

**What's in a Word**

Niacin, a water-soluble B vitamin, comes in two forms: *nicotinic acid* and *niacinamide* (also sometimes called nicotinamide). To avoid confusion with nicotine, the addictive substance in tobacco, the name nicotinamide isn't used very often (actually, niacin has nothing to do with nicotine). The word niacin is generally used to mean both forms. Niacinamide is the form usually found in supplements.

Niacin works closely with all its B relatives, but it's especially close to riboflavin and pyridoxine. All three work together to keep you in overall good health. They're especially important for your skin, nervous system, and digestion.

In very large amounts—much, much more than the RDA—niacin can be a valuable treatment for lowering high cholesterol. The research in this area is so exciting that we'll discuss it a lot more later on in this chapter. We'll point out now, however, that taking a lot of niacin doesn't keep you from getting high cholesterol.

Another interesting new role for niacin may be in helping people with the severe form of diabetes called insulin-dependent diabetes mellitus, or IDDM. Again, we'll talk about this in more depth later in the chapter.

# The RDA for Niacin

The RDA for niacin is based mostly on how many calories you eat—but which foods those calories come from is also part of the picture. The calorie part is easy: At a bare minimum, you need 6.6 mg of niacin for every 1,000 calories you eat. This ratio assumes that you eat 2,000 calories a day and get at least 13 mg of niacin a day. If you don't eat that much (say, you're dieting), you still need the same amount of niacin.

Here's where the food part comes in. You probably think your niacin comes straight from your food. Well, most of it does, but some is also made in your body from the proteins you eat. It works like this: When you eat animal or plant protein, your body breaks the proteins down into their building blocks—amino acids (and we'll spend all of Chapter 22 talking about them). One of those building blocks is the amino acid tryptophan.

Your body uses about half your *tryptophan* for making some of the 50,000-plus proteins you need. The other half gets converted to niacin. In fact, only about half your niacin comes directly from the foods you eat; the other half is converted from tryptophan. You need about 60 mg of tryptophan to make 1 mg of niacin. Because most people eat somewhere between 500 to 1,000 mg of tryptophan a day, they make about 8 to 17 mg of niacin.

The RDA chart ignores tryptophan and only counts the niacin you get as preformed niacin from your food. That's why, even though studies show that most Americans get only about 11 mg of niacin from their diet, very few people are actually deficient—they make up the rest of the RDA from tryptophan. To be on the safe side, though, try to get your full RDA from foods rich in niacin.

**What's in a Word**

WHAT'S THAT ME AN?

*Tryptophan* is one of the nine essential amino acids—you can only get it from your food. Your body uses half the tryptophan it gets to help make the thousands of complicated proteins that keep you running. The rest is converted to niacin. The best way to get your tryptophan is through the proteins in your food (see Chapter 22 for why you can't buy tryptophan supplements).

## The RDA for Niacin

| Age/Sex | Niacin in mg |
|---|---|
| *Infants* | |
| 0–0.5 year | 5.0 |
| 0.5–1 year | 6.0 |
| *Children* | |
| 1–3 years | 9.0 |
| 4–6 | 12.0 |
| 7–10 | 13.0 |
| *Adults* | |
| Men 11–14 years | 17.0 |
| Men 15–18 | 20.0 |
| Men 19–50 | 19.0 |
| Men 50+ | 15.0 |
| Women 11–18 | 15.0 |
| Women 19–50 | 15.0 |
| Women 50+ | 13.0 |
| Pregnant women | 17.0 |
| Nursing women | 20.0 |

# Are You Deficient?

Because you don't really need all that much niacin to begin with, and because you can make niacin from the tryptophan in protein, real niacin deficiency is very rare in the developed world today. That hasn't always been the case. Starting in the eighteenth century, when corn became a staple food for many poor people in Europe, Africa, and North America, pellagra, the deficiency disease caused by lack of niacin, was a common problem. Corn is low in niacin and tryptophan. It wasn't until well into the 1940s that the cause of pellagra was fully understood.

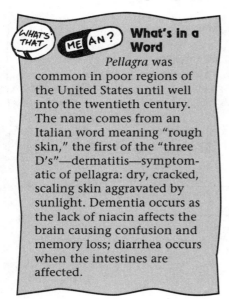

**What's in a Word**

*Pellagra* was common in poor regions of the United States until well into the twentieth century. The name comes from an Italian word meaning "rough skin," the first of the "three D's"—dermatitis—symptomatic of pellagra: dry, cracked, scaling skin aggravated by sunlight. Dementia occurs as the lack of niacin affects the brain causing confusion and memory loss; diarrhea occurs when the intestines are affected.

Today pellagra is almost unknown in the developed world, although it unfortunately still happens in impoverished areas of Asia and Africa. You are very unlikely to get pellagra or even be slightly deficient in niacin, unless:

➤ You abuse alcohol. Alcohol blocks your uptake of all B vitamins, including niacin. Also, alcohol abusers eat very badly and don't get enough vitamins in general.

➤ You're a strict vegetarian or a vegan. If you don't eat a lot of high-quality protein (protein from animal sources such as eggs, milk, fish, and meat), you might be on the low side for niacin—this is especially true for kids. Vegetarian or vegan children should probably take niacin as part of an overall B vitamin supplement.

Usually, someone who's low on niacin is low on all the B vitamins. The reason is almost always poor diet. To solve the problem, eat more protein and take a supplement that includes all the B vitamins.

**Food for Thought**

Pellagra was a widespread problem throughout the South until well into the twentieth century—some 200,000 people were affected every year. For a long time, doctors thought a germ of some sort caused pellagra. It was only in the 1920s that a dedicated public health physician, Dr. Joseph Goldberger, showed that a poor diet was the cause.

# Eating Your Niacin

Niacin is found in lots of common foods, especially meat, fish, poultry, eggs, and whole grains. It's also added to breakfast cereals, rice, bread, and many baked goods. Tryptophan is found in just about every protein food, especially milk, dairy foods, and eggs. Most people can easily get their RDA for niacin and tryptophan from their diet. Strict vegetarians and vegans need to eat plenty of nuts and whole grains such as oatmeal to meet their RDAs. Check the charts to find the foods that give you the niacin and tryptophan you need.

## The Niacin in Food

| Food | Amount | Niacin in mg |
| --- | --- | --- |
| Almonds, roasted | 1 ounce | 0.8 |
| Asparagus | 1/2 cup | 1.0 |
| Avocado | 1/2 medium | 1.5 |
| Bagel | 1 | 1.9 |
| Beef, ground | 3 ounces | 4.0 |
| Beef liver | 3 ounces | 10.0 |
| Bread, whole wheat | 1 slice | 1.0 |
| Chicken breast | 3 ounces | 8.5 |
| Chick peas | 1 cup | 0.9 |
| Corn, kernels | 1/2 cup | 1.2 |
| Cottage cheese, low-fat | 1 cup | 0.3 |
| Cream of wheat | 3/4 cup | 1.1 |
| Flounder | 3 ounces | 2.5 |
| Kidney beans | 1 cup | 1.0 |
| Milk, low-fat | 1 cup | 0.2 |
| Mushrooms, cooked | 1/2 cup | 3.5 |
| Navy beans | 1 cup | 1.0 |
| Nectarine | 1 medium | 1.3 |
| Peanut butter | 2 tablespoons | 3.8 |
| Peanuts, dry roasted | 1 ounce | 3.8 |
| Peas | 1/2 cup | 1.6 |
| Pork, roasted | 3 ounces | 5.5 |
| Potato, baked | 1 medium | 3.3 |
| Rice, brown | 1 cup | 3.0 |
| Rice, white | 1 cup | 3.0 |

*continues*

## The Niacin in Food  Continued

| Food | Amount | Niacin in mg |
|---|---|---|
| Rice, wild | 1 cup | 2.1 |
| Salmon, canned | 3 ounces | 5.0 |
| Spinach, cooked | 1/2 cup | 0.4 |
| Sunflower seeds | 1 ounce | 1.1 |
| Sweet potato | 1 medium | 0.7 |
| Tomato | 1 medium | 0.8 |
| Tuna, canned in water | 3 ounces | 11.3 |
| Turkey breast | 3 ounces | 8.5 |
| Wheat germ | 1/4 cup | 2.0 |

Remember that about half of the tryptophan you consume is converted into niacin. The rest of this amino acid is used to help make the proteins that keep you going.

## The Tryptophan in Food

| Food | Amount | Tryptophan in mg |
|---|---|---|
| Avocado | 1 medium | 45 |
| Banana | 1 medium | 14 |
| Beef, ground | 3 ounces | 243 |
| Beef liver | 3 ounces | 301 |
| Black beans | 1 cup | 181 |
| Cheddar cheese | 1 ounce | 91 |
| Chicken breast | 3 ounces | 326 |
| Corn | 1/2 cup | 19 |
| Cottage cheese, lowfat | 1 cup | 312 |
| Dates, dried | 10 | 42 |
| Egg | 1 large | 76 |
| Flounder | 3 ounces | 230 |
| Milk | 1 cup | 113 |
| Oatmeal | 1 cup | 84 |
| Peanuts, dry roasted | 1 ounce | 64 |
| Pear | 1 medium | 17 |
| Tuna, canned in water | 3 ounces | 243 |
| Turkey, without skin | 3 ounces | 267 |

# Getting the Most from Niacin

Although you might not get enough niacin in your diet to meet the RDA, the tryptophan you eat will probably boost you over the top. Not too many people need supplements of niacin alone—if you're low on niacin, you're almost also certainly low on the other B vitamins and should take a complete B supplement.

## Food for Thought

The Native Americans ate a lot of corn, which is low in both niacin and tryptophan, but they never got pellagra. Why? They soaked dried corn kernels in water mixed with wood ashes. The mixture—really a weak form of lye—softened the kernels and made it easy to slip off the tough outer skin. This made the corn easier to digest and also made the niacin and tryptophan easier to absorb. Corn kernels prepared this way are called hominy. Grits, that Southern breakfast favorite, are made from ground hominy.

If you really feel you need a niacin supplement due to inadequate diet, you can buy tablets or capsules containing 100 mg, 250 mg, or 500 mg. You'll have a choice of niacinamide or nicotinic acid. If you just want to supplement your niacin level, choose niacinamide in the smallest dose. Don't overdo—even 100 mg of niacinamide can cause heartburn, nausea, and headaches for some people.

The only real reason to take nicotinic acid at all is to treat high blood cholesterol under a doctor's supervision. There are some nasty side effects from the large doses you need to take—and some very good reasons why some people shouldn't take it at all. We'll talk about this in detail later in this chapter.

## Warning!

Do not take any sort of niacin supplement if you also take any medicine for high blood pressure! The niacin could make your blood pressure drop way too low!

If you have diabetes, niacin supplements could raise your blood sugar levels too high. If you have gout, niacin could raise your uric acid levels and cause an attack.

# Producing Energy

The members of the B team work together to turn the fats, carbohydrates, and proteins you eat into energy you can use. Niacin plays its role by being an essential part of two coenzymes: nicotinamide adenine dinucleotide (NAD) and nicotinamide adenine dinucleotide phosphate (NADP). You need both enzymes working in sync to use fats and sugar properly. Without them, your cells can't make enough energy to keep going.

Your body needs just enough niacin—20 mg a day tops—and no more. Although you'll feel weak and tired if you don't get enough niacin, taking extra won't give you extra energy.

# Lowering High Cholesterol

You can't open a newspaper or magazine today without seeing big ads that trumpet drugs to treat high cholesterol. The ads tell you how well the drugs work and how they even help prevent heart attacks. If you look more closely at those ads, though, you'll see paragraph after paragraph of tiny type describing the side effects in scary detail.

The one thing that's not mentioned in the ads is the cost. These drugs are expensive. A month's supply of pravastatin (Pravachol®) costs about $70—and you'll probably be taking it for the rest of your life.

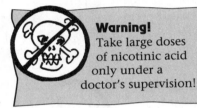

**Warning!**
Take large doses of nicotinic acid only under a doctor's supervision!

For some people, there's a better and cheaper way: niacin. Doctors have known for many years that large doses of nicotinic acid—between 2 and 3 grams a day—lower LDL ("bad") cholesterol and triglycerides and raise HDL ("good") cholesterol (refer to Chapter 1 for more information about cholesterol).

Lowering your LDL cholesterol and triglycerides, and raising your HDL cholesterol, definitely decreases your risk of a heart attack. In fact, a major study that went on for 15 years showed not only that the group who took niacin had lower cholesterol and fewer heart attacks, they also had fewer deaths for any reason.

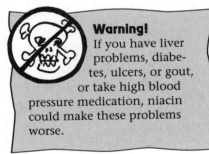

**Warning!**
If you have liver problems, diabetes, ulcers, or gout, or take high blood pressure medication, niacin could make these problems worse.

Niacin works on high cholesterol pretty well by itself. Many people need a combination of drugs to really make a dent in their high cholesterol, though. Niacin can work well here too, especially when it's combined with drugs such as lovastatin (Mevacor®), pravastatin (Pravachol®), or simvastatin (Zocor®). The one-two punch can bring your cholesterol way down.

*Do not try niacin supplements on your own to lower your choles-terol.* The doses needed are so high that the niacin stops being a supplement and becomes a drug. You must work with your doctor and have your cholesterol and liver functions checked often. If you are already taking a cholesterol drug, don't stop taking it and switch to niacin. Also, don't keep taking your cholesterol drug and start taking niacin as well. Discuss your cholesterol and the drugs you take with your doctor before trying niacin.

Not everyone with high cholesterol should take niacin. If you have diabetes, extra niacin could cause your blood sugar to go up. If you have gout, extra niacin could trigger an attack. If you take medicine for high blood pressure, niacin could make your blood pressure drop too low. And if you have liver disease or ulcers, niacin could make these problems worse.

# Boy, Was My Face Red

Large (and even not-so-large) doses of nicotinic acid cause a nasty side effect called the niacin flush. About 15 to 30 minutes after you take it, your face and neck get really red and hot—you blush so badly it reminds you of being back in junior high. The flush can go on for half an hour or longer and then wears off.

## Food for Thought

Back in the days before drug regulation, nicotinic acid was an ingredient in a lot of worthless medicines peddled by snake-oil salesmen. The flush from the nicotinic acid showed that the medicine was "working." The grain alcohol and opium in "patent medicines" probably also did a lot to make whoever took them feel better, at least temporarily. Unfortunately, these potions often also contained dangerous amounts of arsenic, mercury, antimony, iodine, quinine, and other harmful substances. The Pure Food and Drug Act of 1906 was designed to put an end to such deception. The Food and Drug Administration (FDA) was formed in 1928 to make sure all new drugs are safe, effective, and honestly labeled.

You can build up a tolerance to niacin flushing by starting with smaller doses and gradually taking bigger ones. You can usually also prevent the flush by taking an aspirin about half an hour before you take the niacin. Taking the niacin on a full stomach also seems to help.

Another way to avoid flushing is to use the sustained-release (SR) form of nicotinic acid. SR nicotinic acid is good for lowering your LDL cholesterol and triglycerides, but it doesn't do much to raise your HDL level. Also, it can also cause serious liver problems. Don't take it.

## What's in a Word

*Inositol hexaniacinate* (IHN) is a form of nicotinic acid that also includes inositol, one of the unofficial B vitamins (see Chapter 12 for more on inositol). It works just as well or better than nicotinic acid, but doesn't cause flushing or other side effects.

The best way to avoid flushing may be to avoid nicotinic acid and take niacin in the form of *inositol hexaniacinate* (*IHN*). Doctors in Europe have been prescribing IHN for more than 30 years, but it's only become available in the United States recently. IHN works on cholesterol just as well as nicotinic acid, but without the side effects. If you'd like to try IHN, talk to your doctor.

# Niacin and Diabetes

A serious form of diabetes called insulin-dependent diabetes mellitus (IDDM or Type I) strikes children and young people. This disease is pretty mysterious, but we do know that something destroys the part of the pancreas that makes insulin, the hormone that controls your blood sugar. It's possible that the diabetic's own immune system has something to do with causing the destruction. Powerful drugs that suppress the immune system can sometimes slow down or stop the destruction in the pancreas.

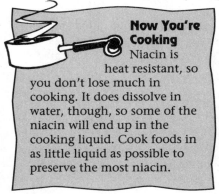

**Now You're Cooking**
Niacin is heat resistant, so you don't lose much in cooking. It does dissolve in water, though, so some of the niacin will end up in the cooking liquid. Cook foods in as little liquid as possible to preserve the most niacin.

Recently researchers have turned to niacinamide to try to stop IDDM soon after it starts. The results of several trials have been encouraging, but there's still a long way to go before this becomes standard treatment.

Another approach is to use niacin to prevent IDDM in kids who are at high risk for it. A major study in New Zealand showed that this can reduce the number of cases by half or more.

IDDM is not the same thing as non-insulin-dependent diabetes, also called adult-onset or Type II diabetes. If you have Type II diabetes, niacin will not help it, it will make it worse!

# Other Problems Helped by Niacin

Niacin in the form of niacinamide seems to help several other common health problems. Talk to your doctor about niacin for:

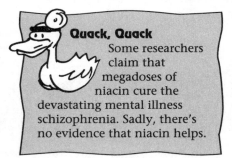

**Quack, Quack**
Some researchers claim that megadoses of niacin cure the devastating mental illness schizophrenia. Sadly, there's no evidence that niacin helps.

➤ **Intermittent claudication.** This is a circulatory problem that makes your legs ache and your calf muscles cramp up when you walk. The reason is that your leg muscles aren't getting enough oxygen because your circulation is poor. Niacin makes your blood vessels widen, which brings more blood to your legs.

➤ **Dizziness (vertigo) and ringing in the ears (tinnitus).** Niacin sometimes helps these problems, although doctors aren't quite sure why.

➤ **PMS headaches.** B vitamins in general help some women with PMS. Niacin seems to help PMS headaches.

Niacin may not cure any of these problems, but it may be worth a try if nothing else is helping. Be sure to discuss niacin supplements with your doctor before you try them.

# The Least You Need to Know

➤ Niacin, also called Vitamin $B_3$, works closely with all the other B vitamins, especially riboflavin and pyridoxine.

➤ You need niacin to release energy within your cells and for about 50 other body processes.

➤ The RDA for niacin is up to 20 mg a day for adults.

➤ Niacin is found in many different foods, especially meat, fish, poultry, eggs, nuts, and whole grains. It's also added to breakfast cereals, bread, and many baked goods.

➤ Your body makes some of the niacin it needs from the amino acid tryptophan.

➤ Most people get the RDA from their diet and don't need supplements.

➤ Niacin supplements in very large doses can help lower high cholesterol—but talk to your doctor before you try it.

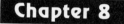

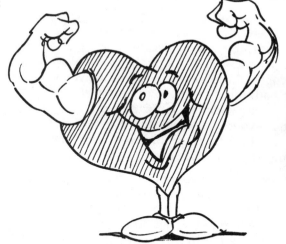

# Chapter 8

# Pyridoxine: Have a Healthy Heart

## In This Chapter

➤ Why you need pyridoxine (Vitamin B$_6$)

➤ Foods that are high in pyridoxine

➤ How pyridoxine helps prevent heart disease

➤ How pyridoxine helps asthma

➤ How pyridoxine boosts your immune system

➤ Why pyridoxine is important for diabetics

It's hard to believe that just two milligrams a day of anything could make a big difference to your health—but that's all the pyridoxine you need to make more than 60 different enzymes, help your immune system stay in top gear, keep your red blood cells red, and help your nerves communicate with the rest of you. All that, and we haven't even gotten to what a little *extra* pyridoxine could do for you.

When pyridoxine teams up with folic acid and cobalamin, your risk of heart disease drops. You don't need a lot of extra pyridoxine to get the benefit. Just doubling your pyridoxine intake—to a whopping four milligrams—could make a big difference. Not only will your heart be healthier, you might also help some other health problems. People with asthma and diabetes often benefit from pyridoxine, and it may also help high blood pressure and PMS.

# Why You Need Pyridoxine

The Institute of Medicine (the people who bring you the RDA) says you need *pyridoxine* as a coenzyme in the transamination process, for the decarboxylation and racemization of amino acids, and as the essential coenzyme for glycogen phosphorylase. Just in case you've forgotten your advanced organic biochemistry, we'll simplify: You need pyridoxine to turn the proteins you eat into the proteins your body needs and you need it to convert carbohydrates from the form you store them in into the form you can use for energy.

What sort of proteins does your body need? For starters, hemoglobin—the stuff that carries oxygen in your red blood cells. Pyridoxine is needed to make lots of other proteins including hormones, neurotransmitters, and enzymes. You also need it to make prostaglandins, hormone-like substances that regulate things like your blood pressure.

Pyridoxine is crucial for converting the foods you eat into carbohydrates or fat your body can store—and for the stored forms into forms you can use when you need extra energy.

Normal amounts of pyridoxine keep your body working normally. What do extra amounts of pyridoxine do? A lot, especially for your heart and immune system, and for asthma and diabetes. You need to be cautious here, though—pyridoxine can be toxic in very large doses.

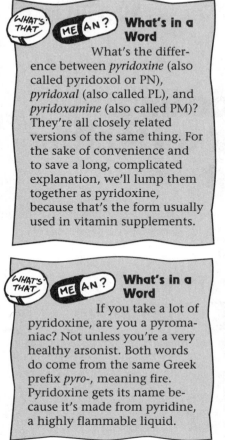

**What's in a Word**

What's the difference between *pyridoxine* (also called pyridoxol or PN), *pyridoxal* (also called PL), and *pyridoxamine* (also called PM)? They're all closely related versions of the same thing. For the sake of convenience and to save a long, complicated explanation, we'll lump them together as pyridoxine, because that's the form usually used in vitamin supplements.

**What's in a Word**

If you take a lot of pyridoxine, are you a pyromaniac? Not unless you're a very healthy arsonist. Both words do come from the same Greek prefix *pyro-*, meaning fire. Pyridoxine gets its name because it's made from pyridine, a highly flammable liquid.

# The RDA for Pyridoxine

You need pyridoxine to turn your amino acids into all the other proteins your body needs. That's why the RDA for pyridoxine is based on how much protein the average person eats. You need to get 0.016 mg of pyridoxine for every gram of protein you take in. The RDA assumes that an average adult male eats about 126 grams of protein a day, which would make the RDA about 2 mg. The protein assumption for an adult woman is about 100 grams a day, which would make the RDA for women about 1.6 g. (To help you get a handle on this, there's about 30 grams of protein in a chicken leg; a quarter-pound hamburger has about 23 grams.)

Even if you eat less protein than the RDA assumes, you still need the RDA for pyridoxine. If you eat a lot more protein (you're a body-builder, for example), you need to increase your pyridoxine intake to keep up with the extra protein. Check the chart to see how much you need.

## The RDA for Pyridoxine

| Age/Sex | Pyridoxine in mg |
|---|---|
| *Infants* | |
| 0–0.5 year | 0.3 |
| 0.5–1 year | 0.6 |
| *Children* | |
| 1–3 years | 1.0 |
| 4–6 | 1.1 |
| 7–10 | 1.4 |
| *Adults* | |
| Men 11–14 years | 1.7 |
| Men 15+ | 2.0 |
| Women 11–14 | 1.4 |
| Women 15–18 | 1.5 |
| Women 19+ | 1.6 |
| Pregnant women | 2.2 |
| Nursing women | 2.1 |

# Are You Deficient?

Like the other B vitamins, pyridoxine is found in many common foods, especially high-protein foods like meat, fish, milk, and eggs. It's also added to flour, breakfast cereals, and many baked goods. You get so much from your food that you're not very likely at all to be deficient.

If you're low on pyridoxine, you're probably also low on the other B's, usually from poor diet. More than 40 different prescription drugs affect your pyridoxine levels, though, and there are some other reasons for being low on pyridoxine:

➤ You're pregnant or breastfeeding. Your baby is taking up a lot of your pyridoxine, so you need about 0.5 to 0.6 mg extra every day.

➤ You're a strict vegetarian or vegan. Milk and dairy products are relatively poor sources of pyridoxine. Most fruits and vegetables have little or no pyridoxine, so vegans have to get theirs mostly from nuts and whole grains. Kids who don't eat any animal products are especially at risk.

➤ You take birth control pills. Your pyridoxine level could be 15 to 20 percent below normal. Talk to your doctor about taking a complete B supplement.

➤ You abuse alcohol. About a third of all alcoholics are deficient in pyridoxine.

➤ You smoke. Tobacco blocks your use of pyridoxine.

➤ You take certain prescription drugs that make you excrete more pyridoxine, including: hydralazine (Apresoline®), used to treat high blood pressure; isoniazid (Laniazid®), used to treat tuberculosis; and penicillamine (Cuprimine®), used to treat rheumatoid arthritis. Talk to your doctor about taking a complete B supplement.

➤ You take theophylline to treat asthma. This drug is so widely prescribed that we'll discuss it more in the section on asthma a little later on.

Pyridoxine is needed for a lot of different roles in your body, but the first place a deficiency shows up is usually your immune system—you get sick more. That might be blamed on a lot of things, but the next common symptom, *anemia,* or red blood cells that aren't carrying enough oxygen, is the clincher. There are different kinds of anemia (and we'll tell you more about them in Chapter 10), but your doctor can tell from a blood test if yours is caused by pyridoxine deficiency. The cure? Supplements and a better diet with more protein.

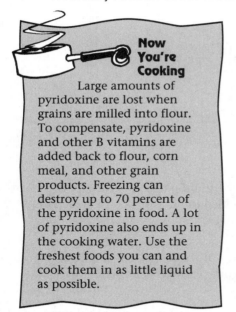

**Now You're Cooking**

Large amounts of pyridoxine are lost when grains are milled into flour. To compensate, pyridoxine and other B vitamins are added back to flour, corn meal, and other grain products. Freezing can destroy up to 70 percent of the pyridoxine in food. A lot of pyridoxine also ends up in the cooking water. Use the freshest foods you can and cook them in as little liquid as possible.

# Eating Your Pyridoxine

The best source of pyridoxine in your food is high-quality protein: chicken, pork, beef, fish, milk, dairy products, and eggs. Milk, dairy products, and eggs have less pyridoxine than fish and other meats, but they're still good sources. Also, pyridoxine is added to flour, corn meal, breakfast cereals, and many baked goods.

Here's a rare case where we can't tell you to eat more fresh fruits and vegetables: most of them don't have much or any pyridoxine. Even broccoli, our old standby, has only 0.15 mg in a half cup. The best plant choices are avocados, bananas, mangos, and potatoes. Whole grains are also good: a three-ounce serving of oatmeal has 0.74 mg. Look at the food chart to find other good sources of pyridoxine.

| The Pyridoxine in Food | | |
| --- | --- | --- |
| Food | Amount | Pyridoxine in mg |
| Apricots, dried | 10 halves | 0.06 |
| Avocado | 1/2 medium | 0.40 |
| Banana | 1 medium | 0.66 |
| Beef, ground | 3 ounces | 0.17 |

| Food | Amount | Pyridoxine in mg |
|---|---|---|
| Beef liver | 3 ounces | 0.78 |
| Black beans | 1 cup | 0.12 |
| Cheddar cheese | 1 ounce | 0.02 |
| Chicken breast | 3 ounces | 0.34 |
| Chick peas | 1 cup | 0.23 |
| Corn, kernels | 1/2 cup | 0.26 |
| Cottage cheese, low-fat | 1 cup | 0.15 |
| Flounder | 3 ounces | 0.20 |
| Kidney beans | 1 cup | 0.21 |
| Lentils | 1 cup | 0.35 |
| Mango | 1 medium | 0.28 |
| Milk, low-fat | 1 cup | 0.10 |
| Navy beans | 1 cup | 0.30 |
| Pork, roasted | 3 ounces | 0.39 |
| Potato, baked with skin | 1 medium | 0.70 |
| Prunes, dried | 10 | 0.22 |
| Raisins, golden | 2/3 cup | 0.32 |
| Rice, brown | 1 cup | 0.28 |
| Rice, white | 1 cup | 0.19 |
| Sweet potato, baked with skin | 1 medium | 0.28 |
| Tuna, canned in water | 3 ounces | 0.30 |
| Turkey breast, with skin | 3 ounces | 0.28 |
| Wheat germ | 1/4 cup | 0.38 |
| Yogurt, low-fat | 8 ounces | 0.11 |

# Getting the Most from Pyridoxine

The RDA for pyridoxine is in most multivitamin supplements; it's also in B vitamin formulas, usually in amounts anywhere from 10 to 50 mg. Supplements of pyridoxine alone come in tablets or capsules in sizes ranging from 25 to 500 mg.

Be very, very cautious about taking pyridoxine supplements. This is one of the few water-soluble supplements that you can actually overdose on. Too

**Warning!**
Large doses of pyridoxine can make the drug phenytoin (Dilantin®), which helps control epilepsy, break down too quickly in your system. If you take this drug, talk to your doctor about taking any vitamin supplements before you try them.

much pyridoxine causes neurological problems such as numbness or tingling in the hands and feet and trouble walking. The symptoms usually go away if you cut back on the dose, but sometimes they're permanent.

Neurological symptoms usually only happen when you're taking really big doses of over 2,000 mg a day. Most people can take up to 500 mg a day without any problems, but even 200 mg a day could cause trouble. To be on the safe side, take no more than 50 mg a day of pyridoxine.

You need to have good levels of magnesium—at least the RDA—for pyridoxine to work properly (see Chapter 18 on magnesium for more information).

| Thumbs Up/Thumbs Down | |
| --- | --- |
| **Pyridoxine is helped by:** | **Pyridoxine is hurt by:** |
| Riboflavin | Alcohol |
| Vitamin C | Birth-control pills |
| Magnesium | Some prescription drugs for asthma, tuberculosis, high blood pressure, and rheumatoid arthritis |
| Selenium | |

# Help for Heart Disease

Coming up in Chapter 9, we'll talk a lot about how folic acid combines with pyridoxine and cobalamin to fight heart disease by breaking down homocysteine. You need all three working together for the maximum effect.

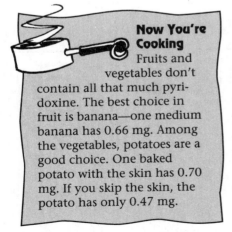

**Now You're Cooking**
Fruits and vegetables don't contain all that much pyridoxine. The best choice in fruit is banana—one medium banana has 0.66 mg. Among the vegetables, potatoes are a good choice. One baked potato with the skin has 0.70 mg. If you skip the skin, the potato has only 0.47 mg.

On its own, pyridoxine plays some other roles that also help prevent heart disease. One of the most important is keeping your red blood cells from getting "sticky" and clumping together, or aggregating. When that happens, the cells release powerful chemicals that eventually cause atherosclerosis—deposits that clog up your arteries and could lead to a heart attack or stroke.

(Check back to Chapter 2 for more information about atherosclerosis.) If enough cells clump together, they form a clot that blocks an artery. Again, the result is a heart attack or stroke. If you're at risk for atherosclerosis or already have it, taking pyridoxine supplements could slow the process down. Talk to your doctor before you try it, however.

Here's another interesting fact: People who have just had heart attacks have low levels of pyridoxine. Is this a cause or an effect? Nobody knows, but researchers are looking into it.

Pyridoxine supplements in fairly high doses—about 500 mg a day—can lower your blood pressure. It's cheaper than prescription drugs and doesn't have their side effects, but you do have to worry about the possible side effects of the large dose. Don't try this on your own, especially if you already take medicine to lower your blood pressure. If you want to try pyridoxine, talk to your doctor first.

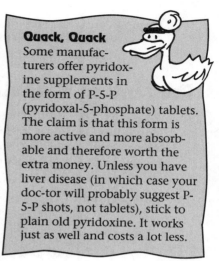

**Quack, Quack**
Some manufacturers offer pyridoxine supplements in the form of P-5-P (pyridoxal-5-phosphate) tablets. The claim is that this form is more active and more absorbable and therefore worth the extra money. Unless you have liver disease (in which case your doctor will probably suggest P-5-P shots, not tablets), stick to plain old pyridoxine. It works just as well and costs a lot less.

## Immune Booster

You need all the B vitamins for your immune system to work right, but pyridoxine is the key. Without it, you can't produce enough of the special infection-fighting cells that fend off illness. People with low immunity—alcoholics, the elderly, cancer patients, and others—also usually have low pyridoxine levels.

Elderly people are very vulnerable to illness—and up to a third of all elderly people have low pyridoxine levels. In part, that's because you just absorb less of the B's from your food as you grow older. It's also because many elderly people don't eat well, especially if they live alone or in a nursing home. The lack of pyridoxine makes them more likely to get sick and also makes them take longer to get better. If you're over age 60 or if your immune system isn't working well for some reason, be sure to get plenty of B's in your diet every day. To be sure you're getting enough, take a good daily multivitamin as well.

## Helping Asthmatics

Some people with asthma benefit from pyridoxine supplements, possibly because their bodies don't use it properly to begin with. Taking extra may bring their pyridoxine level closer to normal, which reduces their wheezing and cuts back on how often they have attacks.

A drug called theophylline is widely prescribed for asthma—and also for bronchitis and emphysema. It's an effective treatment, but it has a lot of bad side effects, including headaches, nausea, irritability, tremors, sleeping problems, and even seizures. The side effects are caused because theophylline blocks the way your body uses pyridoxine. Even if you're taking in enough through your food, the drug is

**Warning!**
Even mild asthma is a serious health problem, because it can suddenly get much worse. If you think you have asthma, see your doctor as soon as possible. If you already take medicine for asthma—even nonprescription drugs—don't stop! Talk to your doctor about taking pyridoxine and other supplements before you try them.

keeping you from using it. Pyridoxine supplements have been shown to reduce the side effects of theophylline, especially tremor. If you're taking this drug, talk to your doctor about pyridoxine supplements before you try them.

# Preventing Diabetic Complications

People with diabetes sometimes get diabetic neuropathy, a painful nerve condition. The symptoms are similar to the symptoms you would get with severe pyridoxine deficiency—and many diabetics are low on pyridoxine. Is there a connection? Some researchers say yes. They feel diabetic neuropathy could be prevented by taking 150 mg of pyridoxine daily.

If you have diabetes and want to try pyridoxine to treat or prevent diabetic neuropathy, talk to your doctor first.

# Relief for Carpal Tunnel Syndrome

Your wrist is a marvel of engineering. To make this joint flexible, bones, ligaments, and muscles all come tightly together, leaving only a narrow passage—the carpal tunnel—for the nerves leading to your hand. If anything swells up in your wrist, even a little, it presses on the passage and squeezes the nerves. The result? Carpal tunnel syndrome (CTS), a painful problem that is becoming very common. Symptoms include pain, numbness, and tingling in the fingers, wrist, or hand. Women seem to get CTS more often than men.

### Food for Thought

Carpal tunnel syndrome is caused by repeatedly doing the same thing with your hands—working at a keyboard, operating a cash register, turning a screwdriver. Injuries from this sort of work are called *repetitive strain injuries*. RSI is the fastest-growing category of occupational injury in America. In 1995, there were over 32,000 new cases of RSI—72 percent of all the occupational injuries reported. If you think you have a repetitive strain injury, see a doctor at once—and talk to your boss. You need to treat the injury—and you also need to change how and where you work to keep it from happening again.

A lot of people claim that pyridoxine supplements help or even "cure" CTS. Is there any evidence for this? Not really. Careful studies show that hardly anyone with CTS is deficient or even low in pyridoxine. The studies also show no real benefit from treating CTS just with large doses of pyridoxine—and as we discussed earlier, large doses could be dangerous. It's possible that pyridoxine can help, however, if it's taken in moderate doses (150 mg a day) along with other treatments, such as physical therapy and drugs to relieve the swelling.

# Pyridoxine for PMS

Researchers have been looking into pyridoxine for treating PMS ever since the early 1970s. There have been more than a dozen serious studies, and none of them have proved that pyridoxine does much one way or the other. In the studies, women who took pyridoxine felt that their symptoms, including depression, irritability, headaches, and fluid retention, got better. The problem is that the women who thought they were taking pyridoxine, but were actually taking sugar pills, also felt their symptoms got better.

So should you take pyridoxine for PMS? Studies aside, many of Dr. Pressman's patients really have benefited from this, so we suggest you try taking 50 mg a day in the days before your period. It won't hurt and there's a good chance it might help.

# Other Problems and Pyridoxine

Depending on who you ask, a long list of ailments, from autism to vomiting, is helped by pyridoxine. Not all these claims hold up, but here's a few that do:

➤ **Melanoma.** Pyridoxine may help stop the growth of *melanoma*, a very dangerous type of skin cancer. This is an exciting new development, because right now melanoma is hard to treat. It's still experimental, though—stay tuned.

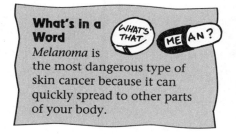

**What's in a Word**
*Melanoma* is the most dangerous type of skin cancer because it can quickly spread to other parts of your body.

➤ **Depression.** Some people hospitalized for depression have low pyridoxine levels and seem to get better if they take supplements. The supplements don't help if their pyridoxine is normal to begin with.

➤ **Kidney stones.** If you get the calcium oxalate type of kidney stone, pyridoxine supplements, along with extra magnesium, could keep the stones from coming back. (We'll talk about this more in Chapter 18 on magnesium.) Talk to your doctor before you try this.

➤ **Cancer drug toxicity.** The nasty side effects of some cancer drugs, such as vincristine, are reduced by extra pyridoxine.

➤ **Morning sickness.** A small daily dose of pyridoxine (25 mg) seems to work for about one out of three women. If nothing else is helping your morning sickness, talk to your doctor about trying pyridoxine.

As pyridoxine research continues, we'll probably find more ways it can help health problems. Pyridoxine may help some forms of infertility, for example, and research continues on ways it can help fight cancer.

# The Least You Need to Know

➤ Pyridoxine, also called Vitamin B$_6$, works closely with all the other B vitamins, especially niacin, folic acid, and cobalamin.

➤ You need pyridoxine to convert amino acids into proteins and for turning stored sugar into energy.

➤ Pyridoxine is vital for your immune system and can help prevent heart disease.

➤ The RDA for pyridoxine is about 2.0 mg a day for adults.

➤ Pyridoxine is found in high-protein foods such as eggs, fish, poultry, and meat. It's also added to breakfast cereals, bread, and many baked goods. Fruits and vegetables have little or no pyridoxine.

➤ Pyridoxine supplements in large doses can be toxic.

# Chapter 9

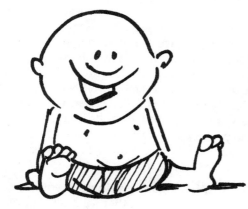

# Folic Acid: Healthy Babies, Healthy Hearts

## In This Chapter

➤ Why you need folic acid (Vitamin B$_9$)

➤ Foods that are high in folic acid

➤ How folic acid can help prevent birth defects

➤ Helping your heart with folic acid

➤ How folic acid can help prevent cancer, especially colon cancer

Popeye the sailorman always eats his spinach so he'll be strong to the finish. Why does Popeye eat spinach instead of one of those other green leafy vegetables we keep talking about, like collard greens, or maybe Swiss chard? Aside from the fact that those vegetables don't rhyme with finish, they don't have anywhere near as much folic acid—and you need folic acid to build muscles and to keep your body strong and in good repair.

Spinach gives Popeye lots of muscles and energy. Does it do the same for Olive Oyl? It sure does—and it helped little Swee'pea, too, because folic acid helps prevent birth defects. Folic acid could even help that big bully Bluto. He's a prime candidate for a heart attack—and the latest research shows that folic acid can help prevent heart disease.

# Why You Need Folic Acid

Researchers in the early 1940s found an interesting substance in spinach leaves. They called it *folic acid* (or folate or folacin) from the Latin word for leaf—"folium." Folic acid is the synthetic form while folate is the natural form found in foods. For practical purposes, they're the same. If you hang out with organic chemists and want to show off, you can call it *pteroylglutamic acid* or *pteroylmonoglutamate*.

You may not realize it, but your body is constantly making new cells to replace old ones that wear out. Your red blood cells are a good example—every day, you make *millions* of new ones to replace old ones that are too beat up to work well anymore. All those new cells are why you need a good supply of *folic acid*. Without it, you can't make enough new cells fast enough or well enough. And folic acid is especially important for cells that wear out and divide rapidly, such as red blood cells, skin cells, and the cells that line your small intestine. What it all comes down to is that you need folic acid for the normal growth and maintenance of every cell in your body.

Folic acid does some other amazing things for your health. In the past few years we've learned that folic acid prevents birth defects, helps prevent heart disease, and may even help prevent cancer. The evidence is so convincing that starting in 1998 many common foods, including bread, breakfast cereal, pasta, and rice, will have extra folic acid, by order of the FDA.

# The RDA for Folic Acid

In 1989, the RDA for folic acid was lowered by about half. The earlier RDA for adult males, for example, was 400 micrograms; this was reduced to 200 micrograms. The RDA for women of childbearing age was also cut in half, from 800 micrograms to 400 micrograms. Studies in the 1980s showed that although the average folic acid intake for all age groups was considerably below the RDA, few people showed any sign of deficiency. So, the reasoning went, the RDA should be lowered to the amount taken in on average by most healthy people, because they all seemed to be OK.

The lowered basic amount is a really good example of how the RDAs give you just the bare minimum needed to prevent deficiency, and not the amount that leads to good health. Today many doctors and nutritionists believe that the RDAs are way, way too low. They recommend that *everyone* get at least 400 mcg of folic acid every day—800 mcg would be even better. When the new RDAs for B vitamins are issued in the spring of 1998, they will probably be raised. The new RDA for folic acid will almost certainly be at least 400 mcg.

| The RDA for Folic Acid | |
|---|---|
| Age/Sex | Folic acid in mcg |
| *Infants* | |
| 0–0.5 year | 25 |
| 0.5–1 year | 35 |
| *Children* | |
| 1–3 years | 50 |
| 4–6 | 75 |
| 7–10 | 100 |
| 11–14 | 150 |
| *Adults* | |
| Men 15+ | 200 |
| Women 15–50 years | 180 |
| Women 50+ | 180 |
| Nursing women | 500 |

# Are You Deficient?

Even after the RDA for folic acid was lowered, studies show that the average American diet contains only about 200 micrograms a day. Not surprisingly, a shortage of folic acid even by the lowered RDA standard is one of the most common vitamin deficiencies, especially among women. One recent study estimated that an astonishing 88 percent of all Americans get less than 400 micrograms a day. You could be deficient in folic acid if:

➤ **You're pregnant.** Because your unborn baby is growing fast, he or she is taking a lot of your folic acid. If you're pregnant, your doctor will prescribe folic acid supplements. And if you're a woman of childbearing age (between 15 and 47), keep reading—in a little while we'll tell you why you need extra folic acid even if you're not pregnant.

➤ **You're breastfeeding.** You're passing a lot of your folic acid on to your baby, so you need some extra for yourself. And if you don't get enough, your baby may not get enough either.

➤ **You abuse alcohol.** Alcoholics have bad nutrition and don't get enough B vitamins in general. Also, alcohol seems to block your absorption of folic acid.

➤ **You smoke cigarettes.** Smokers are low on all the B vitamins, including folic acid.

➤ **You take birth control pills.** If you're on the Pill, you could be low on all the B vitamins, but especially folic acid. Talk to your doctor about taking supplements. And even though you're not interested in babies right now, read the section on folic acid and pregnancy.

➤ **You take drugs such as phenytoin (Dilantin®) for seizures, sulfasalazine (Azulfidine®) for inflammatory bowel disease, or trimethoprim (Proloprim® or Trimpex®) for urinary tract infections.** Many drugs keep you from absorbing enough folic acid (see the chart for a longer list).

➤ **You take methotrexate (Folex® or Mexate®) for rheumatoid arthritis, psoriasis, or inflammatory bowel disease.** This drug blocks your uptake of folic acid. Recent studies have proved that folic acid supplements help you tolerate the drug better. If you take this medicine, talk to your doctor about folic acid supplements.

➤ **You're over age 65.** Many elderly people, especially if they live alone or in a nursing home, don't get enough folic acid from their food. That's partly because their ability to absorb folic acid has dropped, and partly because their food is low in folic acid to begin with.

If you suddenly become deficient in folic acid, it could be an indication that you have cancer. The rapidly growing cancer cells are using up your folic acid to fuel their uncontrolled division.

| **Drugs that Block Folic Acid** | |
| --- | --- |
| **Drug** | **Used For** |
| Anticonvulsants | Preventing seizures |
| Chloramphenicol | Bacterial infections |
| Cortisone drugs | Severe inflammation, arthritis |
| Methotrexate | Rheumatoid arthritis |
| Oral contraceptives | Preventing pregnancy |
| Pyrimethamine | Intestinal parasites |
| Quinine | Malaria |
| Sulfasalazine | Ulcerative colitis |
| Sulfa drugs | Infection |
| Trimethoprim | Urinary tract infections |

Folic acid deficiency affects the growth and repair of your body's tissues. The tissues that have fastest rate of cell replacement are the first ones to be affected, so your blood and digestive tract are where the signs of deficiency will most likely first appear. If you're deficient in folic acid, you might have some of these symptoms:

➤ Anemia

➤ Nausea and loss of appetite

➤ Diarrhea

➤ Malnutrition from poor nutrient absorption

➤ Weight loss

➤ Weakness

➤ Sore tongue

➤ Headaches

➤ Irritability and mood swings

➤ Heart palpitations

Hardly anyone in today's society will be seriously deficient in folic acid just from eating too much junk food. It's much more likely that deficiency symptoms such as anemia, malnutrition, and heart palpitations will appear in someone who is an alcoholic or has some other severe health problem that keeps them from eating or digesting properly.

Mild deficiencies are likely for people who eat only institutional food—nursing home residents, for example. That's because the folic acid in food is easily destroyed by processing, overcooking, or reheating.

In general, if you're deficient in folic acid, you're likely to be deficient in the other B vitamins as well. It's almost always from poor diet or poor absorption, so eating better and taking supplements if needed will usually solve the problem.

# Eating Your Folic Acid

As you can see from the chart, folic acid isn't found in that many animal foods. The only good animal sources are chicken liver and beef liver; there's hardly any in milk and other dairy foods. Beans of all kinds are a great way to get your folic acid. Other good plant sources are spinach and asparagus. On the whole, most fruits don't contain much folic acid. The best choices are bananas, oranges, and cantaloupe.

| The Folic Acid in Food | | |
| --- | --- | --- |
| Food | Amount | Folic acid in mcg |
| Asparagus, cooked | 1/2 cup | 132 |
| Avocado | 1/2 medium | 56 |
| Banana | 1 medium | 22 |
| Beets, cooked | 1/2 cup | 45 |

*continues*

## The Folic Acid in Food  Continued

| Food | Amount | Folic acid in mcg |
| --- | --- | --- |
| Black beans | 1 cup | 256 |
| Black-eyed peas | 1 cup | 123 |
| Bread, whole wheat | 1 slice | 14 |
| Broccoli, cooked | 1/2 cup | 39 |
| Brussels sprouts, cooked | 1/2 cup | 47 |
| Cantaloupe | 1 cup | 27 |
| Chick peas | 1 cup | 282 |
| Collard greens, cooked | 1/2 cup | 65 |
| Corn, kernels | 1 cup | 38 |
| Endive, raw | 1/2 cup | 36 |
| Kidney beans | 1 cup | 229 |
| Lentils | 1 cup | 358 |
| Lima beans, baby | 1 cup | 273 |
| Liver, beef | 3 ounces | 200 |
| Liver, chicken | 3 ounces | 660 |
| Navy beans | 1 cup | 255 |
| Orange | 1 medium | 47 |
| Peanuts, dry roasted | 1 ounce | 41 |
| Romaine lettuce | 1/2 cup | 38 |
| Spinach, raw | 1/2 cup | 54 |
| Spinach, cooked | 1/2 cup | 131 |
| Wheat germ | 1/4 cup | 82 |

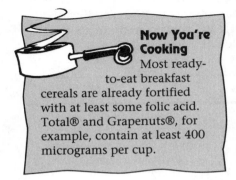

**Now You're Cooking** Most ready-to-eat breakfast cereals are already fortified with at least some folic acid. Total® and Grapenuts®, for example, contain at least 400 micrograms per cup.

Even if you regularly eat lots of beans and fresh vegetables, it's hard to get enough folic acid through your diet alone. That's because you only absorb about half of the folic acid you eat. Also, a lot of it is lost in processing and cooking. Cook fresh veggies lightly in as little water as possible to preserve the folic acid.

Because most Americans don't begin to eat enough beans and fresh vegetables, the FDA has prepared new rules for fortifying enriched breads, flours, corn meal, rice, noodles, pasta, and other grain products with folic acid. As of 1998 all these foods have extra folic acid added to them. The goal is to make sure that everyone gets at least 400 micrograms a day from their food.

# Getting the Most from Folic Acid

Like the other B vitamins, folic acid is water-soluble. That means your body can't really store it, so it's important to get enough every day.

Folic acid works closely with the other B vitamins, especially pyridoxine, cobalamin, and choline. If you're low on any of the B's, you're probably low on folic acid as well—and vice versa. You may need to take a complete B supplement.

Vitamin C prevents folic acid from being broken down too quickly in your body. Most nutritionists today strongly recommend getting at least 500 mg of Vitamin C every day.

Virtually all multivitamin supplements, especially those formulated for women, contain 400 micrograms of folic acid.

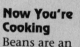

**Now You're Cooking**
Beans are an excellent natural source of folic acid—but there is that embarrassing little problem. Beans produce gas. To reduce the problem, soak dried beans in nine cups of water for every cup of beans. Drain the beans and change the water at least twice during the 24-hour soaking period. Drain and rinse well before using. If you're using canned beans, drain and rinse well before using.

**Food for Thought**

If the government is fortifying common foods so that you're sure to get 400 mcg of folic acid without really trying, do you still need supplements? Maybe not, but if you're a woman in your childbearing years, don't take any chances with your health or the health of your unborn baby. Talk to your doctor about supplements.

It's almost impossible to overdose on folic acid. Any excess just comes out harmlessly in your urine—although if you take a lot, your urine will have a bright yellow color.

Most doctors recommend taking no more than 1 milligram a day in supplements. The reasoning is that taking larger amounts could mask the serious type of anemia caused by a deficiency of cobalamin. If the deficiency isn't discovered in time, you could have permanent nerve damage. It's a good point, but it may be too cautious. Anemia from cobalamin deficiency is actually fairly rare, and it almost always occurs in older adults. Your chances of getting heart

**Warning!**
Folic acid keeps the drug phenytoin (Dilantin®) and most other anticonvulsant drugs from working properly. Do not take folic acid supplements if you take these drugs. Discuss all vitamin supplements with your doctor before you try them.

disease or colon cancer are much higher—and as we'll see, folic acid could really lower those odds.

| Thumbs Up/Thumbs Down | |
|---|---|
| **Folic acid is helped by:** | **Folic acid is hurt by:** |
| All other B vitamins | Alcohol |
| Vitamin C | Anticonvulsant drugs, especially phenytoin (Dilantin®) |
| | Birth control pills |
| | Many other prescription drugs |

# Folic Acid for Healthy Babies

Every year in the United States about 2,500 babies are born with a *neural tube defect (NTD)*. About one to two out of every thousand births—eleven a day—in the United States have a neural tube defect. The most common is the crippling defect spina bifida, or "open spine," which occurs when the vertebrae don't form a complete ring to protect the spine. Sometimes the brain never develops at all, a rare and always fatal condition called anencephaly.

Recent studies have conclusively shown that taking 400 micrograms of folic acid each day *before* getting pregnant can prevent between 50 and 75 percent of all neural tube defects. In 1992, the U.S. Public Health Service recommended that *all* women of childbearing age consume 400 micrograms of folic acid daily. Every agency and organization concerned with birth defects, from the FDA to the March of Dimes, has strongly endorsed this recommendation.

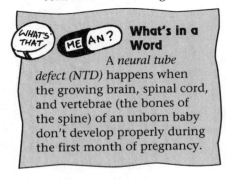

**What's in a Word**

A *neural tube defect (NTD)* happens when the growing brain, spinal cord, and vertebrae (the bones of the spine) of an unborn baby don't develop properly during the first month of pregnancy.

Why does everyone recommend folic acid for all women, not just women who are pregnant? Your unborn baby needs folic acid the most during the first month of pregnancy, when the neural tube is formed—but you might not realize you're pregnant during that critical time, even if you've been trying to have a baby. It's vitally important for every woman to get enough folic acid. If you're a woman between the ages of 15 and 47, the time to start taking folic acid supplements is *now*.

# Folic Acid Forestalls Heart Disease

Like most health-conscious people, you already know that high cholesterol is a warning sign of possible heart disease. The cholesterol clogs your arteries and can eventually lead to a heart attack. So, you've been watching your diet and cutting back on how much fat you eat—and at your last checkup, your cholesterol level was well within the normal range. That's good, you thought, at least I don't have to worry about having a heart attack.

We hate to break the news to you, but you still have to worry. The fact is, most people who have a heart attack have *normal* cholesterol levels—but their arteries are still clogged. If cholesterol isn't causing the problem, what is?

The answer has become very clear in the past few years: High blood levels of *homocysteine,* an amino acid found naturally in your body, damages your arteries. The next question is, What causes the homocysteine to build up to dangerous levels? Here too the answer is very clear: not enough folic acid. Working with pyridoxine and cobalamin, folic acid quickly breaks down the homocysteine and removes it from your body before it can do any damage. Not enough folic acid, and the homocysteine hangs around too long, attacking your artery walls.

> **Now You're Cooking**
> Cooking makes the folic acid in vegetables easier to absorb by breaking down the tough cell walls and releasing the vitamin. On the other hand, once the folic acid is released it dissolves into the cooking water. To get the most folic acid, cook your vegetables gently in as little water as possible.

Here's the really big question: How much folic acid is enough to keep your homocysteine level low? Only 1 to 2 mg a day—not very much, but a lot more than the RDA.

Getting more folic acid, through your diet or with supplements, is simple, safe, and cheap—and it could save your life. By some estimates, just 1 mg a day could be enough to prevent 50,000 heart attacks a year.

Today we've come to realize that high homocysteine levels by themselves are a very accurate warning sign of possible heart trouble—and also raise your chances of a stroke. Your doctor can do a blood test to check your homocysteine level. If it is elevated (above 14 micro-moles per liter for men and 8.5 micromoles per liter for women), discuss ways to raise your folic acid level with your doctor.

> **What's in a Word**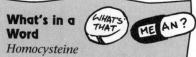
> *Homocysteine* is an amino acid formed when other amino acids in your blood are broken down by normal body processes. Folic acid breaks down the ho-mocysteine into harmless methionine and prevents a toxic buildup. The medical term for too much homocys-teine in the blood is *hyperhomocysteinemia.*

# Preventing Cancer with Folic Acid

For a long time, cancer researchers were so focused on the powerful antioxidant vitamins A, C, and E that they sort of forgot about the B vitamins. Recently, though, folic acid has been getting a lot of attention for its role in preventing cancer of the colon and cervix—and maybe for preventing other cancers as well.

## Folic Acid Helps Prevent Colon Cancer

Recent studies show that people with low folic acid levels are more likely to get colon cancer. If you're a woman and get a lot of folic acid in your diet, for instance, your chances of colon cancer are sharply lower—by as much as 60 percent. (For some reason, this doesn't work as well for men.)

People with ulcerative colitis (UC), a serious chronic disease of the large intestine, have an increased risk of getting colon cancer—and they also often have low folic acid levels. For many patients, the reason is that the drug sulfasalazine (Azulfidine®), which helps UC a lot, also blocks their uptake of folic acid. Recent studies show that UC patients who take 1 mg a day of extra folic acid cut their chances of colon cancer nearly in half. If you have ulcerative colitis, discuss folic acid supplements with your doctor before you try them.

## Preventing Cervical Cancer

> **WHAT'S THAT ME AN? What's in a Word**
>
> Your *cervix* is the neck-shaped structure leading from your vagina to your uterus. *Cervical dysplasia,* or abnormalities in the cells of the cervix, can eventually lead to cervical cancer. The *human papillomavirus (HPV)* causes venereal warts, which can cause cervical dysplasia and cancer of the cervix.

Women with *cervical dysplasia* may later develop cancer of the *cervix*, especially if the problem isn't detected and treated early on. Many women infected with *human papillomavirus (HPV)* have cervical dysplasia. Women who smoke are more likely to have cervical dysplasia, probably because smokers have low folic acid levels.

Recent studies have shown that women with HPV *and* low folic acid levels were five times more likely to have cervical dysplasia. Other studies suggest that minor cervical dysplasia can be effectively treated with large doses (more than 5 milligrams daily) of folic acid. This is not something you should do on your own, however. If you have cervical dysplasia, discuss all your treatment options with your doctor.

# Folic Acid and Depression

Could it be that eating more dark-green leafy vegetables can lift your mood? Quite possibly. A recent study of depressed outpatients at Massachusetts General Hospital showed that low folic acid levels are linked to depression. The most depressed patients in the study had the lowest levels of folic acid—and were the least likely to benefit from antidepressant drugs.

# The Least You Need to Know

➤ Folic acid, also called folate or folacin, is a B vitamin.

➤ Foods high in folic acid include chicken liver, all kinds of beans, spinach, and asparagus.

➤ The adult RDA for folic acid is 180 micrograms for women and 200 micrograms for men—although many researchers now believe these levels are far too low.

➤ All women of childbearing age should be sure to get at least 400 micrograms of folic acid through daily supplements to prevent birth defects.

➤ Folic acid may help prevent heart disease by reducing homocysteine in the blood.

➤ Folic acid may help prevent cancer of the cervix and the colon.

# Chapter 10

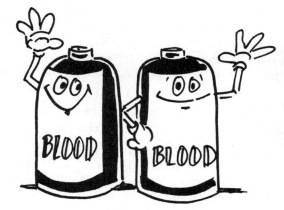

# Cobalamin: The B for Healthy Blood

## In This Chapter

➤ Why you need cobalamin (Vitamin $B_{12}$)

➤ Foods that are high in cobalamin

➤ How cobalamin prevents and treats anemia

➤ Why you need more cobalamin as you get older

Until recently, doctors and nutritionists didn't pay much attention to cobalamin. Sure, we knew you need it to keep your red blood cells healthy, but as long as you didn't actually have anemia, we figured you were getting enough. After all, the amount you need is the tiniest of any vitamin—just a couple of micrograms a day.

Well, we were wrong. Even that tiny amount is essential not just for your blood but for a lot of other things, including preventing heart disease, keeping your mind sharp as you grow older, and keeping your immune system working in top gear. And because so little has to do so much, you need to be absolutely, positively sure you're getting enough.

# Why You Need Cobalamin

Cobalamin does plenty for you, but let's start with its most important role: making healthy red blood cells. If you eat enough *cobalamin*, and if your body can use it properly, you make millions of nice, round, healthy red blood cells every day. If you don't eat enough, or you can't use it properly, you can't make enough red blood cells, and the ones you do make are too large and fragile to work well. When you don't have enough red blood cells to carry oxygen and nutrients around your body, you develop anemia (we'll talk about this a lot more in a little while).

All your cells, not just your red blood cells, need cobalamin to grow and divide properly. For example, you need it to make all the different cells in your immune system, including white blood cells.

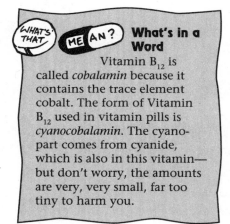

**What's in a Word**

Vitamin $B_{12}$ is called *cobalamin* because it contains the trace element cobalt. The form of Vitamin $B_{12}$ used in vitamin pills is *cyanocobalamin*. The cyano-part comes from cyanide, which is also in this vitamin—but don't worry, the amounts are very, very small, far too tiny to harm you.

Cobalamin's next big role is in making the protective fatty layer, or sheath, that lines your nerve cells—sort of like insulation on electric wires. If the sheath is damaged because you don't have cobalamin, you start getting the equivalent of static on the line. Really bad static can interfere with your mental function—so much that people think you're senile.

Cobalamin is also a team player. Working with the other B vitamins, but especially with pyridoxine and folic acid, it helps you turn the carbos, fats, and proteins in your food into energy in your cells.

The B team also helps protect your heart by removing harmful homocysteine from your blood before it can damage your blood vessels (see Chapter 9 on folic acid for more about this).

# The RDA for Cobalamin

Important as cobalamin is, you need only very small amounts of it. That's why the RDA for an adult is only two micrograms. We're starting to realize that there's a big problem with that RDA, though. It doesn't take into account the fact that you absorb less cobalamin as you get older. (It's quite likely that the new RDA for cobalamin, expected in the spring of 1998, will raise the amounts for older adults.)

We'll talk more about why that's so and what to do about it a little later in this chapter. For now, let's just say that many doctors and nutritionists now feel that people over age 50 need a lot more cobalamin. Doctors usually recommend daily supplements containing 500 to 1,000 micrograms. It's a safe and inexpensive form of health insurance. At the least, check the RDA chart to be sure you're getting the minimum.

| The RDA for Cobalamin | |
|---|---|
| Age | Cobalamin in mcg |
| *Infants* | |
| 0–0.5 year | 0.3 |
| 0.5–1 year | 0.5 |
| *Children* | |
| 1–3 years | 0.7 |
| 4–6 | 1.0 |
| 7–10 | 1.4 |
| *Young Adults and Adults* | |
| 11+ | 2.0 |
| Pregnant women | 2.2 |
| Nursing women | 2.6 |

# Are You Deficient?

That's an important question, because it can be hard to tell. To understand why, we'll have to explain how cobalamin gets into your body. Cobalamin is found only in animal foods such as liver, eggs, fish, and meat—and only in very small amounts that are hard to take in. To get even the small amount of cobalamin you need, your body needs to be really good at absorbing it. In fact, you make a special substance in your stomach, called *intrinsic factor,* just to help you do that—and even that only lets you absorb about half of the cobalamin you eat. Fortunately, most people take in more than twice the RDA through their diet, so they usually get enough.

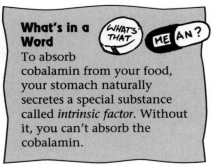

**What's in a Word**
To absorb cobalamin from your food, your stomach naturally secretes a special substance called *intrinsic factor*. Without it, you can't absorb the cobalamin.

Although cobalamin is a water-soluble vitamin, you still store some of it in your liver and kidneys. Also, your body is really good at recycling cobalamin, so you don't use up your body stores very quickly.

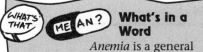

### What's in a Word

*Anemia* is a general term meaning your red blood cells either don't have enough *hemoglobin* (the stuff that carries oxygen) or you have a below-normal number of them. *Megaloblastic anemia* (sometimes called *macrocytic anemia*) happens when you don't get enough cobalamin in your diet. *Pernicious anemia* happens when your stomach, for reasons nobody really understands, stops making intrinsic factor and you are unable to absorb cobalamin from your food.

What we're leading up to here is that if you don't get much cobalamin in your diet, it could take a long time—four or five years—for deficiency symptoms to start showing up. Sometimes people slowly stop making intrinsic factor, but here too it could take several years for real deficiency symptoms to appear.

The most obvious symptom of cobalamin deficiency is *anemia*—in this case, because you don't have enough healthy red blood cells. When the anemia comes from a shortage of cobalamin in the diet, it's called *megaloblastic anemia*. When it comes from a lack of intrinsic factor, it's called *pernicious anemia*. The causes are different, but the result is the same: you don't have enough red blood cells, and the ones you do have are too big and fragile to survive long in your circulation.

## Who's at Risk?

On the whole, most people under age 50 get enough cobalamin from their diet, but older people and some others are at real risk for a deficiency. You might be in that category if:

➤ You're a strict vegetarian or vegan. Because cobalamin is found naturally only in animal foods, people who don't eat these foods can get deficient if they don't take supplements. Kids are especially at risk. (If you don't eat animal foods, be sure to read the section on eating your cobalamin later in this chapter.)

➤ You're over age 50. As you get older, you naturally make less intrinsic factor and absorb less cobalamin. Sometimes you stop making intrinsic factor completely.

### Food for Thought

In the late nineteenth century and well into the twentieth, pernicious anemia suddenly became common, for reasons that to this day no one can really explain. Young women were especially likely to get it. The disease was called "green sickness" because the anemia made victims very pale and gave their skin a greenish cast. Today pernicious anemia is very rare in young people—most people who have it are over 60.

➤ You're pregnant or breastfeeding. Your growing baby is taking a lot of your cobalamin. You need to get extra in your food or through supplements.

➤ You smoke cigarettes. Smokers have low blood levels of cobalamin and all the other B vitamins.

➤ You regularly take the drug omeprazole (Prilosec®) to treat severe heartburn or ulcers. This drug interferes with your absorption of cobalamin—talk to your doctor about supplements.

➤ You've been taking prescription potassium supplements for a long time. These drugs can interfere with your absorption of cobalamin—talk to your doctor about supplements.

➤ You've had part of your stomach surgically removed. You might not be making enough intrinsic factor in what's left of your stomach. Discuss supplements with your doctor.

Long before you actually get anemic, you could be having other cobalamin deficiency symptoms, especially if you're an older adult. Early symptoms often show up in your nervous system, such as:

➤ Tingling or "pins-and-needles" feeling in hands and feet

➤ Numbness in the hands or feet

➤ Moodiness and depression

➤ Trouble sleeping

➤ Memory loss

➤ Dizziness and loss of balance

➤ Dementia

These symptoms can slowly develop even when blood tests show that your cobalamin level is "normal." If you're elderly, they might be mistaken for senility—except great-grandpa might be getting ga-ga not from old age but from a simple vitamin deficiency. That's bad enough, but what's worse is that the damage could be permanent if the deficiency isn't fixed soon.

**Food for Thought**

Cobalamin deficiency is common—way too common—among older people. According to one study, 24 percent of people between the ages of 60 and 69 are deficient. Between the ages of 70 and 79, the number goes up to 32 percent. Among people over 80, nearly 40 percent are deficient.

By the time your cobalamin deficiency shows up on a blood test, you're not doing very well. You're getting sick more often, because you're making fewer infection-fighting white blood cells. You can't replace the cells that line your intestines quickly enough, so you have diarrhea, appetite loss, and vomiting. Finally, you have anemia symptoms. This is unmistakable, because you'll be unbelievably tired and weak. You'll also be very pale and bruise easily. If you start getting more cobalamin, though, your symptoms will quickly disappear.

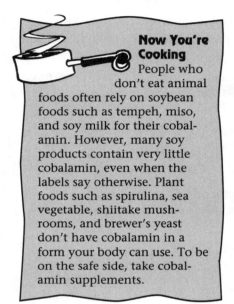

**Now You're Cooking**
People who don't eat animal foods often rely on soybean foods such as tempeh, miso, and soy milk for their cobalamin. However, many soy products contain very little cobalamin, even when the labels say otherwise. Plant foods such as spirulina, sea vegetable, shiitake mushrooms, and brewer's yeast don't have cobalamin in a form your body can use. To be on the safe side, take cobalamin supplements.

# Eating Your Cobalamin

Only animal foods such as meat, fish, and eggs naturally have cobalamin in them (it's added to some breakfast cereals). As you can see from the chart, even then they don't have much—but on the other hand, you don't need much, so most people get enough from their diet.

The big exceptions are people who are strict vegetarians, vegans, or follow a macrobiotic diet. Because they eat no meat and sometimes no animal foods at all, they have to get their cobalamin from some other source. In the diet, that source is usually soybean foods, but these probably don't provide enough, especially for children. If you don't eat meat or animal foods, we strongly suggest you take cobalamin supplements. Which foods in the following list do you eat regularly?

## The Cobalamin in Foods

| Food | Amount | Cobalamin in mcg |
| --- | --- | --- |
| Beef, ground | 3 ounces | 2.1 |
| Beef liver | 3 ounces | 68.0 |
| Cheddar cheese | 1 ounce | 0.23 |
| Chicken leg | 1 medium | 0.35 |
| Chicken liver | 3 ounces | 16.6 |
| Clams, steamed | 3 ounces | 84.06 |
| Cottage cheese, low-fat | 1 cup | 1.43 |
| Egg | 1 large | 0.56 |
| Flounder | 3 ounces | 2.13 |
| Liverwurst | 1 slice | 2.42 |
| Milk, low-fat | 8 ounces | 0.90 |
| Pâté de foie gras | 1 ounce | 2.66 |

| Food | Amount | Cobalamin in mcg |
|------|--------|------------------|
| Swiss cheese | 1 ounce | 0.48 |
| Tuna, light, in water | 3 ounces | 2.54 |
| Yogurt, low-fat | 8 ounces | 1.28 |

# Getting the Most from Cobalamin

Generally speaking, people who are deficient in cobalamin are eating enough of it—the problem is that they're not absorbing it because they don't have enough intrinsic factor.

**Food for Thought**

The role that something in liver—they didn't know what—played in treating pernicious anemia was discovered in the late 1920s by George Minot, William Murphy, and George Whipple. For their achievement, they won the Nobel Prize in medicine in 1934. It wasn't until 1948 that researchers finally isolated cobalamin as the substance in liver that cured anemia. Once cobalamin was isolated, treatment of pernicious anemia became much simpler and more effective.

Back in the 1920s, researchers found that if people with pernicious anemia ate a pound of raw beef liver every day, they got better. Until 1948, when cobalamin was finally isolated, choking down a hefty daily dose of raw liver was the only treatment.

Fortunately, today you can take your cobalamin supplements as tablets or capsules. (If you actually *like* the disgusting taste of slimy raw liver, go right ahead and get it that way instead.) The supplements usually have anywhere from 100 to 500 mcg. Even 100 mcg is a lot more than the RDA, but it's virtually impossible to overdose on cobalamin—any excess is just excreted.

If you're taking supplements because your diet is low in cobalamin, you may also be low in the other B vitamins as well. Folic acid needs cobalamin to work properly, so it's important to be sure you're getting all your B's.

**Warning!**
Large doses of Vitamin C can destroy cobalamin; take these supplements an hour or more apart, not at the same time.

If you're taking cobalamin because you don't make enough intrinsic factor to absorb it from your food, will you be able to absorb it from a pill? Good question. A lot of doctors would say no and make you come in for shots instead. In fact, if the supplement dose is big enough (1,000 to 2,000 mcg), you will absorb enough from it, even if you don't make any intrinsic factor at all. If you have pernicious or megaloblastic anemia, discuss oral cobalamin supplements with your doctor before you try them.

| Thumbs Up/Thumbs Down | |
|---|---|
| **Cobalamin is helped by:** | **Cobalamin is hurt by:** |
| All other B vitamins | Folic acid deficiency |
| Calcium | Iron deficiency |
| | Large doses of Vitamin C |
| | Vitamin E deficiency |

### Food for Thought

Some people prefer to take cobalamin supplements sublingually—that is, under the tongue. Sublingual cobalamin supplements are usually flavored nuggets containing 1,000 or even 5,000 micrograms. You put one under your tongue and let it slowly dissolve; the cobalamin is absorbed straight into your bloodstream through the network of tiny blood vessels under your tongue. If you have pernicious anemia, talk to your doctor about sublingual cobalamin supplements before you try them. When you're first diagnosed with the problem, you may need weekly shots for eight weeks or so to raise your cobalamin level back to normal.

## The Least You Need to Know

➤ Cobalamin, also called Vitamin $B_{12}$, is a water-soluble B vitamin.

➤ You need cobalamin for healthy red blood cells, to make the outer coverings of your nerves, and for a healthy immune system.

➤ Cobalamin is found only in animal foods such as liver, eggs, fish, and meat.

➤ The adult RDA for cobalamin is just 2 micrograms—most people get more than enough from their food.

➤ As you get older, your ability to absorb cobalamin decreases. You may need supplements.

➤ People who don't eat animal foods may need cobalamin supplements.

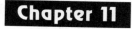

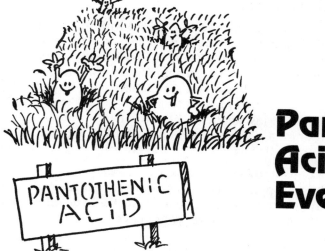

# Chapter 11

# Pantothenic Acid: It's Everywhere

> ### In This Chapter
>
> ➤ Why you need pantothenic acid (Vitamin B$_5$)
> ➤ Foods that are high in pantothenic acid
> ➤ How pantothenic acid produces energy
> ➤ Why athletes need pantothenic acid

It's kind of nice to know that there's one vitamin you can't ever be deficient in—pantothenic acid. At least some pantothenic acid is found in every single food you eat, so there's no way you can't get enough. That's good, because you need pantothenic acid for turning those foods into energy.

Important as pantothenic acid is, it's one of those quiet types that just does its job without much fanfare. The noise about pantothenic acid all comes from people who make a lot of claims for it. Do you need it to make hormones and healthy red blood cells? Definitely yes. Does it boost athletic performance, fix high cholesterol, and stop your hair from turning gray? Definitely maybe.

# Why You Need Pantothenic Acid

The fats and carbohydrates you eat get turned into energy you can use with the vital help of *pantothenic acid*. To be exact, you need pantothenic acid to make two crucial coenzymes: coenzyme A (CoA) and acyl carrier protein (ACP). These enzymes help you use fats and carbos to make energy; you also need them to make some important hormones, for making healthy red blood cells, and for making Vitamin D (we'll talk about that more in Chapter 14). They're so important that just about all the pantothenic acid you get from your food is immediately turned into CoA and ACP—there's not really any left over to do anything else.

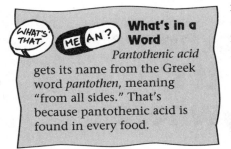

**What's in a Word**

*Pantothenic acid* gets its name from the Greek word *pantothen*, meaning "from all sides." That's because pantothenic acid is found in every food.

A form of pantothenic acid called *pantethine* is now available in supplements. Your body doesn't turn pantethine into coenzymes, so it's available to do other useful things, like help lower your high cholesterol.

# Safe and Adequate Intake

Most vitamins and minerals have established RDAs, guidelines that tell you the amount you need for basic good health. Pantothenic acid is an exception. It's the first (but not the last) supplement without an RDA that we'll discuss in this book.

Why isn't there an RDA for pantothenic acid? The Institute of Medicine scientists (the people who decide these things) have found that the average American gets between 4 and 10 mg of pantothenic acid every day. That must be enough to keep you healthy, because nobody's ever been deficient in it. And if nobody's deficient, why bother figuring out an RDA? Instead, pantothenic acid has Safe and Adequate Intakes, as you can see from the chart.

| Safe and Adequate Intakes for Pantothenic Acid | |
| --- | --- |
| Age | Pantothenic acid in mg |
| *Infants* | |
| 0–0.5 year | 2.0 |
| 0.5–1 year | 3.0 |
| *Children and Adults* | |
| 4–6 years | 3.0–4.0 |
| 7–10 | 4.0–5.0 |
| 11+ | 4.0–7.0 |

# Are You Deficient?

You'd have to deliberately work at it to be deficient in pantothenic acid. It's never been reported in humans, except for test subjects. In fact, there isn't even a lab test for detecting it. The only people really at risk for a deficiency are long-term alcoholics. Anyone else who's a little low also is almost certainly low on the other B's as well.

# Eating Your Pantothenic Acid

Some pantothenic acid is found in just about every food you eat, animal or vegetable—the chart just gives a sample. Organ meats, salmon, eggs, beans, milk, and whole grains are the best sources. As with the other B vitamins, a lot of pantothenic acid is lost when grains are milled into flour. Although the other B's are added back, pantothenic acid isn't, so processed grain foods such as bread, pasta, rice, breakfast cereal, and baked goods aren't good sources.

### The Pantothenic Acid in Food

| Food | Amount | Pantothenic Acid in mg |
| --- | --- | --- |
| Beef, ground | 3 ounces | 0.23 |
| Beef liver | 3 ounces | 3.9 |
| Black beans | 1 cup | 0.42 |
| Broccoli, cooked | 1/2 cup | 0.40 |
| Chicken leg, with skin | 1 medium | 1.32 |
| Chicken liver | 3 ounces | 4.63 |
| Chick peas | 1 cup | 0.72 |
| Corn | 1/2 cup | 0.72 |
| Egg | 1 large | 0.70 |
| Lentils | 1 cup | 1.26 |
| Lima beans | 1 cup | 0.79 |
| Milk | 1 cup | 0.77 |
| Mushrooms, cooked | 1/2 cup | 1.69 |
| Oatmeal | 1 cup | 0.47 |
| Potato, baked with skin | 1 medium | 1.12 |
| Sweet potato | 1 medium | 0.74 |
| Tomato | 1 medium | 0.30 |
| Tuna, canned in water | 3 ounces | 0.18 |
| Wheat germ | 1/4 cup | 0.66 |
| Yogurt, low-fat | 1 cup | 1.34 |

# Getting the Most from Pantothenic Acid

Pantothenic acid is one of the lesser-known members of the B team. It works best when you also have plenty of the other B's, especially thiamin, riboflavin, niacin, pyridoxine, and biotin.

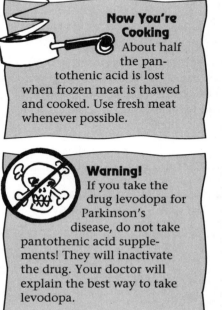

**Now You're Cooking**
About half the pantothenic acid is lost when frozen meat is thawed and cooked. Use fresh meat whenever possible.

**Warning!**
If you take the drug levodopa for Parkinson's disease, do not take pantothenic acid supplements! They will inactivate the drug. Your doctor will explain the best way to take levodopa.

Pantothenic acid is sometimes called the "anti-stress" vitamin. That's because you make more of some hormones that need pantothenic acid, such as adrenalin, when you're under a lot of stress. If that's the case for you, some nutritionists suggest taking extra pantothenic acid. It can't hurt, but we don't think it will really help.

Pantothenic acid supplements usually contain calcium pantothenate in tablets or capsules. Just as there's no RDA for pantothenic acid, there's no real overdose level. People who take very large doses (10 to 20 grams a day) may get diarrhea, but there's no other known side effects. Any excess is excreted in your urine.

Pantethine supplements are also very safe, with no known side effects or overdose level. They're expensive, though, and so far there really aren't any good reasons to take them.

Another form of pantothenic acid called *panthoderm* is available in skin creams and lotions. It's useful for soothing cuts, scrapes, and mild burns.

# Helping High Cholesterol

Pantothenic acid doesn't do a thing for high cholesterol, but it's possible that pantethine does. The research is still in the early stages, but it seems that pantethine can lower your overall cholesterol and triglycerides—if your levels are high to begin with. The research is promising, because even really large doses of pantethine have no side effects, but we're a long way from being able to recommend it.

# Pantothenic Acid for Pentathletes

If you're already an athlete in really good shape—and we mean ready for the Olympics—pantothenic acid might improve your performance just a little bit. Body-builders, long-distance runners, and other serious athletes claim that pantothenic acid helps them train harder. There's only one serious study to back them up, but that one showed that long-distance runners who took 2 grams a day out-performed those who didn't, though not by a lot. If you're just an ordinary weekend warrior, taking pantothenic acid won't help at all.

# Quack, Quack, QUACK!

We usually have only one or two examples of real quackery for a particular supplement, but there are so many silly claims for pantothenic acid that we need a whole section.

➤ **Boosts immunity.** Actually, there might be something to this for pantethine, but it's still way too soon to tell.

➤ **Stops balding and gray hair.** Pantothenic acid deficiency in lab rats causes gray hair and hair loss. Based on that shaky connection, some hair products now contain a form of pantothenic acid called *pantothenyl alcohol*, or *panthenol*. Will putting this stuff on your hair stop you from balding or turning gray? Maybe—if you're a lab rat.

➤ **Stops aging.** In a study many years ago, lab mice were given megadoses of pantothenic acid and supposedly lived 20 percent longer. Since then, some people have claimed that pantothenic acid megadoses can slow aging in humans by "re-energizing" your cells. It's total quackery (or should we say squeakery?).

➤ **Helps arthritis.** The evidence here is pretty thin—just one study of people with a very severe form of arthritis. Skip it.

➤ **Cures allergies.** Some patients claim this works, but there's no evidence one way or the other. Skip it.

# The Least You Need to Know

➤ Pantothenic acid, also called Vitamin $B_5$, is a water-soluble vitamin.

➤ You need pantothenic acid to turn carbohydrates and fats in your food into energy and to make a number of hormones.

➤ There's no RDA for pantothenic acid. The Safe and Adequate Intake is between 4 and 7 mg a day for adults.

➤ Some pantothenic acid is found in almost every food. Good sources are organ meats, salmon, eggs, beans, milk, and whole grains.

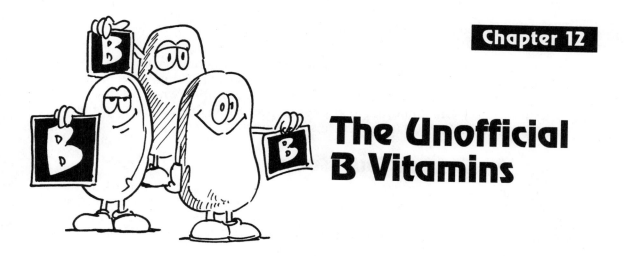

# Chapter 12

# The Unofficial B Vitamins

## In This Chapter

➤ Why you need biotin, choline, inositol, and PABA

➤ Foods that are high in the unofficial B's

➤ How biotin and PABA help your skin and hair

➤ How inositol and choline help you use fats and protect your liver

➤ Why you need inositol and choline for your nervous system

More B vitamins? Yes, sort of. Technically speaking, biotin is a full member of the B family, but choline, inositol, and PABA are more like first cousins. They're important, but you don't absolutely have to have them in your diet. You make all you need in your body and also get some from your food.

The good thing about the unofficial B's is that you don't have to worry about them. You can't really be deficient in them—in fact, they don't even have RDAs.

## When Is a B Not a B?

All the B vitamins work together, in complicated ways, to help you turn your food into energy and to make the vast array of chemical substances your body needs to work properly. They're also important for helping your cells grow and divide properly.

The only way you can get your official B vitamins is by eating them—you can't make them in your body.

Inositol and choline do things that are similar to what B vitamins do, but you can get them from your food and also by assembling them in your body from other foods. So, even though they act like B vitamins, technically speaking, they're not, because you don't have to get them from your food. You still need them, though, and sometimes there are good reasons for taking them in supplements.

# Biotin: The B from Your Body

Biotin is definitely a full-fledged member of the B family, but with a twist. You need it to properly use fats and amino acids from your foods. Like any good member of the family, biotin works closely with other B's, especially folic acid, pantothenic acid, and cobalamin. You don't necessarily have to eat biotin, though. That's because all the biotin you need is made for you in your intestines by the billions of friendly bacteria that live there. It's like having your own little vitamin factory—without having to meet the payroll or even go to the office.

> **Food for Thought**
>
> Biotin was "discovered" a number of times. In 1901, researchers found a substance in animals cells they called "bios," from the Greek word for life. They didn't know what it did, though, and they quickly lost interest in it. Decades later, other researchers found the same substance but called it "coenzyme R"; still other researchers also "discovered" it and called it "protective factor X" or "Vitamin H" (they couldn't make up their minds about whether it was really a vitamin). Science isn't as straightforward as you might think, so it took a while to sort out the confusion. Finally, everyone realized that they had all "discovered" the same thing: a type of B vitamin they agreed to call biotin.

## Getting Your Biotin

There's no RDA for biotin, mostly because almost nobody is ever deficient in it—your intestinal bacteria make pretty much all you need. In fact, most people excrete more biotin than they take in through their diet. In other words, your intestinal bacteria actually make more than you need, so you excrete not only the biotin you eat but also some that you make. You don't really need to worry about how much biotin you get, but we'll give you the Safe and Adequate Intake chart anyway.

| Safe and Adequate Intakes for Biotin | |
|---|---|
| Age | Biotin in mcg |
| *Infants* | |
| 0–0.5 year | 10 |
| 0.5–1 year | 15 |
| *Children and Adults* | |
| 1–3 years | 20 |
| 4–6 | 25 |
| 7–10 | 30 |
| 11+ | 30–100 |

## Are You Deficient?

Biotin deficiency is rare, but there are some special cases:

➤ **Very low calorie diets.** If you go on a really low-calorie diet for a long time, you can become deficient in biotin. You'll know, because your hair starts to fall out.

➤ **Raw eggs.** If, for some really strange reason, you ate a whole lot of raw eggs—like 15 or 20 a day—for a long time, you might become deficient. A substance in the egg white binds with the biotin and keeps you from absorbing it. Cooked eggs don't have the same effect.

➤ **Antibiotics.** People who have to take antibiotics such as tetracycline or sulfa for a long time might become deficient because the antibiotics kill all bacteria, including the beneficial ones that make biotin.

Biotin supplements are available, but few people really need them. You can't overdose on them—large doses of biotin have no known toxic effects.

## Eating Your Biotin

Biotin is found in many foods, but the best sources are beef liver and brewer's yeast. Egg yolks, nuts, and whole grains are also good sources. Check the chart to see everyday foods you consume that contain biotin.

## The Biotin in Food

| Food | Amount | Biotin in mcg |
| --- | --- | --- |
| Banana | 1 medium | 6 |
| Beef liver | 3 ounces | 82 |
| Brewer's yeast | 3 ounces | 73 |
| Eggs | 1 large | 10 |
| Oatmeal, cooked | 1 cup | 9 |
| Peanut butter | 2 tablespoons | 12 |
| Rice, brown | 1/2 cup | 9 |
| Rice, white | 1/2 cup | 2 |

## Biotin for Your Hair and Nails

Some hair care products now contain biotin, claiming that it helps make healthy hair and prevent balding and graying. It's true that you need biotin for healthy hair and that severe biotin deficiency causes hair loss. The biotin in a shampoo or conditioner isn't likely to do much for you, though. Hair lost from biotin deficiency grows back when you fix the problem, but hair lost from natural balding is gone for good.

**Quack, Quack!**
Sadly, there's no cure for male pattern baldness. That doesn't stop some unscrupulous marketers, though, who sell biotin supplements as a way to stop your hairline from receding or to restore lost hair. Save your money for a toupee instead.

Horse breeders have known for decades that biotin helps make hooves harder. Does it also make human fingernails stronger? Possibly. You need a large dose—between 1,000 and 3,000 mcg a day—and it may not work. If you have brittle nails, it might be worth a try, because you can't overdose on biotin.

Biotin is also sometimes suggested for newborns who have cradle cap, an inflammation of the skin on the scalp. The logic is that infants don't yet have the bacteria to make biotin, so they need supplements. Talk to your pediatrician about biotin before you try it.

## Choline: Brain Food

Choline isn't exactly a B vitamin, because you can make it in your body. On the other hand, it isn't exactly not a B vitamin, because you have to have it and it works in complicated ways with folic acid and cobalamin. You especially need it to make the neurotransmitter *acetylcholine,* which is crucial for brain functions, and to make *phosphatidylcholine (PC),* which is crucial for making the membranes of your cells. Choline also moves fats from your liver and keeps them from building up there. Because you make cholesterol in your liver, some people claim that choline lowers high cholesterol. There's some evidence that it might help.

Choline's not a vitamin, so there's no RDA for it and you can't really be deficient in it. Most people get anywhere from 300 to 1,000 mg a day from their diet.

## Eating Your Choline

Boy, does this get complicated! You get choline in your diet from foods that contain *lecithin*. What's lecithin? Chemically, it contains phosphatidylcholine, which is in turn about 15 percent choline. When you eat lecithin, your body breaks it down into the choline and other stuff, then uses the choline to make more phosphatidylcholine and also acetylcholine as you need it.

Some choline is found in all animal and plant foods. The best sources are foods that contain lecithin—but some lecithin is found in all animal and plant foods too! The best animal sources are eggs, red meat, liver, and caviar. Good vegetable sources are cabbage, cauliflower, soybeans, chickpeas, lentils, and rice.

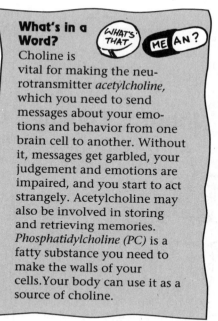

**What's in a Word?**
Choline is vital for making the neurotransmitter *acetylcholine*, which you need to send messages about your emotions and behavior from one brain cell to another. Without it, messages get garbled, your judgement and emotions are impaired, and you start to act strangely. Acetylcholine may also be involved in storing and retrieving memories. *Phosphatidylcholine (PC)* is a fatty substance you need to make the walls of your cells. Your body can use it as a source of choline.

## Choline for Your Liver

You need choline to metabolize fats properly. Without it, the fats can get trapped in your liver. You also need phosphatidylcholine to make your cell membranes—and the densely packed cells of your liver have over 39,000 square yards of them. Doctors in Germany are allowed to prescribe phosphatidylcholine to treat liver problems such as hepatitis or liver damage from toxins. Similar supplements are available at health-food stores, but talk to your doctor before you try them.

## Help for Alzheimer's Disease?

People with Alzheimer's disease usually have low levels of acetylcholine in their brains. Can choline or phosphatidylcholine supplements help? There's been a lot of research into this, and so far the answer is maybe yes, in some cases. Some researchers think that choline could help *prevent* Alzheimer's, but the evidence is pretty thin—it probably can't.

## Choosing a Choline Supplement

Hardly anybody ever really needs a choline supplement, but if you want to take some extra you have a few options. You can buy choline capsules or tablets; you can also get a purer form of phosphatidylcholine called PC-55. The traditional source of choline is lecithin granules made from soybean oil. These contain anywhere from 10 to 20 percent phosphatidylcholine. They go rancid quickly—store the container in the refrigerator.

You can't overdose on choline, but very large doses—over 10 grams—give you an unpleasant fishy body odor. It's harmless, but you may find cats following you down the street. Stick to doses in the 500 to 1,500 mg range.

# Inositol: Choline's Close Cousin

Inositol and choline work very closely together to make neurotransmitters and the fatty substances in your cell membranes; they also combine to move fats out of your liver.

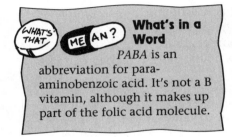

**Now You're Cooking**
Picking the right choline supplement can be a little tricky. For the best results, choose a high-quality supplement that is at least 90 percent phosphatidylcholine.

There's no RDA for inositol, but most people get about 1,000 mg a day from their food. Doses as high as 50 grams have no side effects.

You get inositol from your food in two ways. Phytic acid, a substance found in the fiber of plant foods, gets turned into inositol when bacteria in your intestines digest it. You also get it directly from most foods in the form of myo-inositol. Literally, myo- means "muscle," but it's found in both plant and animal foods. Good sources include organ meats, citrus fruits, nuts, beans, and whole grains. Some manufacturers make supplements that contain myo-inositol or myo-inositol and choline.

Inositol is said to help liver problems, diabetic neuropathy, depression, panic attacks, and even Alzheimer's disease. We can't make any recommendations—there just isn't enough evidence to back them up.

# PABA: Protecting Your Skin

A lot of extravagant claims have been made for PABA. When you read them, it's like reading about the fountain of youth: PABA is said to extend your life, cure arthritis, even turn gray hair back to its original color. Does it really do any of these things? Only in the catalogs of the less scrupulous vitamin makers and health food stores.

**What's in a Word**
*PABA* is an abbreviation for para-aminobenzoic acid. It's not a B vitamin, although it makes up part of the folic acid molecule.

*PABA* is actually part of the folic acid molecule, but taking it by itself doesn't boost your folic acid levels. It's found naturally in some foods, including liver, wheat germ, brown rice, and whole grains. PABA supplements are available, but we don't recommend them. Aside from the fact that they don't do anything for you, they are potentially dangerous. Large doses of a gram or more can make you nauseous and give you diarrhea, a fever, or a skin rash; they might also damage your liver. If you're taking an antibiotic containing sulfa, PABA will keep it from working.

The one thing PABA does for sure is block ultraviolet radiation from sunlight. That's why it's an ingredient in sunscreens—it works well without clogging your pores.

## The Least You Need to Know

➤ Biotin, choline, and inositol work closely with other B vitamins to turn the foods you eat into energy you can use.

➤ Biotin is a B vitamin made in your body by bacteria in your intestines.

➤ Choline, inositol, and PABA are similar to B vitamins but are made in your body from other building blocks.

➤ Choline and inositol work closely together to make your cell membranes and some brain chemicals.

➤ PABA blocks ultraviolet rays in sunlight and is an important ingredient in sunscreens.

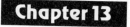

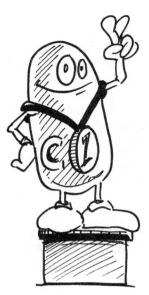

# Chapter 13

# Vitamin C: The Champion

## In This Chapter

➤ Why you need Vitamin C

➤ Foods that are high in Vitamin C

➤ Choosing the right supplement for you

➤ How Vitamin C can help prevent heart disease and cancer

➤ How Vitamin C can help other health problems such as the common cold

Half of all American adults take extra Vitamin C. Can 50 million people be wrong? Not in this case, anyway. Those people know that a daily dose of Vitamin C helps keep them healthy—and they also know that when they're sick, Vitamin C can help them feel better faster. It may even help them live longer. A recent study shows that men who take Vitamin C supplements live, on average, six years longer than those who don't.

Is Vitamin C really that magical? Well, yes. What seemed like wild claims only twenty years ago are now proven medical facts. Vitamin C really does help protect you against cancer, heart disease, cataracts, and other serious health problems. Doctors once scoffed at the health claims for Vitamin C. Now many advise their patients to take Vitamin C supplements.

# Why You Need Vitamin C

There's not much Vitamin C *doesn't* do for you. You need it for more than 300 different purposes in your body. Just for starters, Vitamin C is needed to make *collagen,* the strong connective tissue that holds your skeleton together, attaches your muscles to your bones, builds strong blood vessels, and keeps your organs and skin in place. Collagen is the glue that holds your body together—and you can't make it unless you have enough Vitamin C. (The next time someone tells you to pull yourself together, maybe you should reach for the C supplements!)

Because you need collagen to fix damage to your body, it stands to reason that Vitamin C helps heal wounds of all sorts. Broken bones, sprained joints, cuts, and other injuries all heal a lot faster if your body gets plenty of Vitamin C.

Vitamin C is your body's top antioxidant. Not only does it mop up those nasty free radicals, it helps many of your body's other antioxidants do their work better. And without Vitamin C, you can't use some other vitamins and minerals, like folic acid and iron, properly.

Your immune system needs a lot of Vitamin C to run at peak levels. If you don't get enough, you're likely to get sick more often and to stay sick longer. You also need Vitamin C to manufacture many of your body's hormones.

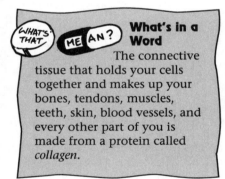

**What's in a Word**
The connective tissue that holds your cells together and makes up your bones, tendons, muscles, teeth, skin, blood vessels, and every other part of you is made from a protein called *collagen.*

Vitamin C also does things, like curing some types of male infertility and helping diabetics, that make it seem more like a miracle drug than a plain old vitamin. People with high levels of Vitamin C have lower blood pressure, which makes them less likely to have a stroke or heart attack. And although Vitamin C can't cure heart disease or cancer, it could help keep you from getting them in the first place.

What about the common cold? Not even Vitamin C prevents or cures that. If you do catch a cold, though, Vitamin C may help you feel better sooner.

# The RDA for Vitamin C

Humans, unlike almost all other animals, can't manufacture Vitamin C in their bodies. Because Vitamin C is water-soluble, you also can't store it in your body for very long. Both these facts mean that you need to have a new supply on a regular daily basis through the foods you eat and the supplements you take.

The RDA for Vitamin C is quite low (far too low in the opinion of many nutritionists), mostly because it's based on a compromise. On the one hand, you need only about 10 mg a day to prevent *scurvy,* a deficiency disease caused by lack of Vitamin C. On the other hand, if you take in more than 200 mg at a time, you pass the rest out of your body in your urine within a few hours. Because the spread between the minimum dose needed and the maximum you can handle is fairly large, the Institute of Medicine came down in the middle. It decided that the RDA should be set at an amount that would keep you from getting scurvy if, for some strange reason, you suddenly got absolutely no Vitamin C for several weeks.

Today many researchers believe that the RDA is the absolute bare minimum for Vitamin C intake. A study by the National Institutes of Health (NIH) in 1996 found that 200 mg of Vitamin C a day—more than three times the RDA—is optimal. Many other researchers believe that even 200 mg a day is too low. The Institute of Medicine may well raise the RDA in the future.

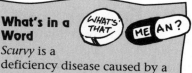

**What's in a Word**

*Scurvy* is a deficiency disease caused by a prolonged lack of Vitamin C in the diet. Among the symptoms are sore and bleeding gums, loose teeth, fatigue, bruising, sore joints, slow wound healing, and anemia. Another name for Vitamin C is *ascorbic acid*, which literally means "acid that prevents scurvy."

These amounts prevent disease, but they don't do much to promote health. Decades of research plainly show that people who take large amounts of Vitamin C on a regular basis are healthier than those who don't. The research also clearly shows that large doses of Vitamin C help many health problems, such as asthma, as well as or better than strong prescription drugs—at less cost and without nasty side effects. Finally, extensive research shows that large doses of several thousand milligrams a day (or even more) are perfectly safe for almost everyone. Not surprisingly, today many doctors suggest taking at least 500 mg daily.

**Food for Thought**

Scurvy is the oldest known vitamin deficiency disease. For centuries, scurvy was a big problem for sailors on ocean voyages, who often had to go for many weeks with no fresh fruits or vegetables. In 1753, Dr. James Lind, the chief doctor for the British Navy, proved that lime juice prevented and cured the problem—although he didn't know why. After that, British sailors were given lime juice every day to prevent scurvy, which is why they have the nickname "limeys."

The major argument against larger Vitamin C doses is that you excrete anything beyond 200 mg a day. By that logic, taking more means you flush away the cost of the supplements. This isn't quite true. In fact, a healthy person's body contains about 5,000 mg of Vitamin C. You'll start excreting the excess only after you reach this saturation point—and only if you're in perfectly good health. Any sort of stress or illness increases your need for Vitamin C. During illness or stress your body draws down its reserves and needs a refill quickly. Aside from that, many of Vitamin C's beneficial effects, like blocking cancer and heart disease, occur only at levels above 200 mg a day. Find the RDA for your age in the following table.

| The RDA for Vitamin C | |
|---|---|
| Age/Sex | Vitamin C in mg |
| *Infants* | |
| 0–0.5 year | 30 |
| 0.5–1 year | 35 |
| *Children* | |
| 1–3 years | 40 |
| 4–6 | 45 |
| 7–10 | 50 |
| 11–14 | 50 |
| *Adults* | |
| Men 15+ | 60 |
| Women 15+ | 60 |
| Pregnant women | 70 |
| Nursing women | 95 |

The RDAs in the table are for people who don't smoke. Smokers have below-normal levels of Vitamin C—as much as 40 percent lower in pack-a-day smokers. Cigarettes rob your body of Vitamin C by breaking it down and excreting it much faster than normal. The Institute of Medicine recommends 100 mg a day for smokers and is considering raising this to 200 mg. We think this number is way too low. If you smoke, consider taking 1,000 mg daily. This amount could also help protect you against two types of cancer smokers often get: cancer of the larynx and cancer of the esophagus.

# Are You Deficient?

After several weeks with no Vitamin C in your diet, you'd start to get scurvy. At first you'd just feel a little tired and irritable, but soon you'd have sore and bleeding gums, loose teeth, fatigue, bruising, sore joints, slow wound healing, and anemia. In the days before canning and refrigeration, mild scurvy was quite common, especially in the winter when fresh fruits and veggies were scarce.

Luckily, Vitamin C is found in so many common fruits and vegetables that almost everyone in our modern society gets about 100 mg a day without even trying. You only need about 10 mg a day to prevent scurvy, but even so, the RDA is far from what most nutritionists consider the optimal amount of at least 250 mg. Even though almost everyone gets the RDA, that's often not enough. If you fall into any of these categories, you may need more Vitamin C than you're actually getting:

> **Warning!**
> Admit it—you started smoking as a teenager so you'd look older. Keep smoking and you'll *really* start to look older. We all get facial lines as we age, but cigarette smokers get more of them—lots more—and sooner. Smoking robs your body of the Vitamin C it needs to build collagen. Without strong collagen to support it, the skin on your face sags, bags, and wrinkles.

➤ **You smoke.** As mentioned earlier, cigarette smoke breaks down your Vitamin C quickly. Also, you need extra Vitamin C to combat the damage smoking does to your cells. Studies show that people exposed to passive smoke—smoke other people create—also need extra Vitamin C.

➤ **You have diabetes.** Vitamin C doesn't get into your cells very well if you have diabetes (we'll talk about this more later in the chapter).

➤ **You have allergies or asthma.** Fighting allergic reactions and asthma attacks uses up a lot of your Vitamin C (we'll talk about this more later in the chapter).

➤ **You're sick with an infectious illness such as a cold or flu.** Your immune system needs plenty of Vitamin C, especially when it's in high gear fighting off an illness. (We'll discuss this some more later on.)

➤ **You've just had surgery.** Vitamin C helps heal wounds and fight infection.

➤ **You're under a great deal of stress—physical or psychological.** When you're under stress, your body's systems go into overdrive and use up your Vitamin C extra fast.

➤ **You're an older adult.** Older people need more C's in general, especially if they take drugs that interfere with Vitamin C absorption. If you're elderly and live alone or in a nursing home, you might not be eating well or getting enough fresh foods, which means you might not be getting enough C's.

➤ **You're pregnant or breastfeeding.** You're passing a lot of your Vitamin C on to your baby.

➤ **You regularly take aspirin, birth-control pills, antibiotics such as tetracycline or sulfa drugs, or certain other drugs such as cortisone.** These drugs either block Vitamin C from being absorbed into your body or break it down too fast.

➤ **You abuse alcohol.** People who abuse alcohol don't eat properly in general. Also, alcohol may destroy Vitamin C.

Your teeth won't fall out if you have a mild Vitamin C deficiency, but you might have these symptoms: fatigue and tiring easily; appetite loss; muscle weakness; bruising easily; and frequent infections.

Fatigue, appetite loss, and weakness could all be caused by other things, but the clincher is bruising easily. A shortage of Vitamin C weakens the walls of your blood vessels. They break easily, causing bruises and even nosebleeds. If you think low Vitamin C is the problem, try supplementing with 500 mg a day. You should feel a lot better and stop getting bruises within a week.

Low Vitamin C can lead you into a downward spiral of bad health. The deficiency means you're tired all the time—too tired to eat properly. So you eat poorly and get sick more often, which means that you take in even less Vitamin C and use up that lower amount to help fight the infection, which means you stay deficient and eat less and get sick more often, which means....you get the picture. Break out of the cycle with a better diet and Vitamin C supplements.

# Eating Your C's

You know from all those OJ ads that oranges and other citrus fruits are a great way to get your C's. But did you know that there's as much Vitamin C in one kiwi as there is in an orange? Or that a tangerine has less than half the Vitamin C of an orange?

### Food for Thought

Even though citrus fruits are a great way to get your Vitamin C, in recent years we've been eating less of them. According to the Department of Agriculture, per capita consumption of fresh oranges in 1970 was 16.2 pounds; in 1995, it was only 12.2 pounds. On the other hand, we drink a lot more orange juice. Per capita consumption in 1971 was 3.81 gallons; in 1995, it was 5.45 gallons. (In the same period, prune juice consumption dropped from 0.12 gallons to 0.04 gallons.) Citrus fruit is big business. In 1994, farmers in Florida, California, Arizona, and Texas produced 247,000,000 boxes of oranges and tangerines. The crop's value was $1.68 billion.

There's some Vitamin C in just about every fruit and green vegetable. Strawberries, melons, and cranberries are high in Vitamin C. Tropical fruits such as guavas, mangos, and papayas are all high in Vitamin C—as high as oranges or higher.

The food that's richest of all in Vitamin C is acerola, a large red berry that's native to the West Indies. One cup of raw acerola berries has a whopping 1,600 mg of Vitamin C, compared to just 80 mg for a medium-sized orange. Don't ask the produce manager at your supermarket where the acerola is. Ripe acerola berries have a pleasantly tart taste, but they're not really grown to be eaten. Instead, juice from the berries is made into a powder that's used as a supplement or added to other foods to raise their Vitamin C level.

Dark-green leafy vegetables such as spinach and kale are fairly good sources of Vitamin C. Vegetables such as broccoli, Brussels sprouts, potatoes, turnips, and tomatoes are also good dietary sources. Peppers of all sorts—from sweet to ultrahot—are high in Vitamin C. In fact the average american now eats about seven pounds of peppers a year. Half a cup of chopped green bell (sweet) pepper has 45 mg. Half a cup of chopped red bell pepper has 95 mg, while an equal amount of chopped yellow bell pepper has a whopping 341 mg. If you're planning to get your Vitamin C from peppers, stick to the sweet ones—we defy anyone to eat half a cup of Scotch bonnets!

## Food for Thought

His research on the role of Vitamin C in human health brought Albert Szent-Györgi (1893–1986) the Nobel Prize in 1937. Hungarian by birth, Szent-Györgi was the first to isolate Vitamin C from food. Naturally, the food he chose was the sweet red peppers used to make paprika.

There's some, though not a lot, of Vitamin C in meat, poultry, fish, milk, and dairy products. Beans generally have little or no Vitamin C, and there's none in grains such as oats or wheat. Check the fruits and veggies you eat in the following table.

## The Vitamin C in Food

| Food | Amount | Vitamin C in mg |
|---|---|---|
| Acerola | 1 cup | 1,644 |
| Apple | 1 medium | 8 |
| Banana | 1 medium | 10 |
| Blueberries (fresh) | 1 cup | 19 |
| Broccoli (cooked) | 1/2 cup | 58 |
| Brussels sprouts | 1/2 cup | 48 |
| Cabbage (raw) | 1/2 cup | 17 |
| Cantaloupe | 1 cup pieces | 68 |
| Carrot | 1 medium | 7 |
| Cauliflower (raw) | 1/2 cup | 36 |
| Collard greens (cooked) | 1 cup | 15 |

*continues*

## The Vitamin C in Food   Continued

| Food | Amount | Vitamin C in mg |
|---|---|---|
| Cranberry juice | 6 oz. | 67 |
| Grapefruit (pink) | 1/2 medium | 47 |
| Grapefruit (white) | 1/2 medium | 39 |
| Guava | 1 medium | 165 |
| Honeydew melon | 1 cup pieces | 42 |
| Kale (cooked) | 1/2 cup | 27 |
| Kiwi | 1 medium | 75 |
| Lemon | 1 medium | 31 |
| Lime | 1 medium | 20 |
| Mango | 1 medium | 57 |
| Orange (navel) | 1 medium | 80 |
| Orange juice (fresh) | 8 oz. | 97 |
| Papaya | 1 medium | 188 |
| Peach | 1 medium | 6 |
| Pear | 1 medium | 7 |
| Pepper (green bell) | 1/2 cup | 45 |
| Pepper (yellow bell) | 1 medium | 341 |
| Pineapple | 1 cup pieces | 24 |
| Potato (baked) | 1 medium | 26 |
| Spinach (cooked) | 1/2 cup | 9 |
| Strawberries | 1 cup | 85 |
| Tangerine | 1 medium | 26 |
| Tomato | 1 medium | 24 |
| Turnips (cooked) | 1/2 cup | 9 |

Most people, even those who seem to live on junk food, easily manage to get enough Vitamin C to meet the RDA and then some. That's mostly because a lot of prepared foods are fortified with extra C's. Orange Tang®, the breakfast drink of the astronauts, has 60 mg of Vitamin C in a six-ounce serving—all artificially added.

## Citrus for C's

| Citrus Fruit | Amount | Vitamin C in mg |
|---|---|---|
| Grapefruit (pink) | 1/2 medium | 47 |
| Grapefruit (white) | 1/2 medium | 39 |

| Citrus Fruit | Amount | Vitamin C in mg |
|---|---|---|
| Grapefruit (canned) | 1/2 cup | 42 |
| Grapefruit juice (canned) | 8 oz. | 72 |
| Grapefruit juice (fresh) | 8 oz. | 94 |
| Lemon | 1 medium | 31 |
| Lemon juice | 1 tablespoon | 7 |
| Lime | 1 medium | 20 |
| Lime juice | 1 tablespoon | 5 |
| Orange (mandarin) | 1/2 cup canned | 43 |
| Orange (navel) | 1 medium | 80 |
| Orange (valencia) | 1 medium | 59 |
| Orange juice (concentrate) | 8 oz. | 97 |
| Orange juice (fresh) | 8 oz. | 124 |
| Orange peel | 1 tablespoon | 8 |
| Pummelo | 1 cup pieces | 116 |
| Sunny Delight® | 6 oz. | 60 |
| Tang® powder | 6 oz. | 60 |
| Tangerine | 1 medium | 26 |

If you eat five servings of fresh fruits and vegetables every day, you'll easily reach 250 mg of Vitamin C or even more. When figuring out your Vitamin C intake for a day, be cautious how you count the fruits and vegetables you get from a salad bar. Although the salad bar is a healthier lunch choice than the chicken nuggets and fries, you may not be getting as much Vitamin C as you think. Up to half of it is lost when fruits and vegetables are prepared in advance and left out for a few hours.

Freezing preserves most of the Vitamin C in vegetables. In fact, frozen vegetables have almost as much Vitamin C as fresh. Canned vegetables are cooked and then packed in water, which pretty much destroys the Vitamin C. Finally, a good excuse not to eat those mushy green vegetables from the cafeteria steam table!

Frozen fruits have somewhat less Vitamin C than fresh, but canned fruits have almost none. Most canned fruits also have a lot of added sugar, which most of us don't really need, so go for the fresh fruits whenever you can.

**Now You're Cooking**
To help preserve the Vitamin C in foods, buy the freshest fruits and vegetables you can, store them in a cool, dark place, and use them as soon as possible. A lot of Vitamin C is lost when foods are cooked. Try to cook vegetables very lightly in as little water as possible.

**Food for Thought**

Pickled cabbage is found in many ethnic cuisines, from German sauerkraut to pungent Korean kim chee. Why? Because half a cup of cabbage has about 20 mg of Vitamin C. In earlier times, during the long winter months when fresh fruits and vegetables were scarce, pickled cabbage staved off scurvy.

# Getting the Most from Vitamin C

Because Vitamin C is water soluble, it's almost impossible to overdose or reach toxic levels even when you take large doses—the excess passes harmlessly out in your urine. The usual safety range is from 500 to 4,000 mg a day. Large doses sometimes cause stomach upsets, diarrhea, and cramping, however. The problem usually starts at doses over 2,000 mg, but children and some adults are more sensitive. If you want to take large amounts of Vitamin C, start with smaller doses and gradually build up until you get diarrhea. Cut back until the problem goes away and then stick with that dose. Nutritionists call this "reaching bowel tolerance."

**Warning!**
Too much Vitamin C can give you the runs—especially if you take more than 2,000 mg a day or take a large dose all at once. If this happens to you, cut back on your daily dose until you return to normal. If you want to increase your daily dose, do it gradually over several weeks.

Take your total Vitamin C dose in several small doses spread throughout the day. Each dose is gone from your body within four hours, so spreading them out helps keep your level steady. We suggest taking your supplements with each meal and before bed.

You'll get the most out of your Vitamin C supplements if you take them along with a good daily supplement that contains all the other vitamins and minerals. You need all of them, but especially calcium and magnesium, to use Vitamin C most effectively. Flavonoids also help Vitamin C work better—we'll discuss that more in Chapter 25.

Alcohol and many common drugs such as aspirin and birth-control pills either block Vitamin C in your body or make it break down too fast. Baking soda (sodium bicarbonate), found in some antacids such as Alka-Seltzer®, blocks your absorption of C's. If you take any of these drugs, take your Vitamin C a few hours later to help avoid interference. Also, if you take aspirin and Vitamin C together, you're more likely to get stomach irritation from the aspirin.

Large doses of Vitamin C can interfere with medical tests for sugar and calcium oxalate in the urine, for blood in the stool, and for hemoglobin levels in the blood. If you are scheduled for a medical checkup, cut back on your C supplements for a few days before to avoid false readings.

If you've ever had a kidney stone or if you have kidney disease, your doctor will probably advise against taking large doses of Vitamin C. Doses up to a 1,000 mg a day are unlikely to cause kidney stones, but if you have kidney problems, discuss Vitamin C supplements with your doctor before trying them.

> **Warning!**
> If you've been taking large doses of Vitamin C for a long time and suddenly stop, you could temporarily get the symptoms of mild scurvy (rebound scurvy) as your body adjusts to the change. Taper off slowly over two to four weeks instead.

| Thumbs Up/Thumbs Down | |
|---|---|
| **Vitamin C works better with:** | **Vitamin C is blocked by:** |
| All other vitamins and minerals | Alcohol |
| B vitamins | Some antibiotics |
| Calcium | Some antihistamines |
| Flavonoids | Aspirin |
| Magnesium | Baking soda (sodium bicarbonate) |
| | Barbiturates such as phenobarbital |
| | Birth-control pills |
| | Cortisone |
| | Estrogen |

# Which Type Should I Take?

The Vitamin C shelves have got to be the most confusing place in any health-food store. Do you want to take your C's in capsules, tablets, or chewable tablets? Or do you prefer powder, crystals, or liquid, or maybe chewing gum or syrup? Should you buy your C's as ascorbic acid or buffered ascorbic acid? How about those pricey "all-natural" tablets made from rose hips? And what exactly is esterized Vitamin C? Read on—it's not as complicated as it seems.

Vitamin C is ascorbic acid and ascorbic acid is Vitamin C, whether it's synthesized in a lab or extracted without solvents from rose hips or acerola. In fact, most of the Vitamin C sold today is made from corn and it's all pretty much the same. Stick to a reliable, inexpensive brand and don't waste your money on the stuff that claims it's better because it's "organic" or "natural."

Vitamin C breaks down when it is exposed to light, heat, water, or air. Buy just a few weeks' worth at a time from a store that turns over its stock quickly. Store your C's in a cool, dark, dry place.

Pick the form of Vitamin C that's most convenient for you. Here's a rundown of the various versions:

➤ **Ascorbic acid tablets and capsules.** These usually contain 500 mg and are meant to be swallowed whole. For most people, the most convenient and economical way to take your C's.

➤ **Chewable tablets.** These usually contain 250 mg. They have a pleasant, mildly tart taste that kids usually like. A few drawbacks: They're more expensive and they often have sweeteners and flavors added. Also, sodium ascorbate is often added to reduce the acidity (which could damage your tooth enamel)—avoid if you're on a sodium-restricted diet.

➤ **Ascorbic acid crystals.** Kids (and plenty of adults too) don't like to swallow pills. Crystals can be stirred into fruit juice or sprinkled on applesauce or fruit. They have a slightly acid or sour taste. (Don't add crystals to milk—it will curdle.) A level teaspoon of crystals has about 4 grams (4,000 mg), so just a large pinch is all you need to get 1,000 mg.

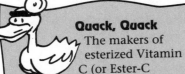

**Quack, Quack**
The makers of esterized Vitamin C (or Ester-C ascorbate) say it is absorbed faster, used better, and excreted slower. It also costs more than plain ascorbic acid. Save your money. There's no major difference.

Some nutritionists tout ascorbyl palmitate, the fat-soluble form of Vitamin C, saying it stays in your body longer. Perhaps—researchers disagree. But it will cost a whole lot more for no real

➤ **Sodium or calcium ascorbate tablets and crystals.** If plain ascorbic acid bothers your stomach, try switching to a buffered version that's made from sodium ascorbate or calcium ascorbate. Don't take large doses (over 3,000 mg) of these—you'll get too much sodium or calcium. You could also try time-release tablets of plain ascorbic acid. These don't kick in until they reach your intestines, so you avoid stomach upsets. You may not absorb that much, though.

➤ **Potassium ascorbate crystals.** A spoonful of this stuff mixed with an ounce or two of water makes a bubbly, pleasant-tasting drink that has 4,000 mg of Vitamin C. It also has 700 mg of potassium—an amount that could kill a child or someone with a heart or kidney condition. If you want to take Vitamin C this way, talk to your doctor first.

➤ **Other forms.** If you want, you can get Vitamin C in liquid, wafer, chewing gum, syrup, and other forms. If you have a practical reason for choosing these pricier products, go ahead. Read the labels to figure out how much C you're actually getting.

# Front-Line Antioxidant

It's this simple: *Vitamin C is the most important antioxidant in your body.* You need Vitamin C as your front-line defense against free radicals (remember those destructive molecules from chapter 1?). Job one for Vitamin C is to capture free radicals and neutralize them before they can do any damage to your cells.

Dealing with free radicals is the main job of lots of other vitamins and minerals in your body. What makes Vitamin C so important? First, because it's water-soluble, it's everywhere in your body—inside all your cells and in the spaces in between. Because free radicals are also everywhere, Vitamin C is always on the spot to track them down. Second, and just as important, other powerful antioxidants such as Vitamin E and antioxidant enzymes such as superoxide dismutase (SOD) and glutathione need Vitamin C to work properly.

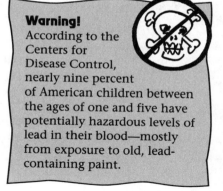

**Warning!**
According to the Centers for Disease Control, nearly nine percent of American children between the ages of one and five have potentially hazardous levels of lead in their blood—mostly from exposure to old, lead-containing paint.

Vitamin C is also needed to make other enzymes that round up and remove toxins such as lead and environmental pollutants in your body. In today's society, environmental pollutants of all sorts are almost impossible to avoid. The faster the toxins are booted out, the less damage they can do. Your best protection is a high level of Vitamin C.

# Preventing Cardiovascular Disease

According to some pretty careful studies of data from the National Center for Health Statistics, if every adult in the United States took an extra 500 mg of Vitamin C a day, about 100,000 of them wouldn't die of heart disease every year. Not only would all those people still be alive and kicking, they wouldn't be costing *billions* of dollars in health care costs every year. Here's where Vitamin C pays dividends in both better health and in real dollars and cents. A year's supply of Vitamin C costs under $45; a coronary bypass operation costs about $45,000.

Let's look a little closer at how Vitamin C helps your heart.

## Lowering Cholesterol Levels

Studies show that people with high levels of Vitamin C have lower total cholesterol levels. (We went into the details of cholesterol in Chapter 1—if you skipped it, go back and read it now.) They also have lower LDL cholesterol (that's the bad stuff) and higher HDL cholesterol (that's good). So if your total cholesterol is high, can you lower it by taking Vitamin C? It depends. If your C level is low to begin with, raising it will probably help your total cholesterol level by raising your HDL level. If your C level is already high because you're taking 2,000 mg a day, it's not certain that taking more will help—although it definitely won't hurt.

If your total cholesterol is borderline high (above 220 mg/Dl but below 240 mg/Dl), Vitamin C supplements, along with a low-fat diet, exercise, and weight loss, could bring it down. If your cholesterol is above 240 mg/Dl, or if you're already taking a drug such as Mevacor®, Pravachol®, or Zocor® to lower your cholesterol, talk to your doctor about taking extra Vitamin C before you try it.

## Lowering Blood Pressure

High blood pressure (above 140/90) is a big risk factor for heart disease—and also for stroke and kidney disease. (We'll talk about this in detail in Chapter 18 on magnesium and Chapter 26 on Coenzyme $Q_{10}$.) Numerous studies show that people with high levels of Vitamin C have blood pressure readings that are slightly lower than people with low C levels. The difference is about four points in the diastolic (when your heart is relaxed between beats) reading. That may not sound like much, but lowering your diastolic blood pressure by just two points reduces your chance of heart disease by eight percent. It's the main reason people with high Vitamin C levels live longer—they have fewer heart attacks and strokes.

If you have borderline high blood pressure, Vitamin C, along with exercising, losing weight, and quitting smoking could help bring it down. If you have high blood pressure or if you're already taking a drug such as Corgard®, Inderal®, or Lopressor® to lower your blood pressure, talk to your doctor about Vitamin C before you try it.

# Enhancing Your Immune System

Your immune system protects you against infection. To do that, it makes several different kinds of white blood cells and a whole lot of complicated chemical messengers that tell the white blood cells where to go and what to do. When you're healthy, you have about a *trillion* white blood cells in your body. When you're sick, you make millions more every hour to fight off the illness. All those cells, and all the chemical messengers they rely on, need plenty of Vitamin C to work right. We still don't know for sure if Vitamin C can keep you from getting sick in the first place, but we do know that it can help you get better faster. If you're sick or have an infection, taking extra Vitamin C will help your immune system fight back efficiently.

## Curing the Common Cold

Does Vitamin C keep you from catching a cold, flu, bronchitis, or pneumonia? No. Does it help you get better faster if you do? Yes. If you're basically healthy and take 1,000 to 2,000 mg of extra Vitamin C, your cold symptoms will probably be less severe and you'll get better a little faster. The older you are, the more the extra Vitamin C seems to help.

If you're one of those people who seems to get one soggy cold after another all winter long, or maybe just one bad cold that you can't seem to shake off, low Vitamin C could be causing the problem. Which comes first, the cold or the deficiency? It doesn't really matter—each problem is making the other worse. Low Vitamin C makes you more susceptible to illness, and fighting off an illness uses up a lot of Vitamin C. To break the cycle and give your immune system a much-needed boost, try supplementing with 1,000 mg of Vitamin C a day.

### Food for Thought

The idea of treating colds and other illnesses with megadoses of Vitamin C started with Dr. Linus Pauling in the 1970s. Pauling was the only person ever to win two unshared Nobel Prizes (for chemistry in 1954 and for peace in 1962). Pauling believed passionately in the value of vitamins. He claimed, "We could add an extra twelve to eighteen years to our lives by taking from 3,200 to 12,000 milligrams of Vitamin C a day." Vitamin C certainly worked for him: Pauling took as much as 16 grams a day and lived to 93.

# Healing Wounds and Recovering from Surgery

One sign of scurvy is wounds that won't heal or old wounds that reopen. That's because you need Vitamin C to make collagen, which is what makes scar tissue and heals wounds. Extra Vitamin C will help you heal faster if you have a cut, scrape, broken bone, burn, or any other sort of wound.

If you have an operation, your Vitamin C levels will probably be low right after the surgery. We don't know exactly why that happens, but it's just the opposite of what you want. To help you heal and fight off infections, your Vitamin C level needs to be high. We strongly suggest taking 1,000 mg a day for at least two weeks before the operation and four weeks after it. Not only will you heal faster from the operation, you'll be less likely to get bed sores because the collagen under your skin will be stronger.

# Fighting Allergies and Asthma

Does summer mean carefree days in the sun to you? Or does it mean days of sneezing and sniffling from pollen allergies? If you're in the sneezing group, it's because your body thinks the pollen is an invading germ that has to be attacked. To do that, your immune system releases chemicals called histamines into your blood. The major casualty of the battle against the "invaders" is you. Your own histamines make you sneeze, wheeze, sniffle, cough, itch, and be generally miserable. Don't you wish you could explain the difference between pollen and germs to your inner self?

Drugs that counteract your natural histamines are called, not surprisingly, antihistamines. There's a lot of different kinds, including many you can buy over the counter in any drugstore. The long lists of cautions and side effects on these drug labels are more than a little scary. Most antihistamines can make you dangerously drowsy. If you have a health problem such as high blood pressure, heart disease, kidney problems, prostate disease, or lung disease, you shouldn't take them. Recently Seldane® (terfenadine) has been taken off the market because it caused heart problems for some people.

There's an easier, more natural—and cheaper—way to cope with respiratory allergies: Vitamin C. Try taking 1,000 to 2,000 mg a day for several weeks. Your allergies should calm down noticeably and stay that way as long as you keep taking extra C's. Why? Because Vitamin C keeps your immune system from making as many histamines to begin with and helps you get them out of your bloodstream faster.

# Fighting Asthma Attacks

Some people react to pollen and irritants such as air pollution or chalk dust by having an asthma attack. The airways in their lungs swell up, making them wheeze and have trouble breathing. The airways clog up with extra mucus and the muscles that surround them go into spasms, which makes breathing even harder. If you have asthma, you're not alone. Nearly ten million Americans have it—and the numbers are on the rise, especially among children.

**Warning!**
Even mild asthma is a serious health problem, because it can get suddenly much worse. If you think you have asthma, see your doctor as soon as possible. If you already take medicine for asthma—even nonprescription drugs—don't stop! Talk to your doctor about taking Vitamin C and other supplements before you try them.

Many nutritionists today believe that taking 1,000 to 2,000 mg a day of extra Vitamin C can help reduce the number of asthma attacks you have and also make them less severe. This works for two reasons. First, as we discussed previously, Vitamin C lowers your histamine production, so your allergies won't trigger an asthma attack as often or as severely. Second, the antioxidant effect of Vitamin C protects your lungs and airways against damage from your own free radicals and from outside air pollution.

Vitamin C is even more helpful for asthma if you also take extra magnesium—we'll talk about that more in Chapter 18.

# Diabetes and Vitamin C

Diabetics, especially those with non-insulin dependent, adult-onset (Type II or NIDDM) diabetes, often have low Vitamin C levels. Diabetics also often have gum disease, slow wound healing, frequent infections, and problems with the tiny blood vessels of the circulatory system. Sounds a little like scurvy, doesn't it? In a way, it is—and Vitamin C can help.

The hormone insulin, which is made in your pancreas, carries glucose into your cells, where you use it for energy. Insulin also carries Vitamin C into your cells. People with Type II diabetes, however, are resistant to their own insulin. Not enough insulin enters their cells, so not much Vitamin C does either. Diabetics need to take in much more than the RDA to be sure enough reaches their cells. If you have diabetes, your doctor will probably recommend that you take 500 or 1,000 mg a day of extra Vitamin C. Some diabetics say that their circulatory problems and other complications get a lot better when they take larger doses, as high as 3,000 mg a day or even more. They also say that they can control their blood sugar better when they take large doses. It's also possible that extra Vitamin C could help prevent diabetic cataracts.

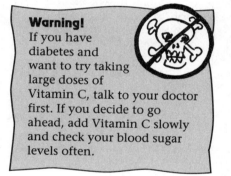

**Warning!**
If you have diabetes and want to try taking large doses of Vitamin C, talk to your doctor first. If you decide to go ahead, add Vitamin C slowly and check your blood sugar levels often.

Talk to your doctor before you start taking large doses of Vitamin C for diabetes. One possible drawback is that you will have a lot of Vitamin C in your urine, which could give a false negative reading on a glucose urine test. If you are at risk for diabetes or already have it and are taking extra Vitamin C, ask your doctor if you should skip the supplements for a day or two before an office visit.

# Cancer and Vitamin C

Before we go any further into Vitamin C and cancer, let's clear up a few things. Yes, Vitamin C can definitely help prevent cancer. No, Vitamin C does not cure cancer. Maybe, Vitamin C helps treat cancer. Let's take these one at a time.

## Preventing Cancer

Study after study after study proves that Vitamin C can help protect you against cancer. People with high levels of Vitamin C and other antioxidants are markedly less likely to get cancer of the lung, cervix, colon, pancreas, esophagus, mouth, and stomach. Why? We're still not sure, but it's very likely that the antioxidants gobble up free radicals and damaging toxins before they can damage your cells and trigger cancer. In the case of stomach cancer, Vitamin C blocks the formation of cancer-causing nitrosamines from the nitrates and nitrites found in bacon, hot dogs, and other cured meats.

## Curing Cancer

A study by Dr. Linus Pauling in 1976 showed that some terminally ill cancer patients lived as much as a year longer if they took megadoses (over 10,000 mg) of Vitamin C. A later study backed this up. In both studies, though, all the patients eventually died—none was cured. No study since then has ever shown that megadoses of Vitamin C (or any other vitamin, for that matter) cure cancer.

## Treating Cancer

**Quack, Quack**

There is no evidence that megadoses of Vitamin C—or any other vitamin—cure cancer. Sadly, some unscrupulous people claim otherwise, promising to "cure" your cancer with expensive vitamins and other weird supplements and treatments. Your health and even your life are at stake—don't fall for this sort of quackery.

If you're being treated for cancer, there's no question that Vitamin C can really help you get through this difficult time. As mentioned previously, Vitamin C could help you bounce back from surgery more quickly. Many people getting radiation treatment or chemotherapy have low Vitamin C levels. Part of the reason is that the treatment can make you tired and nauseous, as well as giving you diarrhea. The other part is that the treatment is making you produce huge amounts of free radicals, so any Vitamin C you get from your food is going to mop them up. Unless you take supplements, you won't have any left over for other things, like keeping your immune system active. Cancer treatment lowers your immunity, making you more likely to get sick or pick up an infection.

Discuss nutrition and supplements, especially Vitamin C, with your doctor *before* you start your cancer treatment. They could make a big difference in how well you do.

# Making Babies with Vitamin C

OK, guys, stop snickering and pay attention. If you and your partner want a baby and nothing's happening, the problem could be the quality of your sperm. Don't panic—there's a good chance that Vitamin C can make you a father.

Your seminal fluid contains lots of Vitamin C—much more even than your blood. It's there to protect the delicate genetic material in your sperm from free radical damage. If your Vitamin C level in general is low (because you smoke, for example), your sperm count is probably low as well. Studies show that taking 1,000 mg of Vitamin C daily can raise your sperm count by quite a bit.

**Food for Thought**

If your sperm count is low, taking just 1,000 mg of Vitamin C a day for few weeks could raise it by 100 percent or more.

Another common cause of male infertility is antibodies that cling to your sperm, making them clump together instead of swimming freely to their destination. You probably have the antibodies because you have a chronic infection such as prostatitis. Even after you take antibiotics to clear up the infection, you'll still be making the antibodies. Here's where Vitamin C can help. Taking 1,000 mg daily for two to three months is quite likely to stop those antibodies from hitching rides. In one study, every participant had a pregnant wife at the end of sixty days.

# C-ing Is Believing

Vitamin C can help prevent cataracts—clouding of the lens in your eye that can lead to blindness—as you grow older. A 1997 study by researchers at Tufts University and Harvard University School of Medicine found that taking Vitamin C supplements over a long period—ten years or more—lowered the risk of cataracts among older women by an amazing 77 percent. Even women who had other risk factors for cataracts, such as smoking, were protected if they took Vitamin C supplements. The researchers believe the antioxidant powers of Vitamin C are the key here. The extra C's mop up free radicals in your eyes before they can damage the delicate lens. How much Vitamin C do you need for eye protection? The study suggests 250 mg a day does the trick.

# Other Health Problems Helped by Vitamin C

We could go on—and on and on—about the wonders of Vitamin C, but let's just hit a few highlights instead:

➤ **Preventing premature births.** In about one out of every ten pregnancies, the membrane that holds the amniotic fluid breaks weeks or even months too soon, leading to a premature baby. A recent study shows that this is a lot more likely to happen to women whose C levels are low. Could taking Vitamin C supplements help prevent the problem? Research continues—stay tuned.

➤ **Treating lead poisoning.** Vitamin C helps you excrete lead faster. High lead levels have recently been linked to high blood pressure in adults, another reason Vitamin C may help blood pressure.

➤ **Gum disease (gingivitis).** You may be more at risk for getting gum disease if you have even a slight Vitamin C deficiency. Remember, bleeding gums are an early sign of scurvy.

➤ **Parkinson's disease.** High doses of antioxidant vitamins such as Vitamin C and Vitamin E could slow down the progress of Parkinson's disease in the early stages. If you have Parkinson's, discuss taking antioxidants and other supplements with your doctor before you try them.

Other health problems that may be helped by Vitamin C supplements include herpes, eczema, hepatitis, gallbladder disease, chronic fatigue syndrome, and many others. There aren't many studies of Vitamin C for these problems, so we can't say for sure that it helps. It doesn't hurt, though, and many patients do feel better when they take extra C's.

# The Least You Need to Know

➤ Vitamin C is your body's main antioxidant vitamin.

➤ You need Vitamin C to build connective tissue, heal wounds, and keep your immune system running properly.

➤ Although the adult RDA for Vitamin C is 60 mg, most doctors and nutritionists believe the RDA is far too low and recommend 250 to 500 mg of Vitamin C a day.

➤ Foods high in Vitamin C include citrus fruits, strawberries, melons, cranberries, tomatoes, peppers, dark-green leafy vegetables, potatoes, turnips, and broccoli.

➤ Vitamin C can help diabetes, high blood pressure, and high cholesterol, and can help prevent cancer and heart disease.

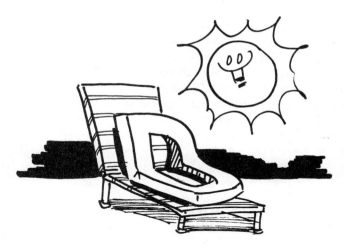

# Chapter 14

# Vitamin D: Look on the Sunny Side

## In This Chapter

➤ Why you need Vitamin D

➤ How your body makes Vitamin D from sunshine

➤ Foods that are high in Vitamin D

➤ How Vitamin D builds strong bones

➤ How Vitamin D helps prevent colon cancer

Go out in the sun without sunscreen? Are you kidding? Risk sunburn, wrinkles, or even skin cancer? Go on, live dangerously—but just for ten minutes a day. On a nice afternoon in July, that's all the sunshine you need to get your daily dose and then some of Vitamin D. Your body makes this important vitamin from sunlight on your skin.

Vitamin D is essential for keeping your bones and your immune system healthy—and it could also keep you from getting colon cancer and some other types of cancer as well. So the next time you sneak out early from the office to go to the beach, don't feel guilty, feel healthy! But remember to put your sunscreen on as soon as you've gotten enough rays for your Vitamin D.

## Why You Need Vitamin D

It's the calcium in milk that helps make your bones strong, right? Right—but without the Vitamin D that's also added to milk, the calcium won't work. Vitamin D's most important role is to regulate how much calcium you absorb from your food. Most of that

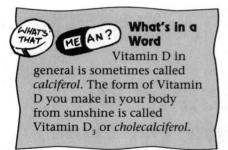

**What's in a Word**

Vitamin D in general is sometimes called *calciferol*. The form of Vitamin D you make in your body from sunshine is called Vitamin D₃ or *cholecalciferol*.

calcium goes to build strong bones and teeth. You also need calcium to send messages along your nerves and to help your muscles contract (like when your heart beats). Vitamin D regulates the amount of calcium in your blood and makes sure you always have enough. We're just starting to realize that Vitamin D also plays a role in a lot of other body functions. Your immune system needs Vitamin D, and it may help prevent cancer, especially colon cancer. The future for this vitamin looks very sunny!

## The Sunshine Vitamin

Vitamin D is the eccentric uncle of the vitamin family—it does things its own way. To get all the other vitamins, you have to eat them. To get Vitamin D, all you have to do is go outside. That's because you actually make Vitamin D when the sun shines on your skin. How? Basically, the ultraviolet light in the sunshine makes a type of cholesterol that's found just under your skin turn into something called Vitamin $D_3$ or *cholecalciferol*. The Vitamin $D_3$ gets carried to your liver, where it gets changed into a more active form; from there, it goes to your kidneys, where it becomes even more active. Some of the Vitamin $D_3$ stays in your liver and kidneys, where it helps you reabsorb calcium from your blood. Some goes to your bones to help them hold on to their calcium. The rest goes to your intestines to help you absorb calcium from your food.

Even eccentric uncles act normal sometimes, though—and so does Vitamin D. It's found naturally in a few foods, but in a slightly different form called Vitamin $D_2$, or *ergocalciferol*. Your body can use this just as well—in fact, it's the form that's used in most Vitamin D supplements.

**Food for Thought**

The form of Vitamin D you get from foods or supplements is called Vitamin $D_2$ or *ergocalciferol* (it's also sometimes called calcifidiol or calcitrol). The *ergo-* part comes from ergot, a fungus that grows on rye plants. Substances in ergot cause hallucinations—in fact, LSD was first made from ergot. It also contains ergosterol, which is converted by ultraviolet light into Vitamin $D_2$. Don't worry—Vitamin D was first discovered in ergot, but your daily supplement is made from yeast or fish liver and can't cause hallucinations.

# The RDA for Vitamin D

For years, many researchers said the RDA was too low for older people. You just naturally make less Vitamin D in your skin as you get older—which is one of the reasons older people tend to have fragile bones. In 1997, the recommended amounts for Vitamin D were changed to account for age changes. The Institute of Medicine decided not to set an RDA or DRI, though. Instead, the Vitamin D amounts are now called Adequate Intakes (AI) and are based on the amounts needed "to sustain a defined nutritional status." In other words, the AI is the amount you need to maintain a basic level of good health.

Although the AI is given in micrograms, the Vitamin D in food and supplements is generally measured in International Units (IU). One microgram equals 40 IU.

| Adequate Intakes for Vitamin D | | |
|---|---|---|
| Age/Sex | Vitamin D in mcg | Vitamin D in IU |
| *Infants, Children, and Adolescents* | | |
| 0–18 years | 5 | 200 |
| *Adults* | | |
| 19–50 years | 5 | 200 |
| 51–70 | 10 | 400 |
| 70+ | 15 | 600 |
| Pregnant women | 5 | 200 |
| Nursing women | 5 | 200 |

Many nutritionists and doctors feel that you need even more Vitamin D as you get older to keep your bones strong and avoid osteoporosis (bones that are thin, brittle, and break easily). An important study published in *The New England Journal of Medicine* in 1997 backs them up. The study showed that men and women over age 65 can cut their risk of a bone fracture in half if they take 700 IU of Vitamin D and 500 mg of calcium every day. (We'll talk more about osteoporosis in Chapter 17 on calcium.)

# Are You D-ficient?

You might be, if you're D-prived of sunlight. As a rule of thumb, an average person needs to get sunlight on the face for about two hours a day in the winter to make enough Vitamin D. On a really bright summer day, ten minutes is enough.

If you never go outdoors, you won't get any ultraviolet light from sitting by a sunny window—it's blocked by window glass.

Vitamin D is fat-soluble, so when you make a lot (by spending a day at the beach, for example), some of it gets stored in your fatty tissues and your liver. Once you've made enough to last for while, your body automatically stops making more. If you're outside a lot in the nice weather, you probably store enough D's to carry you well into the winter.

On the other hand, it's hard to tell if you're getting the AI every day, because you can't really know how much Vitamin D you're making from sunshine. If you live in a sunny climate like Florida or Arizona, you probably get plenty year-round just from your normal outdoor activities. If you live in a very rainy, foggy, or overcast climate, or in an area that has a lot of air pollution, you might not, because the ultraviolet light from the sun is blocked. You also might not be getting enough Vitamin D if your skin is very dark.

You might be deficient in Vitamin D if:

➤ You're an older adult. You're now making only about half as much Vitamin D in your skin as when you were younger.

➤ You don't get any sunlight. People who are housebound or live in nursing homes are especially at risk.

➤ You have kidney or liver disease. You can't convert Vitamin $D_3$ into its more active forms. Talk to your doctor about supplements.

➤ You take drugs such as cholestyramine (Cholybar® or Questran®) or colestipol (Colestid®) to lower your cholesterol. These drugs block your absorption of Vitamin D and other fat-soluble vitamins. Talk to your doctor about supplements.

➤ You take corticosteroid drugs such as cortisone, prednisone, or dexamethasone for allergies, asthma, arthritis, or some other health problem. These drugs can deplete your Vitamin $D_3$ level. Talk to your doctor about supplements.

➤ You take anticonvulsant drugs such as phenytoin (Dilantin®) or phenobarbital. These drugs interfere with how you use your Vitamin D. Talk to your doctor about supplements.

➤ You're a strict vegetarian or vegan. There's very little Vitamin D in plant foods. If you don't drink milk and also don't get outside much, you—and your vegan kids—might not be getting enough Vitamin D.

➤ You abuse alcohol. Alcohol blocks your ability to absorb Vitamin D in your intestines and store it in your liver.

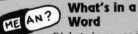

**What's in a Word**

*Rickets* is caused by a crippling shortage of Vitamin D. Without enough Vitamin D, bones can't absorb enough calcium to grow straight and strong. Bowed legs and other bone deformities are the result. Today, because of good nutrition, rickets is rare in the developed world. *Osteomalacia* happens to older adults who don't get enough Vitamin D and can't absorb enough calcium to keep their bones strong.

Kids who don't get enough Vitamin D develop *rickets*—their bones don't grow and harden properly. Fortunately, most kids get plenty of Vitamin D and rickets is pretty rare. Today, older adults, especially people who don't get much sun because they're in nursing homes or can't get out much, are the ones most likely to be short on Vitamin D. The deficiency shows up as osteomalacia—soft, weak, and painful bones. (Osteoporosis, or bones that are brittle and break easily, is caused mostly by a shortage of calcium—we'll talk a lot more about that in Chapter 17.)

## Food for Thought

Rickets in children is unusual today, but starting about 150 years ago it became very common, especially in northern Europe and the northern United States. At that time, poor young children were often put to work in factories, spending long days indoors and eating a diet low in protein foods such as eggs. When they did get a chance to be outside, the smog from the factories blocked the sunlight. Fortunately, the days of child labor are long over. Rickets now happens very rarely, usually to babies who are fed only breast milk (which is low in Vitamin D) and also never get any sunshine.

# Eating Your D's

Long before anyone knew what caused rickets (Vitamin D wasn't discovered until the 1930s), they knew that choking down a daily spoonful of awful-tasting cod-liver oil prevented it. Fish oil contains a lot of Vitamin D, so you get some from eating fish liver, mackerel, herring, sardines, salmon, tuna, and other oily fish.

There aren't that many other foods that naturally have Vitamin D. Beef liver, egg yolks, butter, and margarine all have some, though not a lot. Plant foods have almost none, but Vitamin D is added to a lot of breakfast cereals. Take a look at the chart to find the foods that are naturally high in Vitamin D.

Today almost all the Vitamin D people get from their diet comes from *fortified milk*. There isn't naturally

## What's in a Word

*Fortified milk*—milk that has Vitamin D and (sometimes) Vitamin A added to it—has been around ever since the 1930s. As part of a public health drive to eliminate rickets, milk producers began adding 400 IU of Vitamin D to every quart of milk. The program worked—rickets soon became rare. It's still very rare today, mostly because 90 percent of all milk producers in the United States fortify their milk.

much Vitamin D in milk, but milk producers have been adding 400 IU of it to every quart of milk—whole, skim, low-fat, and nonfat—for decades. It's the reason rickets has practically disappeared. There's no Vitamin D in most milk products, though. Cheese, yogurt, cottage cheese, and other dairy foods aren't made with fortified milk, so they don't have much or any Vitamin D. Also, raw milk, most organic milk, and goat's milk don't have added Vitamin D. Margarine, however, is fortified with Vitamin D. How much of your Vitamin D requirement do you get from food?

| The Vitamin D in Foods | | |
| --- | --- | --- |
| Food | Amount | Vitamin D in IU |
| Butter | 1 pat | 2 |
| Cheddar cheese | 1 ounce | 2.8 |
| Cod-liver oil | 1 teaspoon | 460 |
| Egg | 1 large | 25 |
| Herring, fresh | 3 ounces | 270 |
| Liver, beef | 3 ounces | 26 |
| Mackerel, fresh | 3 ounces | 943 |
| Margarine | 1 tablespoon | 21 |
| Milk | 8 ounces | 100 |
| Salmon, fresh | 3 ounces | 350 |
| Sardines, canned | 3 ounces | 1,000 |
| Shrimp | 3 ounces | 129 |

# Getting the Most from Vitamin D

If you spend a lot of time outdoors in the sun, your body automatically stops making Vitamin D after you've stored up enough. In other words, you can't overdose on yourself.

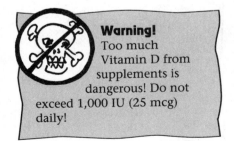

**Warning!** Too much Vitamin D from supplements is dangerous! Do not exceed 1,000 IU (25 mcg) daily!

The same definitely isn't true of Vitamin D supplements. Of all the vitamins, this is the one you need to be most careful with. Large doses can make calcium build up in your blood, which could have serious consequences—although this is very unlikely in doses under 1,000 IU. Too much Vitamin D might also increase your risk of a heart attack or kidney stones.

If you fall into one of the risk categories we talked about earlier, you probably need Vitamin D supplements. How about if you don't? Most people get only about 50 to 70 IU in their diet, so if you're not outside much, supplements might be a good idea—especially in the winter.

Most multivitamin supplements have 200 IU, which meets the AI for people under 50 even if you never get any sun or drink any milk. If you decide to take additional supplements, be on the safe side and keep your total daily dose to no more than 1,000 IU. Talk to your pediatrician before giving Vitamin D supplements to babies and children.

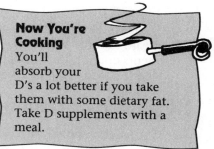

**Now You're Cooking**
You'll absorb your D's a lot better if you take them with some dietary fat. Take D supplements with a meal.

## Vitamin D and Cancer

We've known for a long time that colon cancer and breast cancer are more common among people in northern climates—places where it's too cold for part of the year to get much sun. Is there a Vitamin D connection?

Yes, when it comes to colon cancer—and maybe also breast and prostate cancer. According to recent studies, people who get a lot of Vitamin D from their food and supplements are much less likely to get colon cancer. To get the protection, you only need to get 200 IU from your diet—the amount in just two cups of milk. Do you get the same protection if you just stay outside in the sun longer? Probably, but it's really hard to say exactly how much Vitamin D you make from sunshine. To be sure you're getting enough, take supplements.

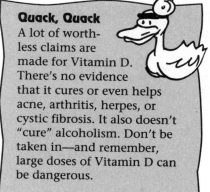

**Quack, Quack**
A lot of worthless claims are made for Vitamin D. There's no evidence that it cures or even helps acne, arthritis, herpes, or cystic fibrosis. It also doesn't "cure" alcoholism. Don't be taken in—and remember, large doses of Vitamin D can be dangerous.

Vitamin D not only helps prevent cancer, it can help treat it. The powerful anticancer drug tamoxifen, which is widely used to treat cancer of the ovaries, uterus, and breast, seems to work even better when it's combined with small doses of Vitamin D. It's also possible that Vitamin D can help treat leukemia and lymphoma, but there's not enough research yet to be sure.

## Other Health Problems Helped by Vitamin D

Vitamin D can help strengthen your immune system in general. In particular, you need it to make monocytes, special white blood cells that fight off infections. About five percent of your white blood cells are monocytes, so a shortage of Vitamin D could leave you wide open to infection.

## Helping Psoriasis

Psoriasis is a chronic skin disease that makes your skin get itchy red flaky patches. Sunshine seems to help clear up the patches for some people. Likewise, a prescription skin cream that has Vitamin D in it seems to help. Just taking a lot of Vitamin D in supplements doesn't, though—and it could be dangerous. If you have psoriasis, talk to your doctor about Vitamin D creams.

## Helping Your Hearing

The smallest bones in your body are in your ears. In each ear, three tiny bones transmit sounds from your eardrum to another tiny bone called the cochlea. The snail-shaped cochlea sends the sounds on to your brain. If any of the tiny bones are damaged, the sound doesn't get sent on very well.

Many adults lose some of their hearing as they grow older. In fact, more than one out of every four adults over age 65 has some hearing loss. In some cases, a shortage of Vitamin D may have damaged the delicate ear bones—and it's possible that taking Vitamin D supplements can help restore some hearing. This doesn't work in every case, of course, so talk to your doctor before you try it.

## The Least You Need to Know

➤ Vitamin D is a fat-soluble vitamin.

➤ Vitamin D is essential for strong bones.

➤ Vitamin D may also help prevent cancer, especially colon cancer.

➤ The adequate intake (AI) for Vitamin D is 5 mcg or 200 IU for people under age 50. You need more Vitamin D as you get older. For people aged 51 to 70, the AI is 10 mcg or 400 IU; for people over age 70, the AI is 15 mcg or 600 IU.

➤ Your body makes Vitamin D from sunshine on your skin. You also get some from your food.

➤ Most foods don't have much Vitamin D. The best source is fortified milk.

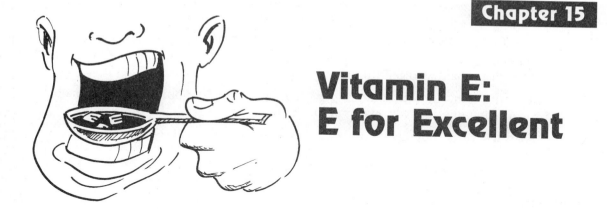

# Chapter 15

# Vitamin E: E for Excellent

**In This Chapter**

➤ Why you need Vitamin E

➤ How Vitamin E prevents heart disease

➤ Boosting your immunity with Vitamin E

➤ How Vitamin E helps prevent cancer

➤ Why you need extra Vitamin E as you get older

On the vitamin report card, E stands for excellent. Vitamin E is at the head of the class for heart health. It's an honor student in cancer prevention. And it's an A+ student in immune system improvement. All that, and it plays well with others, too. Vitamin E teams up with Vitamin A and Vitamin C to give you maximum antioxidant protection.

When it comes to heart disease, Vitamin E isn't just excellent, it's exciting. That's because the latest research proves that Vitamin E can really help prevent heart disease—safely, easily, and cheaply. And for those who already have heart trouble, the exciting news is that Vitamin E can help keep it from getting worse.

## Why You Need Vitamin E

You need Vitamin E for one big reason: free radicals. We know, we know—we're always talking about these dangerous little vandals. What makes Vitamin E so special? Vitamin E is special because it's especially good at protecting your cell membranes against free radicals—and damage to your cell membranes is often the first step down a slippery slope that can lead to cancer, heart disease, and other health problems.

Vitamin E works so well as an antioxidant because it's a fat-soluble vitamin—and your cell membranes are made up mostly of fat. Vitamin E gets into the membrane and lassos any free radicals that try to get through.

Vitamin E also teams up with Vitamin A, beta carotene, and Vitamin C, the other major antioxidant vitamins, to give you extra protection.

In the past few years, a number of important studies on the benefits of Vitamin E supplements have been in prestigious medical publications like the *Journal of the American Medical Association.* Mainstream medicine is catching on to something nutritionists have known for a long time: Vitamin E really does help prevent heart disease—and if you already have disease, Vitamin E can help keep it from getting worse. The studies also show that Vitamin E can help prevent cancer, boost your immunity, and help problems such as diabetes. Best of all, Vitamin E supplements, even in large doses, are very safe.

## The Alpha, Beta, and Gamma of E

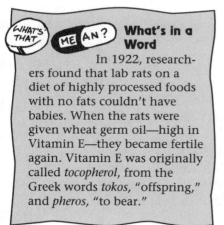

**What's in a Word**

In 1922, researchers found that lab rats on a diet of highly processed foods with no fats couldn't have babies. When the rats were given wheat germ oil—high in Vitamin E—they became fertile again. Vitamin E was originally called *tocopherol,* from the Greek words *tokos,* "offspring," and *pheros,* "to bear."

Vitamin E is a family of different compounds, all working together to protect you against roaming free radicals. The family is divided into two branches: the *tocopherols* and their cousins the *tocotrienols.*

The tocopherol clan has four members. They're named alpha, beta, gamma, and delta tocopherol (aren't scientists imaginative?). For a long time, we thought that only alpha tocopherol was really important and that the others were just along for the ride. That's because alpha tocopherol is the most common and the most active form, the one that works the hardest to fend off free radicals. It turns out, though, that the other forms of tocopherol also help fend off free radicals pretty well. Gamma tocopherol, for example, seems to protect you best against free radicals from nitrogen oxides. (That's the stuff that makes acid rain—imagine what it can do to your cell membranes!)

But just as your mother always compares you unfavorably to your well-behaved older brother, nutritionists compare all the other Vitamin E family members to alpha tocopherol. Gamma tocopherol, for example, is only about 20 percent as active as alpha tocopherol.

The four tocotrienol cousins (also called alpha, beta, gamma, and delta) are members of the E family found in some plant foods such as rice and barley. They're not as active as the tocopherols, but on their own they have antioxidant powers. In fact, they may be even better than the tocopherols at protecting you against some types of free radicals, especially that pesky peroxyl radical. Tocotrienols may also help in cancer prevention and in keeping your cholesterol down.

# The RDA for Vitamin E

It's hard to figure out exactly what the RDA for Vitamin E is for that mythical average person. That's because how much you need depends in part on your body size: The heavier you are, the more you need. It also depends in part on how much fat you get in your diet from plant foods and fish. Here too, the more fat you eat, the more Vitamin E you need. There are probably some other things about your diet that affect how much Vitamin E you need, but we're not sure yet what they are—stay tuned for more news.

The RDA is based on natural alpha tocopherol, because that's the most active form of Vitamin E. Nutritionists often count the Vitamin E in food in milligrams, because foods contain mixed tocopherols. Scientific types like to count the Vitamin E in terms of International Units (IU) of alpha tocopherol, because that's the most common and active form. One milligram of Vitamin E is equal to 1.49 IU. The RDA is shown both ways in the chart.

| The RDA for Vitamin E | | |
| --- | --- | --- |
| Age/Sex | Vitamin E in mg | Vitamin E in IU |
| *Infants* | | |
| 0–1 year | 3–4 | 4.5–6.0 |
| *Children* | | |
| 1–10 years | 6–7 | 9.0–10.5 |
| *Young Adults and Adults* | | |
| Men 11+ | 10 | 15 |
| Women 11+ | 8 | 12 |
| Pregnant women | 10 | 15 |
| Nursing women | 12 | 18 |

As with the other RDAs, the amount of Vitamin E is very small. It's the bare minimum you need to avoid deficiency, but more and more solid evidence shows it is far from the real amount you need to reach optimal health. Along with many other nutritionists and doctors, we're going to ignore the RDA and suggest much higher doses—100 IU or even more—in the rest of this chapter. Fortunately, doses this large and even much larger are safe.

## Are You Deficient?

Vitamin E deficiency doesn't have any dramatic effects—your teeth don't fall out, you don't go blind. If you don't get the RDA for a long time—several months or even years—you eventually get nerve damage, especially to the nerves in the spinal cord, and sometimes damage to the retina of your eye. The damage is hard to spot, though, and it takes a long time to show up. It's also very rare, because almost everyone gets somewhere between 7 and 11 mg of Vitamin E just from the foods they eat.

There are a few medical conditions that can make you deficient in Vitamin E:

➤ You have cystic fibrosis. You can't digest fats well, so you don't absorb enough Vitamin E. Talk to your doctor about supplements.

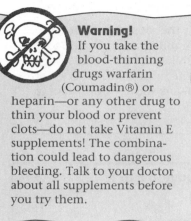

**Warning!**
If you take the blood-thinning drugs warfarin (Coumadin®) or heparin—or any other drug to thin your blood or prevent clots—do not take Vitamin E supplements! The combination could lead to dangerous bleeding. Talk to your doctor about all supplements before you try them.

➤ You have Crohn's disease. You can't absorb Vitamin E well through your intestines. Talk to your doctor about supplements.

➤ You have liver disease. You can't use Vitamin E properly. Talk to your doctor about supplements.

➤ You're on a very low-fat, low-calorie diet. You might not be getting enough Vitamin E from your food. Also, you need a little fat in your food to absorb Vitamin E.

➤ You take drugs such as cholestyramine (Cholybar® or Questran®) or colestipol (Colestid®) to lower your cholesterol. These drugs block your absorption of Vitamin E and other fat-soluble vitamins. Talk to your doctor about supplements.

You almost certainly get all the Vitamin E you need to meet the RDA. The real question is, is that enough for long-term good health. We'll explain why it isn't and why you need more when we come to the sections on health problems later in this chapter.

## Eating Your E's

There just aren't that many foods with Vitamin E in them. The only ones that really have any are vegetable oils, seeds, wheat germ, and nuts. There's a little Vitamin E in plant foods such as avocados, asparagus, mangos, and sweet potatoes, but it's hardly worth mentioning. Animal foods such as meat and milk have practically no Vitamin E. Here's the breakdown:

## Foods High in Vitamin E

| Food | Amount | Vitamin E in mg |
|------|--------|-----------------|
| Almond oil | 1 tablespoon | 5.30 |
| Almonds, dry roasted | 1 ounce | 6.72 |
| Apple | 1 medium | 0.81 |
| Asparagus, cooked | 4 spears | 0.81 |
| Avocado | 1/2 medium | 2.32 |
| Corn oil | 1 tablespoon | 1.90 |
| Hazelnuts | 1 ounce | 6.70 |
| Mango | 1 medium | 2.32 |
| Olive oil | 1 tablespoon | 1.67 |
| Peanut butter | 2 tablespoons | 3.00 |
| Peanut oil | 1 tablespoon | 1.60 |
| Peanuts | 1 ounce | 2.56 |
| Safflower oil | 1 tablespoon | 4.60 |
| Sunflower oil | 1 tablespoon | 6.30 |
| Sunflower seeds | 1 ounce | 14.18 |
| Sweet potato | 1 medium | 5.93 |
| Wheat germ | 1/4 cup | 4.08 |
| Wheat germ oil | 1 tablespoon | 20.30 |

Vegetable oils in general have Vitamin E, but there's a lot of variation. About 90 percent of the Vitamin E in safflower oil is alpha tocopherol, but it's only about 10 percent in corn oil. The Vitamin E in soybean oil, which is used in a lot of prepared salad dressings, is mostly gamma tocopherol.

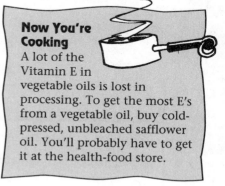

**Now You're Cooking**
A lot of the Vitamin E in vegetable oils is lost in processing. To get the most E's from a vegetable oil, buy cold-pressed, unbleached safflower oil. You'll probably have to get it at the health-food store.

## Getting the Most from Vitamin E

The benefits of Vitamin E really kick in only at daily amounts over 100 IU. There's no way you can eat that much Vitamin E—in fact, it's hard to eat even 25 IU. To get 100 IU from food, you'd have to eat about 15 ounces of almonds (which would have over 2,500 calories) or swallow five tablespoons of wheat germ oil (600 calories) or 22 tablespoons of safflower oil (over 2,600 calories). Supplements are the way to go. But which kind?

## Natural or Synthetic?

Natural Vitamin E is made from vegetable oil, usually from soybeans or safflower seeds; synthetic Vitamin E is made chemically. Natural Vitamin E is about twice as expensive, but it's also more active. You absorb it better and it stays in your system longer. Natural E is definitely the best choice.

When you look at the label on the vitamin jar, you can easily tell the difference. Natural Vitamin E is called d-alpha-tocopherol, while the synthetic version is called dl-alpha-tocopherol. Look for supplements that have just the d- prefix.

## I'm All Mixed Up

Vitamin E isn't just Vitamin E—it's the whole family. To make sure you're getting every-thing the family has to offer, choose a mixed supplement that has all the tocopherols; you can also get supplements that have tocotrienols. Most of the E's in a mixed supple-ment will still come from alpha-tocopherol, because it's the most active form.

## Wet or Dry?

Vitamin E supplements are available in "dry" and "wet" forms. In the dry form, the alpha-tocopherol is chemically bound to succinate; in the wet form, it's bound to acetate.

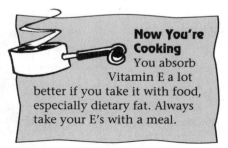

**Now You're Cooking**
You absorb Vitamin E a lot better if you take it with food, especially dietary fat. Always take your E's with a meal.

Acetate and succinate are weak acids found naturally in your body—they're added to keep the Vitamin E from reacting with oxygen in the air and don't affect you in any way.

Dry Vitamin E is made into tablets or capsules. Wet Vitamin E is more like an oil, so it's usually sold as soft gel capsules or as a liquid. If you have trouble digesting fats or oils, pick the dry succinate form. Otherwise, choose the wet form—you'll absorb the E's better.

| Thumbs Up/Thumbs Down | |
|---|---|
| **Vitamin E works better with:** | **Vitamin E is harmed by:** |
| Small amounts of dietary fat | Antacids |
| Selenium | Some cholesterol-lowering drugs |
| Vitamin A | |
| Beta carotene | |
| Vitamin C | |

# What About Selenium?

The trace mineral selenium helps Vitamin E work better and longer in your body. (We'll talk more about selenium in Chapter 21 on the trace minerals.) You need only very tiny amounts of it—the amount in your daily multivitamin/mineral supplement is usually plenty. If you think you're not getting enough selenium, though, try one of the Vitamin E supplements that has added selenium.

# E-vading Heart Disease

In the past few years, three really important studies have shown that people who take Vitamin E supplements have less heart disease. One of the studies, the Cambridge Heart Antioxidant Study (CHAOS), looked at 40,000 men who already had heart disease and found that Vitamin E kept their heart disease from getting worse. In fact, the men who took at least 400 IU of Vitamin E cut their chances of a nonfatal heart attack by an amazing 77 percent. Another study looked at a group of over 87,000 women nurses and found that those who took Vitamin E cut their overall risk of heart disease by about two-thirds. Finally, a long-term study of over 34,000 postmenopausal women showed that those who ate the most foods high in Vitamin E but didn't take E supplements had strikingly less heart disease.

### Food for Thought

Since the CHAOS study first appeared in 1993, a number of other, smaller studies have backed up the findings. Two recent studies are very interesting, because they show that Vitamin E helps heart disease even after it is pretty far along. The studies looked at patients who needed heart surgery for blocked arteries. When these people took daily Vitamin E supplements after their surgery, their arteries were a lot less likely to clog up again.

The explanation for this excellent news about evading heart disease? Vitamin E helps prevent *atherosclerosis* (hardening of the arteries) caused by atheromas or *plaque* on the walls of the arteries that lead to your heart. And how does Vitamin E prevent this? By its powerful antioxidant action, which helps keep cholesterol in your blood from oxidizing into those artery-clogging deposits in the first place—and helps keep the deposits you may already have from getting worse.

### What's in a Word

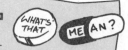

*Atherosclerosis* is the medical term for hardening of the arteries. Atherosclerosis starts with fatty deposits called *atheromas* in your arter-ies. The atheroma slowly gets bigger and harder and turns into a waxy substance called *plaque*. The plaque narrows or even blocks the artery.

Vitamin E works because it is a powerful antioxidant that keeps your LDL ("bad") cholesterol from being oxidized. Less oxidized cholesterol, less plaque, less heart disease.

There's another way Vitamin E helps prevent heart disease. If your arteries are narrow and clogged, tiny blood cells called platelets are likely to get stuck in the plaque. Red blood cells then get stuck in the platelets and form a blood clot. If the clot gets big enough, it blocks the artery and causes a heart attack. Vitamin E helps keep the platelets from sticking, so clots don't form as easily.

### Food for Thought

Atherosclerosis is a long, slow, complex process. It starts when the smooth lining of an artery (usually an artery feeding your heart) gets damaged—we still don't really know how. Your body sends cholesterol to fix it, but the process goes haywire—we still don't know exactly why. Instead, the cholesterol reacts with oxygen in your blood—it oxidizes—and forms a fatty deposit or streak (an atheroma) in the artery. The atheroma gradually gets bigger and harder and turns into plaque. All this makes the artery get stiffer and narrower, and less and less blood flows through; sometimes blood clots block the flow even more. If the artery is so blocked with plaque or a blood clot that no blood gets through, you have a heart attack.

## Is It Really that E-Z?

Amazingly, a lot of doctors still aren't convinced about the benefits of Vitamin E—they want more studies. They also point out that giving up smoking, drinking less alcohol, getting exercise, and eating better all help prevent heart disease. The docs have a good point: Your lifestyle counts. Vitamin E isn't a miracle drug or an excuse to keep smoking.

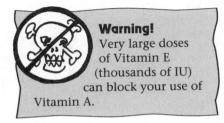

**Warning!**
Very large doses of Vitamin E (thousands of IU) can block your use of Vitamin A.

Even so, the patients in the CHAOS study took either 400 or 800 IU of Vitamin E a day. They didn't have any problems from the large doses and their hearts were helped—even when they didn't change any unhealthy habits.

Why wait? The possible benefits of Vitamin E supplements for your heart are very clear, and there isn't really a down side. Vitamin E is safe even in large doses of 5,000 IU a day—and many researchers believe that just 400 IU a day will go a long way to help protect you against heart disease.

# E-luding Cancer

The evidence that Vitamin E helps prevent cancer isn't as dramatic as for heart disease, but it's still pretty strong. Researchers have known for many years that people with cancer have low Vitamin E levels. But do they have cancer because they have low Vitamin E? Maybe, said the skeptics, they have low Vitamin E because they have cancer.

We now know that people with low Vitamin E levels are more likely to get cancer—in other words, low Vitamin E could be a cause, not an effect. We also now know that people with high Vitamin E levels are less likely to get cancer. Vitamin E's antioxidant effect seems to provide the protection. It mops up free radicals before they can do the sort of cell damage that leads to cancer.

Here's a good example. A recent study at the National Cancer Institute looked at oral and throat cancer. People who took Vitamin E supplements cut their chances of getting these types of cancer in half. Another good example: In a 1997 study, men who had the highest intake of Vitamin E had the least chance of getting one common type of colon cancer. The protection was especially good for men over 60, who are at higher risk anyway. Their risk was cut an amazing 80 percent compared to the men who had the lowest intake. Here's a surprise, though: Vitamin E didn't do that much to protect women against colon cancer. Why? We don't know yet.

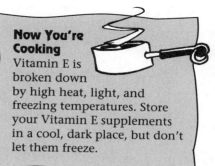

**Now You're Cooking**
Vitamin E is broken down by high heat, light, and freezing temperatures. Store your Vitamin E supplements in a cool, dark place, but don't let them freeze.

Vitamin E may also help protect against cancer of the cervix and breast cancer. We're a little less sure about lung cancer. Extra E's probably help protect you, but only if you don't smoke.

# Excellent for the Elderly

As you get older, your immune system naturally slows down. That makes you more likely to get sick with something serious that you can't fight off, like pneumonia or cancer.

There's recently been some excellent news for older adults about Vitamin E and immunity—and it comes from the prestigious *Journal of the American Medical Association*. In a 1997 article, researchers showed that taking Vitamin E can give your immune system a real boost. Healthy volunteers, all over age 65, took Vitamin E supplements for 33 weeks. Tests at the end of that time showed that their immune systems were much more active. The best results came from taking 200 mg a day; taking more didn't seem to help more.

If you're over age 60, it's probably time to start taking those extra E's—but talk to your doctor first, especially if you have any chronic health problems.

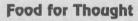

**Food for Thought**

Let's get down to dollars and cents here: Vitamins cost money. But so does being sick—and a whole year's supply of Vitamin E costs a heck of a lot less than just one day in the hospital because you have pneumonia.

The news about Alzheimer's disease and Vitamin E is good but not quite excellent. Vitamin E in large doses (2,000 IU) seems to slow down—but not stop or prevent— Alzheimer's. In fact, it works just as well as a more expensive prescription drug. The antioxidant power of the E's is probably what helps, because it seems to slow the breakdown of brain cells. This is a promising area of research for a devastating disease—we'll be watching it carefully.

## Other Health Problems Helped by Vitamin E

Vitamin E can be helpful for a lot of health problems, although it's not a cure for any of them. Here's a rundown of some current medical thinking:

➤ **Male infertility.** Some men are infertile because of free radicals. Why? You probably haven't ever given this much thought, but the cell membranes of sperm are very fatty, so they're especially vulnerable to attack by free radicals. Taking Vitamin E supplements can help mop up enough free radicals to prevent the damage. In one study, five out of 15 infertile men became fathers after just one month of 200 IU a day.

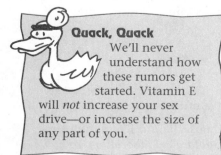

**Quack, Quack**

We'll never understand how these rumors get started. Vitamin E will *not* increase your sex drive—or increase the size of any part of you.

➤ **Benign breast disease.** If you want to make your doctor squirm, ask him or her why this perfectly natural condition is called a disease. Benign breast disease makes your breasts feel "lumpy." They might also swell and become tender when you're getting your period. It's uncomfortable and annoying, but usually benign breast disease isn't dangerous or a sign of breast cancer. We don't know exactly why this works, but taking anywhere from 200 to 600 IU of Vitamin E a day seems to relieve the symptoms for a lot of women.

➤ **Diabetes.** Vitamin E supplements can help diabetics better control their blood sugar. The doses needed are generally on the high side—well over 400 IU—but the benefits are often worthwhile. If you have diabetes and want to try Vitamin E supplements, talk to your doctor first.

➤ **Eye health.** The delicate blood vessels in your eyes are easily damaged by free radicals. A good supply of Vitamin E helps prevent the damage by sopping up the free radicals before they can do any harm. Likewise, Vitamin E helps protect the lens of your eye from free radical damage. People with low levels of Vitamin E are more likely to develop cataracts (clouding of the lens) as they get older. Studies show that people who take in 400 IU of Vitamin E a day could cut their cataract risk in half.

➤ **Intermittent claudication and leg cramps.** Intermittent *what?* This is an annoying circulation problem that's caused by hardening of arteries in the legs. It makes your calf muscles ache and cramp up when you walk even a short distance. Vitamin E seems to help some people. If you want to try it, start with 200 IU daily for a week. If that doesn't help, try slowly increasing the dose, but don't go over 600 IU. Vitamin E also helps another annoying problem, nighttime leg cramps. Small doses of just 200 IU often do the trick. Take it with your evening meal.

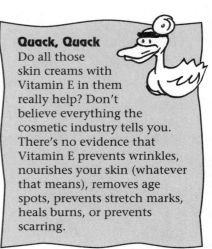

**Quack, Quack**
Do all those skin creams with Vitamin E in them really help? Don't believe everything the cosmetic industry tells you. There's no evidence that Vitamin E prevents wrinkles, nourishes your skin (whatever that means), removes age spots, prevents stretch marks, heals burns, or prevents scarring.

➤ **Parkinson's disease.** A long-term study is looking at whether Vitamin E, along with the drug selegiline (Deprenyl®), slows down the progression of this devastating brain disease. The evidence isn't in yet—if you have Parkinson's, talk to your doctor about Vitamin E and other supplements before you try them.

Some athletes claim Vitamin E improves their performance, although there's no real evidence for this. Other people claim Vitamin E miraculously cures everything from acne to gallstones. Although just about everybody can benefit from getting some extra Vitamin E, use your common sense. Talk to your doctor before you try big doses of Vitamin E for any reason.

# The Least You Need to Know

➤ The adult RDA for Vitamin E is between 8 and 10 mg or 12 and 15 IU.

➤ Many doctors today recommend taking 100 IU to 400 IU of Vitamin E every day.

➤ To get more than the RDA of Vitamin E, you'll need to take supplements.

➤ Vitamin E is safe in large doses.

➤ Vitamin E supplements can help prevent heart disease and cancer and boosts the immunity of older adults.

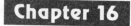

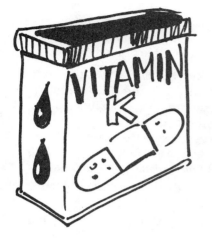

# Chapter 16

# Vitamin K: The Band-Aid in Your Blood

## In This Chapter

➤ Why you need Vitamin K

➤ Foods that are high in Vitamin K

➤ How Vitamin K helps your blood clot

➤ How Vitamin K helps keep your bones strong

When you cut your finger slicing onions in the kitchen, what happens? First, you swear under your breath. Next, you grab a paper towel and press it against the cut. A few minutes later, the bleeding stops. You slap on a band-aid and go back to fixing dinner. But what made the bleeding stop? Without going into all the gory (get it?) details, it's Vitamin K—the same stuff that stopped the bleeding all the other times you got hurt during the day, like when you cut yourself shaving, barked your shins on someone's bike in the driveway, and gave yourself a paper cut at the office.

Life is full of minor injuries, of course, which is why your blood needs to be full of Vitamin K. For most people, that's not a problem—a real shortage of Vitamin K is pretty rare.

# Why You Need Vitamin K

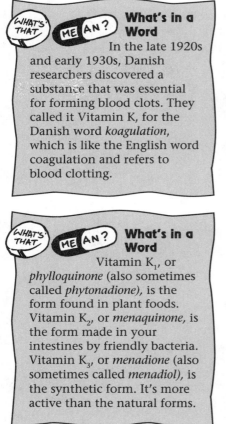

**What's in a Word**
In the late 1920s and early 1930s, Danish researchers discovered a substance that was essential for forming blood clots. They called it Vitamin K, for the Danish word *koagulation*, which is like the English word coagulation and refers to blood clotting.

**What's in a Word**
Vitamin K$_1$, or *phylloquinone* (also sometimes called *phytonadione*), is the form found in plant foods. Vitamin K$_2$, or *menaquinone*, is the form made in your intestines by friendly bacteria. Vitamin K$_3$, or *menadione* (also sometimes called *menadiol*), is the synthetic form. It's more active than the natural forms.

Vitamin K is essential for making the blood clots that quickly stop the bleeding whenever you injure yourself. This fat-soluble vitamin actually comes in three different forms.

First, there's Vitamin K$_1$, or *phylloquinone*. This is the form of Vitamin K found in plant foods. Next, there's Vitamin K$_2$ (you were expecting some other number?), also called *menaquinone*. This is the form friendly bacteria in your intestines make for you. If you guessed that the last form would be called Vitamin K$_3$, you're absolutely right. This is the artificial form, also called *menadione*. All your Vitamin K ends up in your liver, where it's used to make some of the substances that make your blood clot.

Vitamin K is mostly needed to help you stop bleeding, but it has some other jobs as well. The most important is the role Vitamin K$_1$ plays in building your bones. Vitamin K is needed to help you hold onto the calcium in your bones and make sure it's getting to the right place. There's also some interesting research on Vitamin K and cancer.

## The RDA for Vitamin K

There's only been an RDA for Vitamin K since 1989. Up until then, researchers thought that all the Vitamin K you need was made for you by friendly bacteria in your intestines. In fact, though, the bacteria make only half or less of what you need. You get the rest mostly from—you guessed it—green leafy vegetables.

The amount of Vitamin K in the RDA is based on your body weight. It's set at one microgram (mcg) for every kilo (2.2 pounds) you weigh, so the numbers in the chart are for that mythical average person. If you're heavier than average, you might need more. If you're lighter than average, though, you should still get the RDA. Check out the chart to make sure you're getting enough Vitamin K.

| The RDA for Vitamin K | |
| --- | --- |
| Age/Sex | Vitamin K in mcg |
| *Infants* | |
| 0–0.5 year | 5 |
| 0.5–1 year | 10 |

| Age/Sex | Vitamin K in mcg |
| --- | --- |
| *Children* | |
| 1–3 years | 15 |
| 4–6 | 20 |
| 7–10 | 30 |
| *Young Adults and Adults* | |
| Men 11–14 years | 5 |
| Men 15–18 | 65 |
| Men 19–24 | 70 |
| Men 25+ | 80 |
| Women 11–14 years | 45 |
| Women 15–18 | 55 |
| Women 19–24 | 60 |
| Women 25+ | 65 |
| Pregnant women | 65 |
| Nursing women | 65 |

# Are You Deficient?

As a rule, Vitamin K deficiency is rare—almost everyone gets more than enough from their own bacteria and from their food. Sometimes newborn babies don't have enough Vitamin K because they don't yet have any bacteria to make it in their intestines. To make up for that, most newborns are given an injection of a tiny amount of Vitamin K soon after birth.

When adults get Vitamin K deficiency, it's generally because they eat very few green vegetables or because they have been taking oral antibiotics for a long time. The antibiotics kill off the intestinal bacteria that make Vitamin K. Sometimes Vitamin K deficiency is caused by liver disease or a problem digesting fat. You might be deficient if:

➤ You have serious liver disease. You can't use Vitamin K properly. Your doctor will probably recommend Vitamin K shots.

➤ You have Crohn's disease, ulcerative colitis, or some other serious intestinal problem. You can't absorb fats well, so you don't absorb much Vitamin K from your food. Talk to your doctor about supplements.

➤ You've been taking antibiotic pills for a long time (at least several weeks). Tetracycline, neomycin, and cephalosporin kill the bad bacteria—but they also kill the friendly bacteria that make Vitamin K in your intestines. Eating more Vitamin K foods should help, but talk to your doctor first.

➤ You take drugs such as cholestyramine (Cholybar® or Questran®) or colestipol (Colestid®) to lower your cholesterol. These drugs block your absorption of Vitamin K and other fat-soluble vitamins. Talk to your doctor about supplements.

The major symptom of Vitamin K deficiency is that your blood clots very slowly, so you bleed for a long time even from minor injuries. Vitamin K deficiency causes big black-and-blue marks from very slight bruises or even for no reason, nosebleeds, blood in your urine, and intestinal bleeding.

### Food for Thought

About one in 10,000 American males has *hemophilia,* a hereditary blood disease that causes abnormal bleeding. Hemophiliacs can't make clotting factor VIII, one of the factors that doesn't depend on Vitamin K. Several important clotting factors do depend on your Vitamin K level. Prothrombin (also known as clotting factor II) is the most important; clotting factors VII, IX, and X also depend on Vitamin K. If you don't have enough K's, you can't make them.

If you have Vitamin K deficiency symptoms, see your doctor at once. You'll need blood tests to check your clotting time and your prothrombin level (we'll explain about prothrombin a little later in this chapter). If the results show a deficiency, you may need more tests to figure out why. In the meantime, your doctor will probably give you Vitamin K shots. These can take a while to kick in, though, so you may also have to take Vitamin K supplements.

## Eating Your K's

### Now You're Cooking

There are 199 mcg of Vitamin K in an ounce of green tea leaves—but not any other kind of tea. That sounds like a lot, until you realize that it takes a dozen tea bags to make an ounce. In other words, a cup of green tea has only about 16 mcg of Vitamin K.

A lot of foods haven't ever been analyzed to find out how much Vitamin K they have. And in the ones that have been studied, the K amounts are variable—some sources give amounts that are a lot different than others. In general, though, all the dark-green leafy vegetables, like kale, broccoli, and cabbage, are good choices. Strawberries are also good. Some animal foods, including egg yolks and liver, have small amounts of Vitamin K.

Check out the chart for good choices. The amount of K in each food is only approximate, but it's close enough to help you make sure you're getting what you need. The amounts given are for raw foods, but very little Vitamin K is lost in cooking.

## Foods High in Vitamin K

| Food | Amount | Vitamin K in mcg |
|---|---|---|
| Beef liver | 3 ounces | 89 |
| Broccoli, raw | 1/2 cup | 58 |
| Cabbage, raw | 1/2 cup | 52 |
| Cauliflower, raw | 1/2 cup | 96 |
| Egg | 1 large | 25 |
| Milk, skim | 1 cup | 10 |
| Potato, baked | 1 medium | 6 |
| Soybean oil | 1 tablespoon | 76 |
| Spinach, raw | 1/2 cup | 74 |
| Strawberries | 1 cup | 21 |
| Tomato, raw | 1 medium | 28 |
| Turnip greens, raw | 1/2 cup | 182 |
| Wheat germ | 1 ounce | 10 |

# Getting the Most from Vitamin K

Most people get well over the RDA for Vitamin K from their food and don't ever need to take a supplement. Not too many multivitamins have even small amounts of Vitamin K in them, although you can buy K supplements in 100 mcg capsules. In fact, because supplements should be used only if your doctor has diagnosed a real Vitamin K deficiency, you need a prescription for them in some states. If you want to make sure you're getting enough Vitamin K, the best approach is to eat your vegetables.

If you're low on Vitamin K because of an intestinal problem that makes it hard for you to digest fats, you may need supplements to treat or prevent clotting problems.

If your doctor advises Vitamin K supplements, you will probably have to take only 100 mcg a day. Any more than that in the synthetic form could be toxic and might cause liver damage. Talk to your doctor about supplements made with phytonadione, a water-soluble version of Vitamin $K_1$.

**Now You're Cooking**
The best food source of Vitamin K is seaweed. There's about 1500 mcg in 3 ounces of dried dulse or rockweed. Seagrass has about 200 mcg in 3 ounces and kelp (sea lettuce) only has about 60 mcg. Check for seaweed in your health food store.

**Warning!**
Do not take Vitamin K supplements if you also take a blood-thinning drug such as coumarin (Coumadin®) or warfarin. You'll keep the drug from doing its job.

# Vitamin K and Clotting

**What's in a Word**

*Clotting factors* are substances in your blood that help it clot and stop bleeding. You make a lot of different clotting factors, but the most important is *prothrombin*. You need Vitamin K to make prothrombin and several other clotting factors.

Your blood normally has a number of different *clotting factors*—substances that help it form clots to stop bleeding from cuts, bruises, and other injuries. You need Vitamin K to help your liver make *prothrombin* (factor II), the most important of the clotting factors. Some of the other factors, including factors VII, IX, and X, are also made in your liver and also depend on Vitamin K. Without clotting factors, your blood clots very slowly or not at all, so even a small cut can bleed for a long time and even a minor bang can cause a big bruise.

# Vitamin K and Osteoporosis

**Quack, Quack**

Skin creams containing Vitamin K and other "healing compounds" are said to make spider veins on your face and legs "disappear." The cost for these worthless creams? At least $15 an ounce. Save your money.

You need Vitamin K to help your bones grab onto calcium, put it in the right place, and hold onto it once it's there. If you don't have enough K's, you won't be able to form new bone very well. In the long run, a shortage of Vitamin K can lead to osteoporosis, or bones that are brittle and break easily. (We'll talk a lot more about osteoporosis in Chapter 17 on calcium.)

Once osteoporosis starts, researchers think that extra Vitamin K may help slow down the process. This is still being studied, though, so don't start taking supplements just yet.

# K Kills Cancer Cells

But so far, only in the test tube. Vitamin K seems to slow down or kill tumor cells in the lab just as well as powerful drugs. Some studies are looking at combining Vitamin K with standard anticancer drugs to help them work better. We don't know how well this works yet.

# The Least You Need to Know

➤ You need Vitamin K to help your blood clot properly.

➤ The adult RDA for Vitamin K is 60 mcg.

➤ Green leafy vegetables are the best food source of Vitamin K. Friendly bacteria in your intestines also make some of your Vitamin K.

➤ Vitamin K deficiency is very rare, so supplements aren't needed.

# Part 3
# Minerals: The Elements of Good Health

*Ever feel a little rocky? It's not surprising—you have enough different minerals in your body to keep a geologist busy for days!*

*You need the essential minerals every bit as much as you need vitamins. In fact, without the minerals, your vitamins can't do their job, and vice versa. And like vitamins, some minerals have important roles in helping you prevent and treat health problems. All the minerals in your body add up to a market value of just a few dollars. But when it comes to your good health, they're worth more than their weight in gold.*

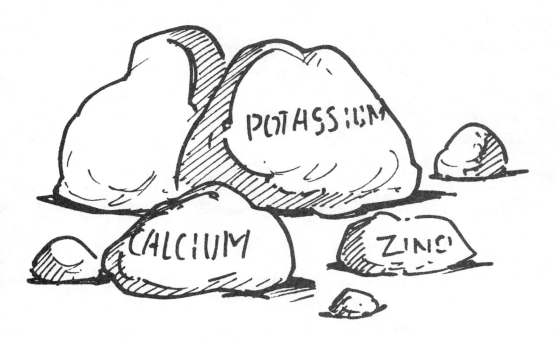

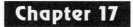
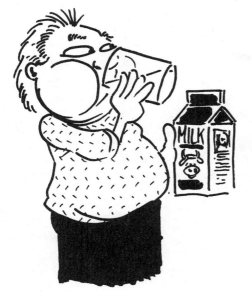

# Chapter 17

# Calcium: Drink Your Milk!

## In This Chapter

➤ Why everyone needs calcium—and why women need extra

➤ How calcium keeps your bones strong all your life

➤ Foods that are high in calcium

➤ Choosing the right calcium supplement

➤ How calcium may help your blood pressure

Close your eyes and think back to your childhood. You can probably still hear your mother saying, "Drink your milk! It's good for you." You might even find yourself saying the same thing to your own kids today. Well, your mom was right—and so are you. Milk is the best food source of calcium, and kids need plenty of calcium to build strong bones.

Close your eyes and think back again, this time to your teen years. You can probably still hear yourself saying to your mother, "Aw, Mom, milk's a kid's drink." Your mom was right—and you were wrong. Milk—or more precisely, the calcium in milk—isn't just for kids. You need calcium all through your life to keep your bones strong.

# Why You Need Calcium

Calcium is by far the most abundant mineral in your body. It makes up about 2 percent of your total body weight, or between 2 and 3 pounds if you're an average adult. Most of your calcium—98 percent of it—is in your bones. Another 1 percent is in your teeth, and the last 1 percent circulates in your blood. Small as the amount of calcium in your blood is, it's very important—so important that your body will pull calcium from your bones to make sure there's enough in your blood. Among other things, calcium helps regulate your heartbeat, control your blood pressure, clot your blood, contract your muscles, and send messages along your nerves. Calcium is needed to make many different hormones and enzymes, especially the ones that control your digestion and how you make energy and use fats. It also helps build your connective tissue and may help prevent high blood pressure and colon cancer.

# Boning Up on Calcium

How many bones are in your skeleton? Give up? You have 206. Every single one of them is made up mostly of calcium phosphate, a very hard, dense mixture made when calcium and phosphorus combine. (We'll talk about phosphorus a little later in this chapter.)

Your bones may be hard, but they're also living tissue. You're constantly breaking down old bone and building new bone. From the time you're born until you get to be about 30 to 35 years old, you build up bone faster than you lose it, so your bones get bigger and denser, and you reach what's called peak bone mass. You could think of it as building up a bone savings account. After about age 35, you start to slowly break down bone faster than you can rebuild it—you start to draw on your saved-up bone. Some slow bone loss is a normal part of getting older, but if you don't get enough calcium, the process can start to happen too fast, especially in older women who've reached menopause. If you lose too much bone, you empty out your bone savings account. At that point, your bones are thin, brittle, and break very easily. You've got *osteoporosis*.

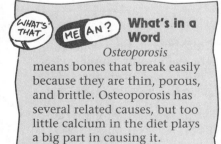

**What's in a Word**

*Osteoporosis* means bones that break easily because they are thin, porous, and brittle. Osteoporosis has several related causes, but too little calcium in the diet plays a big part in causing it.

Here's where calcium comes in. If your bones are strong to begin with, and if you keep giving them plenty of calcium as you get older, you'll help keep your bones strong throughout your life. And even if osteoporosis has already set in, calcium may help slow it down.

We'll be talking a lot about the role of calcium in preventing and treating osteoporosis all through this chapter. That's because osteoporosis is a very serious health problem. It affects some 25 million Americans—four out of five of them older women—and costs nearly $14 billion a year. You need calcium now to avoid the crippling broken bones osteoporosis can cause.

# The DRI for Calcium

In 1994, the National Institutes of Health (NIH) had a major conference on osteoporosis. A panel of experts looked at all the latest information on the importance of calcium and recommended much higher daily intakes of calcium for everyone. Here's the chart with their recommendations:

| NIH Consensus Panel on Optimal Calcium Intake | |
| --- | --- |
| Age/Sex | Calcium in mg |
| 0–0.5 year | 400 |
| 0.5–1 year | 600 |
| 1–10 | 800–1,200 |
| 11–24 | 1,200–1,500 |
| Women, 25–50 | 1,000 |
| Women 50–65, taking estrogen | 1,000 |
| Women 50–65, not taking estrogen | 1,500 |
| Men 25–65 | 1,000 |
| Men and women over 65 | 1,500 |
| Pregnant women | 1,200–1,500 |
| Nursing women | 1,200–1,500 |

In 1997, the Food and Nutrition Board of the Institute of Medicine, the division of the National Academy of Sciences that sets the official standards for nutrients, caught up to the NIH. The old RDA for calcium, set by the Food and Nutrition Board back in 1989, was scrapped in favor of a higher standard, the first of the new Dietary Reference Intakes (DRI) that will gradually replace the old RDAs (check back to Chapter 2 for a more detailed explanation). Here's the new and improved DRI for calcium:

| The DRI for Calcium | |
| --- | --- |
| Age/Sex | Calcium in mg |
| *Infants* | |
| 0–0.5 year | 210 |
| 0.5–1 year | 270 |

*continues*

## The DRI for Calcium  Continued

| Age/Sex | Calcium in mg |
|---|---|
| *Children* | |
| 1–3 years | 500 |
| 4–8 | 800 |
| 9–18 | 1,300 |
| *Adults* | |
| 19–30 years | 1,000 |
| 31–50 | 1,000 |
| 51+ | 1,200 |
| *Pregnant women* | |
| 14–18 years | 1,300 |
| 19–30 | 1,000 |
| 31–50 | 1,000 |
| *Nursing women* | |
| 14–18 years | 1,300 |
| 19–30 | 1,000 |
| 31–50 | 1,000 |

**Now You're Cooking**

Check out some of the new calcium-fortified foods at the supermarket—even Wonder Bread® and Hawaiian Punch® are in on it. Many breakfast cereals (hot and cold) now have extra calcium, and calcium-fortified orange juice (300 mg in 8 ounces) is very popular. You can even try calcium-enriched beer. Regular beer has about 15 mg of calcium, but the Sophie McCall brand has nearly 150 mg.

When you compare the charts, you see that the biggest difference between them is the amounts for older adults and pregnant and nursing women. The NIH suggests somewhat higher amounts for these groups and also suggests different amounts based on your sex and whether or not you take estrogen after menopause. (We'll explain more about estrogen and older women a little later in this chapter.) The overall message is clear from both charts: You need plenty of calcium, especially as you get older.

## Are You Deficient?

Over half of all young people today don't meet the DRI for calcium. That means they're not getting the calcium they need during the crucial childhood, teen, and young adult years to build up their bone mass. If you don't get enough calcium during these critical years, you don't build up your bone savings account, which could lead to big trouble when you're older.

> ### Food for Thought
>
> One reason people today don't get enough calcium is that they don't drink enough milk. We used to drink a lot more. In 1970, the average person drank 31.3 gallons a year; in 1994, that number had dropped to 24.7. At the same time, we started drinking a lot more soda pop, going from 24.3 gallons a year per person in 1970 to 52.2 gallons in 1994. We urge you to follow the advice of the National Osteoporosis Foundation: Drink three glasses of milk a day to get the calcium you need.

It's not just kids who don't get enough calcium. Most women in the United States eat under 600 mg of calcium a day. In fact, calcium is the one nutrient most likely to be missing in the typical American diet. According to U.S. Department of Agriculture surveys, 90 percent of adult women aren't getting even 800 mg of calcium! The numbers aren't much better for teenaged girls: 85 percent of them get only between 300 and 800 mg a day. Men do better, but even so, only four out of every ten men is getting enough calcium. It's no wonder that today we have a virtual epidemic of osteoporosis—and that we'll have even more cases in the future as the population gets older. By one estimate, the number of hip fractures in the United States may triple by the year 2040.

Poor diet is bad enough, but a number of common drugs can rob your body of calcium. This is such an important topic that we have to deal with it separately.

# Calcium-Robbing Drugs

Some common prescription and over-the-counter drugs can rob your body of calcium and lead to osteoporosis. If you regularly take any of these drugs, talk to your doctor about calcium supplements.

## Cortisone and Other Steroid Drugs

A lot of people take drugs called glucocorticoids, which are synthetic versions of the steroid hormones your body naturally produces. This large class of drugs includes cortisone, hydrocortisone, prednisone, and dexamethasone. These drugs are lifesavers for some 30 million Americans who have severe asthma, lupus, rheumatoid arthritis, inflammatory bowel disease, and other medical problems. But—and this is a big but—they can also cause bone loss by breaking down bone faster than you can rebuild it. For a long time, doctors thought you had to worry only if you were taking high doses. Recent studies show, however, that taking even small doses—under 10 mg a day—for a long time can cause osteoporosis. So, if you're taking any sort of steroid drug, talk to your doctor about having a bone density test and taking calcium and Vitamin D supplements. You should also follow all the lifestyle suggestions we'll talk about a little further on to avoid osteoporosis.

# Thyroid Drugs

Many people, especially middle-aged women, don't produce enough hormones from their thyroid gland and need to take supplements (Synthroid® or another drug), usually for the rest of their lives. There's no question that they need the supplements, but large doses over a long period can lead to bone loss. If you take thyroid drugs, check your dose with your doctor once a year—your need may change and you may be able to take less. Also talk to your doctor about calcium supplements.

# Drugs for High Cholesterol

Cholestyramine (Cholybar® or Questran®), a drug used to treat high cholesterol, can block your absorption of calcium and fat-soluble vitamins such as Vitamin D. Talk to your doctor about calcium supplements.

# Aluminum Antacids

If you often take nonprescription antacids that contain aluminum (Maalox®, Rolaids®, Gelusil®, and others), your body may start storing aluminum in your bones instead of calcium. You could end up with weakened bones—especially if you also have kidney problems. If you only take these antacids now and then, you don't have to worry, but if you often take antacids for heartburn, talk to your doctor about other ways to control it.

# Alcohol and Tobacco

**Now You're Cooking**
Great news for caffeine addicts! For a long time, researchers thought caffeine made bone loss worse. The most recent study proves, however, that caffeine has nothing to do with bone loss.

Heavy drinkers and people who smoke have a higher risk for osteoporosis. If you do both, you're at even greater risk. Smokers have lower bone density than nonsmokers (we don't really know why). In fact, a recent study showed that smoking doubles your risk of a hip fracture, even if you don't have osteoporosis. Alcohol interferes with your absorption of calcium. Also, heavy drinkers often don't eat very well and don't get enough calcium in their food. People under the influence tend to fall—and combined with osteoporosis this leads to broken bones.

# Other Prescription Drugs and Calcium

Valuable as calcium supplements are, they can sometimes interfere with prescription drugs you might have to take. Doctors usually recommend taking your calcium supplements two hours apart from any other drugs to prevent problems. There are some cases, thought, where you might even need to skip the supplements. If you take any of these drugs, be very careful about your extra calcium:

➤ **Digitalis.** If you take calcium supplements with this heart medicine, you might get dangerous irregular heartbeats. Try to get enough calcium from your foods and avoid supplements.

➤ **Phenytoin (Dilantin®).** Calcium and phenytoin (a drug used to treat epilepsy and other problems) react to each other. The calcium can keep the phenytoin from working right, while the phenytoin can keep you from absorbing the calcium. Talk to your doctor about calcium supplements before you try them. If you decide to take calcium supplements, take them three hours after you take your phenytoin.

➤ **Antibiotics such as tetracycline and ciprofloxacin (Cipro®).** Calcium from milk, dairy products, and supplements keeps these antibiotics from working well to fight infection. Take them on an empty stomach. Wait at least an hour before drinking milk or eating any dairy products. You usually have to take antibiotics for only a week or ten days, so it's probably best to just skip your calcium supplements for that time. If you take a multi supplement that has calcium, take it a couple of hours apart from your medicine.

➤ **Calcibind® (cellulose sodium phosphate).** This drug is used to prevent kidney stones. If you take it, do not take calcium supplements. In fact, you need to avoid calcium completely, even calcium from food. Your doctor will explain how to take Calcibind and what foods to avoid.

# Eating Your Calcium

The NIH panel says that the preferred way to get enough calcium is through your food. Fortunately, lots of favorite foods are rich in calcium—and a lot of common foods, including orange juice, are now available with added calcium.

Milk and dairy products are by far the best sources of calcium. There's about 300 mg of calcium in one 8-ounce glass of milk. (Milk also has Vitamin D, which you need to absorb calcium better and also to build your bones.) Yogurt usually has even more calcium than milk, and many yogurt makers are now adding extra calcium. The amounts vary from brand to brand, though, so read the labels carefully. An ounce of cheddar cheese has 200 mg, while an ounce of mozzarella has 147 mg and a cup of low-fat cottage cheese has 138 mg.

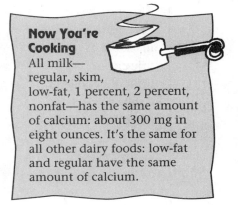

**Now You're Cooking**
All milk—regular, skim, low-fat, 1 percent, 2 percent, nonfat—has the same amount of calcium: about 300 mg in eight ounces. It's the same for all other dairy foods: low-fat and regular have the same amount of calcium.

Here's the best news of all: ice cream is a good source of calcium. There's 85 mg in half a cup of plain vanilla ice cream. So next time you order a double-scoop cone, forget the calories and think of the calcium!

### Food for Thought

Can't drink milk because it gives you gas, cramps, or even diarrhea? You're lactose intolerant—you naturally don't make lactase, an enzyme that helps you digest milk. Lactose intolerance is quite common, but that's no excuse to skip your milk. A lot of people who can't drink regular milk do fine with lactose-reduced or lactose-free milk. You can also add lactase drops to your regular milk or chew some lactase tablets before drinking it. Look for lactase products at your drugstore or health food store. You could also try calcium-fortified soy milk.

Other good dietary sources of calcium are dark-green leafy vegetables, including broccoli, kale, and spinach. Beans, nuts, tofu (bean curd), and fish with soft, tiny bones (canned sardines and salmon are good choices) also give you plenty of calcium. English muffins turn out to be a good source of calcium—there's about 90 mg in each one. Use the chart to pick the calcium-rich foods you need.

### Foods High in Calcium

| Food | Amount | Calcium in mg |
| --- | --- | --- |
| Almonds, dry roasted | 1 ounce | 80 |
| American cheese | 1 ounce | 124 |
| Black beans | 1 cup | 47 |
| Brie cheese | 1 ounce | 52 |
| Broccoli, cooked | 1/2 cup | 36 |
| Cabbage, cooked | 1/2 cup | 25 |
| Cheddar cheese | 1 ounce | 204 |
| Chick peas | 1 cup | 78 |
| Colby cheese | 1 ounce | 194 |
| Collard greens, cooked | 1/2 cup | 15 |
| Cottage cheese, low-fat | 1 cup | 138 |
| Egg | 1 large | 25 |
| English muffin | 1 regular | 90 |
| Ice cream, vanilla | 1/2 cup | 85 |
| Kale, cooked | 1/2 cup | 47 |
| Kidney beans | 1 cup | 50 |
| Milk | 8 ounces | 300 |
| Mozzarella cheese | 1 ounce | 147 |

| Food | Amount | Calcium in mg |
|------|--------|---------------|
| Navy beans | 1 cup | 128 |
| Okra | 1/2 cup | 50 |
| Peanuts | 1 ounce | 15 |
| Potato, baked | 1 medium | 20 |
| Pudding, instant chocolate | 1/2 cup | 149 |
| Ricotta cheese, part skim | 1/2 cup | 337 |
| Salmon (with bones) | 3 ounces | 203 |
| Sardines (with bones) | 3 ounces | 92 |
| Spinach, cooked | 1/2 cup | 122 |
| Sunflower seeds | 1 ounce | 34 |
| Sweet potato, baked | 1 medium | 32 |
| Swiss chard, cooked | 1/2 cup | 51 |
| Swiss cheese, processed | 1 ounce | 272 |
| Tofu, uncooked | 1/2 cup | 130 |
| Turnip greens, cooked | 1/2 cup | 99 |
| Yogurt, plain low-fat | 8 ounces | 415 |

Cooking green veggies and beans breaks down the tough cell walls and releases the calcium so you can absorb it better. Because calcium is a mineral, cooking doesn't affect it. Cook the greens lightly, though, to protect the other vitamins in them.

# Picking the Right Calcium Supplement

Let's face it: The only way a lot of us are going to get enough calcium each day is to take supplements. But just look at how many different supplements are on the shelf at the store. How can you pick the right one for you from all those choices?

It's not as complicated as it looks.

For starters, you need to know that you can't buy pure calcium—for complicated chemistry reasons, it's always combined with another harmless element. Your body breaks this combination down and absorbs the calcium. What this means is that a 500 mg tablet doesn't have 500 mg of calcium—it has a mixture of calcium and something else. The amount of actual calcium in the tablet is the *elemental calcium*. Today

**What's in a Word**

WHAT'S THAT MEAN?

The actual amount of usable calcium in a supplement is called the *elemental calcium*. It's given on the label as a percentage of the total in the supplement. For example, a 1,000 mg tablet of calcium carbonate is 40 percent elemental calcium—so you get only 400 mg of calcium from it. So you don't have to do all that mental arithmetic, many manufacturers now list on the label only the amount of elemental calcium.

You get 300 mg of calcium—at least a quarter of what you need each day—from eight ounces of 1% milk. Here's what else you get:

| | |
|---|---|
| Cobalamin | 0.90 mcg |
| Folic acid | 12 mcg |
| Magnesium | 34 mg |
| Niacin | 0.2 mg |
| Phosphorus | 235 mg |
| Potassium | 381 mg |
| Protein | 8 g |
| Riboflavin | 0.41 mg |
| Vitamin A | 500 IU |
| Vitamin D | 100 IU |
| Zinc | 0.95 mg |

All that nutrition for just 100 calories and 2.5 grams of fat! Skim milk has only 80 calories and no fat (that's why it can now be labeled "fat-free" milk) in an 8-ounce serving. Whole milk has 150 calories and 8 grams of fat in 8 ounces; 2 percent milk (now also called "reduced-fat" milk) has only 120 calories and 5 grams of fat in 8 ounces.

many manufacturers list just the elemental amount on the label, so you can figure out how much calcium you're really getting much more easily. Keeping that in mind, let's look at the different calcium combinations (check out the chart for the quick version):

➤ **Calcium carbonate.** The cheapest supplement, calcium carbonate is also the highest in elemental calcium: 40 percent. This is the form of calcium found in Tums and many generic versions. It has one big drawback: It dissolves slowly in your stomach, so you may not get the full benefit of all the calcium.

➤ **Calcium phosphate (also called tribasic calcium phosphate).** This form is 39 percent elemental calcium. You don't need the extra phosphorus that comes with these tablets—skip them.

➤ **Calcium citrate.** This is the form many doctors and nutritionists recommend. Calcium citrate is only 21 percent elemental calcium, and it's relatively expensive. On the big plus side, it dissolves easily even if you don't have much stomach acid, so you're more likely to absorb all the calcium before the pill passes out of your stomach. Many people naturally produce less acid as they age, so calcium citrate is a good choice for older adults. It's also good for people taking acid-blocking drugs such as ranitidine (Axid®, Pepcid®, Tagamet®, and Zantac®) or omeprazole (Prilosec®).

➤ **Calcium lactate.** This form is found in many generic calcium supplements. It has only 13 percent elemental calcium and is relatively expensive. On the other hand, it dissolves easily even if you're low on stomach acid, so, like calcium citrate, it's a good choice for older adults and people who take acid-blocking drugs.

➤ **Calcium gluconate.** This form is also found in many generics, but it has only 9 percent elemental calcium. It's not a very good choice.

➤ **Calcium glubionate.** This is a concentrated syrup form that contains 6.5 percent elemental calcium. You'd need to take 12 teaspoons a day to get 1,000 mg of calcium. Calcium glubionate is on the expensive side. Take it only if your doctor suggests it.

## The Elemental Calcium in Supplements

| Form | % | Tablet Size in mg | Calcium in mg | # Tablets for 1,000 mg Calcium |
|------|-----|------|------|------|
| Calcium carbonate | 40 | 625 | 250 | 4 |
| | | 650 | 260 | 4 |
| | | 750 | 300 | 4 |
| | | 835 | 334 | 3 |
| | | 1,000 | 400 | 3 |
| | | 1,250 | 500 | 2 |
| | | 1,500 | 600 | 2 |
| Calcium phosphate | 39 | 500 | 115 | 9 |
| Calcium citrate | 21 | 950 | 200 | 5 |
| Calcium lactate | 13 | 325 | 422 | 4 |
| | | 650 | 84 | 12 |
| Calcium gluconate | 9 | | 500 | 45 |
| | 22 | 650 | 58 | 17 |
| | | 1,000 | 84 | 12 |

### Food for Thought

Some chewable antacids contain calcium in the form of calcium carbonate. This isn't a very good way to get your calcium. Ordinarily your stomach acid separates the calcium from the carbonate. Antacid tablets, however, are designed to neutralize your stomach acid—so most of the calcium won't be released and will just pass through your body instead. You'll also get other ingredients you may not want, like aluminum and sugar.

## Calcium Supplements to Avoid

Adding to all the calcium confusion are three forms you should not take, no matter how large the word "natural" is on the label:

➤ **Bone meal.** A powder made from the ground bones of cattle, bone meal has over 1,500 mg of calcium in a 5-gram serving, along with other minerals such as phosphorus and zinc. The FDA warns that bone meal may contain dangerously high amounts of lead.

➤ **Dolomite.** This is a mineral also known as calcium magnesium carbonate. It contains calcium—and also magnesium, which you may not want or shouldn't take. The FDA warns that dolomite may contain dangerously high amounts of lead.

➤ **Oyster shell calcium.** Actually, this is calcium carbonate, but it's made from ground-up oyster shells. These supplements may also contain too much lead and sometimes other contaminants such as mercury and cadmium. Don't use them if you're allergic to shellfish.

# Getting the Most from Calcium

Your body uses calcium around the clock, so try to space out your calcium over the day. If you can, have calcium-rich foods with every meal. If you take supplements, spread them out through the day, and don't more than 600 mg at a time.

Should you take calcium supplements with meals or on an empty stomach? It's hard to say. On the one hand, you need stomach acid to make the supplement dissolve, and you make acid when you eat. On the other hand, the food you eat along with the supplement could block your absorption of the calcium—especially if you eat foods that are high in fiber—while at the same time calcium could block your absorption of other minerals from your food.

We've run out of hands, so do what most doctors recommend: Take your calcium supplements between meals, but with a small protein snack—a few spoonfuls of yogurt, a piece of cheese, or maybe a leftover chicken leg—to make your stomach produce acid.

If milk is good and calcium supplements are good, isn't it even better to take them together? No—take them an hour or two apart so your body can absorb the most calcium from both.

Calcium citrate dissolves faster than calcium carbonate, but it has less elemental calcium. To get the benefits of both forms, you could try a combination formula. Two popular brands are Os-Cal® and Caltrate®.

Most people don't have any side effects from taking calcium supplements even in high doses. To be on the safe side, though, don't take more than 2,000 mg of calcium in a day—that's your total intake, including food and supplements.

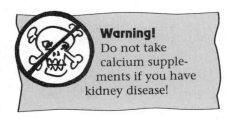

**Warning!**
Do not take calcium supplements if you have kidney disease!

Sometimes people who take calcium supplements get constipation. If this happens to you, space out your supplements more across the day and be sure to drink plenty of water.

In very rare cases, too much calcium (over 2,000 mg a day for a long time) can cause hypercalcemia, or an overload of calcium in the blood. The symptoms include appetite loss, drowsiness, constipation, dry mouth, headache, and weakness. Stop taking the supplements and call your doctor.

## The Dynamic Duo: Calcium and Vitamin D

Vitamin D and calcium work together to keep your blood level of calcium normal. You also need Vitamin D to help your bones hold on to their calcium. For the best protection against osteoporosis, try to get about 200 IU of Vitamin D daily. (Refer to Chapter 14 on Vitamin D for more information.)

Some calcium supplements also contain Vitamin D. These combinations are meant only for people who don't get outside very much. Most people don't need extra Vitamin D, because your body makes it from sunshine—and too much Vitamin D can be toxic.

The dynamic duo has a sidekick: magnesium. This mineral helps you absorb calcium and use Vitamin D properly. The rule of thumb is: half as much magnesium as calcium. So, if you're getting 1,000 mg of calcium a day from food and supplements, you need 500 mg of magnesium. You can get calcium supplements that also have magnesium in them, but that may not be a good idea (see Chapter 18 on magnesium for why).

| Thumbs Up/Thumbs Down | |
| --- | --- |
| **Calcium is helped by:** | **Calcium is blocked by:** |
| Vitamin D | Alcohol |
| Vitamin K | Tobacco |
| Magnesium | High-fiber foods |
| | Foods high in oxalic acid |
| | Cortisone-like drugs |
| | Tetracycline |
| | Thyroid drugs |
| | Aluminum antacids |
| | Some drugs for high cholesterol |

## The Function of Phosphorus

After calcium, phosphorus is the second most abundanh mineral in your body—about 1 percent of your body weight, or between one and 1 1/2 pounds, is phosphorus. Over 80 percent of that is combined with calcium in your bones and teeth; the rest is spread around in every cell of your body.

Phosphorus is needed to build the structure of your bones and teeth, and it also plays important roles in almost every body process. For all its importance, phosphorus doesn't get much attention in books like this. Phosphorus is so widespread in every food you eat that it's almost impossible to be deficient in it. In fact, because phosphorus deficiency is almost unheard of, researchers don't know how much or little you really need. The RDA is based on the rule of thumb that you should get about as much phosphorus as calcium. Because phosphorus is so widely found in foods, most people actually get much more than that—up to twice as much phosphorus as calcium.

Phosphorus is found in protein-rich foods such as meat, poultry, eggs, and fish. It's also found in milk and dairy products, whole grains, beans, most vegetables, nuts, and fruits. Many people get a good dose of phosphorus every day from widely used food additives like monocalcium phosphate and sodium aluminum phosphate. There's also about 30 mg of phosphorus in a 12-ounce can of diet soda.

You're likely to be deficient in phosphorus only in very rare circumstances. If that happens, you need to be under a doctor's care—don't take phosphorus supplements on your own.

# Avoiding Osteoporosis

Are you at risk for osteoporosis? Answer the questions in this chart and add up your Yes answers. The more Yes answers you have, the greater your risk.

---

### Are You at Risk for Osteoporosis?

| | | | |
|---|---|---|---|
| 1. Do you have a small, thin frame? | Yes | No |
| 2. Are you white or Asian? | Yes | No |
| 3. Are you over age 50? | Yes | No |
| 4. Have you passed menopause? | Yes | No |
| 5. Did your mother have osteoporosis? | Yes | No |
| 6. Did you reach menopause early or have a hysterectomy? | Yes | No |
| 7. Do you take thyroid medicine? | Yes | No |
| 8. Do you take cortisone-like drugs? | Yes | No |
| 9. Is your diet low in calcium-rich foods? | Yes | No |
| 10. Are you physically inactive? | Yes | No |
| 11. Do you smoke? | Yes | No |
| 12. Do you drink a lot of alcohol? | Yes | No |

---

## Food for Thought

When a woman reaches menopause, she makes a lot less of the hormone estrogen. But estrogen helps control how quickly you lose calcium from your bones, so when you make less of it, you start losing bone faster—a lot faster if you also have other risk factors. For the first six to ten years after menopause, you could lose bone quickly, as fast as about 3 percent of your total every year. Over ten years, then, you could lose well over 30 percent of your total bone density. By that point, your bones could be so thin that even a hard hug from a grandkid could make a rib break.

If you're at risk, what should you do? Getting more calcium is just one of the steps you need to take at once. Here are the others:

➤ Get regular exercise. Regular weight-bearing exercise—walking, jogging, dancing, bowling, climbing stairs—helps keep your bones strong. (Swimming, yoga, and bike riding are good exercise, but they won't strengthen your bones.) Walking for half an hour just three times a week could make a big difference.

➤ If you smoke, stop.

➤ Limit your alcohol to two drinks a day.

➤ If you're a woman past menopause, talk to your doctor about hormone replacement therapy (HRT). Estrogen, one of the hormones in HRT, slows calcium loss and helps restore lost bone.

➤ If you already show signs of bone loss, talk to your doctor about prescription drugs to slow bone loss and build new bone. Some of the newest drugs are easy to take and very helpful.

➤ Do everything you can to avoid falls that could break bones. For example: Remove scatter rugs and electrical cords you could trip over; put night lights by stairs; install a grab bar and nonskid tape in the shower or tub; wear flat, rubber-soled shoes.

**Warning!**
According to the National Osteoporosis Foundation, osteoporosis affects over 20 million American women. Every year osteoporosis causes about 1.5 million bone fractures in older adults. As a woman, your risk of getting a bone fracture from osteoporosis is equal to your total risk of getting breast, uterine, and ovarian cancer.

# Not for Women Only

Osteoporosis is a problem for all older adults—not just women. The odds are lower if you're a man, but even so, some 2 million men already have osteoporosis and about 3 million are at risk. In fact, a third of all hip fractures from osteoporosis happen to men. And when they do, it's serious—a third of all the men who get these fractures die within a year.

Just as bone loss gets worse in older women when they start producing less estrogen, it gets worse in older men when they naturally start making less of the male hormone testosterone, which your body converts into estrogen.

Even so, hormones don't seem to really be the main reason for osteoporosis in men. Not enough calcium in the diet and not enough exercise are important factors, but medications, smoking cigarettes, and drinking heavily also play big roles.

Because osteoporosis is seen as such a problem for women, doctors sometimes overlook it in older men. If you fall into any of the risk categories, talk to your doctor.

> **Warning!**
> You don't have to wait for a fracture to tell if your bones are thinning. One early warning sign is trouble with your teeth. If your dentures stop fitting right, it might be because of bone loss in your jaw. If you're at risk for osteoporosis, talk to your doctor about having a bone density test. New X-ray techniques make this quick, safe, and easy.

# Calcium and High Blood Pressure

Calcium may help prevent or treat high blood pressure in some people. If you don't eat much calcium, you're more likely to get high blood pressure than someone who gets the DRI or more. In general, the higher the level of calcium in your blood, the lower your blood pressure. According to one study, taking 1,000 mg a day of extra calcium also lowers your diastolic blood pressure (that's the pressure when your heart is relaxed between beats), but it doesn't seem to do anything for your systolic pressure (when your heart is contracting and the pressure is highest).

Other studies show that taking calcium supplements (anywhere from 400 to 1,000 mg) can lower blood pressure for some people, especially African-Americans and people who are sensitive to salt.

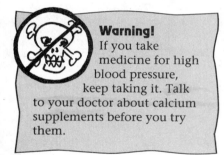

> **Warning!**
> If you take medicine for high blood pressure, keep taking it. Talk to your doctor about calcium supplements before you try them.

If your blood pressure is on the high side but you don't yet need medicine to lower it, take a look at your calcium level. Try to raise your intake to at least 1,000 mg a day. After a few months, you may notice a drop in your blood pressure.

Pregnant women sometimes have trouble with high blood pressure. Calcium supplements seem to help. Because pregnant women need extra calcium anyway, this is another good reason to be sure you're getting 1,000 mg a day—enough for you and your growing baby.

# Calcium and Colon Cancer

The research here is promising. In general, the lower your calcium intake, the more likely you are to get colon cancer, possibly because calcium blocks the growth of cancer cells. If you're at risk (if one of your parents had colon cancer, for example), getting 1,500 to 2,000 mg of calcium a day could help ward it off.

# Calcium and Kidney Stones

For years, doctors warned patients who had kidney stones to avoid calcium. The idea was that the calcium combined with oxalate, a natural substance found in green leafy vegetables such as spinach, to form the painful stones.

In fact, the opposite may be true. In a recent study, women who had the highest calcium intake were the least likely to have kidney stones. If you've ever had a kidney stone, there's no longer really much reason to give up the bone-protecting benefits of calcium. To be on the safe side, though, try to get most of your calcium from food, not supplements. If you do take supplements, take them with meals to block your uptake of oxalates. And be sure to drink plenty of water every day.

# Calcium and Heart Disease

Two important studies in 1997 pointed out a link between atherosclerosis (arteries clogged with fatty deposits called plaque) and osteoporosis. In the first study, researchers found that women who had the most bone loss from osteoporosis were also the most likely to have calcium-containing plaque blocking their carotid arteries. Because the carotid arteries carry blood to the brain, these women were at higher risk of having a stroke. The second study showed that men and women with low Vitamin D levels also had higher rates of calcium-containing plaque in the arteries leading to their hearts, making them more vulnerable to heart attacks. Much more follow-up research needs to be done, of course, but these studies show how important calcium is for every aspect of your long-term health.

# The Least You Need to Know

➤ Calcium is the most abundant mineral in your body.

➤ You need calcium along with Vitamin D to build strong bones and keep them that way throughout your life.

➤ The new adult DRI for calcium is between 1,000 and 1,200 mg.

➤ Milk and other dairy foods are the best source of calcium. Dark-green leafy vegetables such as kale also have calcium. Many foods, including orange juice and breakfast cereals, are now available with added calcium.

➤ Many different kinds of calcium supplements are available. Calcium citrate supplements are best for most people.

➤ Calcium can help prevent osteoporosis, or bones that are thin, brittle, and break easily. Calcium may also help prevent high blood pressure and colon cancer.

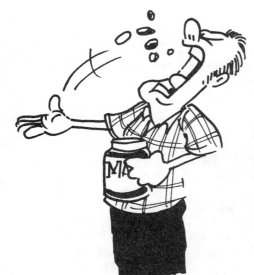

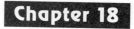

# Chapter 18

# Magnesium: Magnificent for Your Heart

> **In This Chapter**
>
> ➤ Why you need magnesium
>
> ➤ Foods that are high in magnesium
>
> ➤ How magnesium helps your heart
>
> ➤ Helping your blood pressure with magnesium
>
> ➤ Magnesium helps relieve asthma
>
> ➤ How magnesium can help diabetes

If sometimes you feel like a nut, go for it! Nuts are high in magnesium, and this magnificent mineral helps maintain your maximum health. Magnesium makes your muscles relax—and that plays a big role in keeping your heartbeat healthy and holding down your blood pressure.

Today many doctors have realized that magnesium makes a big difference for some patients. Magnesium is getting to be a mainstream medication for people with migraines, asthma, and diabetes. Getting enough magnesium helps these people control their medical problems. Magnesium has one other major mission: Working with calcium, it helps keep your bones strong throughout your life.

# Why You Need Magnesium

Every single cell in your body needs magnesium to produce energy. You also need magnesium to make more than 300 different enzymes, to send messages along your nerves, to make your muscles relax, to maintain strong bones and teeth, help your heart beat, and to keep your blood pressure at normal levels. Magnesium seems to help some health problems, such as asthma and diabetes, and can be very valuable for treating heart rhythm problems.

**Food for Thought**

Magnesium gets its name from a region of Greece called Magnesia. In ancient times, people believed that a white, salty-tasting powder from that area had magical powers, perhaps because it burned very rapidly with a brilliant flame. (That's why old-time photographers used magnesium powder for flash lighting.) Magnesium was first isolated from the powder by the father of modern chemistry, Sir Humphry Davy, in 1808. Davy was also the first to isolate potassium, sodium, barium, boron, and calcium.

You also need magnesium to use other vitamins and minerals properly. Vitamin C and calcium both work better, for example, when there's plenty of magnesium around.

To do all that, you need a fair amount of magnesium. In fact, your body contains about 25 grams of magnesium. Most of it's in your bones and teeth, but you also have a lot in your muscles and blood. The amount in your blood is very important for keeping your body's functions in balance. Just as you need calcium to make your muscles contract—when your heart beats, for example—you need magnesium to make them relax again. That's why the levels of calcium and magnesium in your blood have to be steady and why you need to be sure you're getting enough of both. If you don't have enough of them, your body will pull these minerals from your bones and put them into your blood—which can lead to weakened bones.

# The DRI for Magnesium

In 1989, the RDA for magnesium was lowered somewhat, especially for children and pregnant women. As usual, the reasoning was that most people were getting less than even the lowered amount, but they seemed healthy enough anyway. In 1997, the recommended amounts for magnesium were raised a little as one of the first of the new DRIs. (Remember those from Chapter 2?) Here's a chart with the new guidelines:

**The DRI for Magnesium**

| Age/Sex | Magnesium in mg |
|---|---|
| *Infants* | |
| 0–0.5 year | 30 |
| 0.5–1 year | 75 |
| *Children* | |
| 1–3 years | 80 |
| 4–8 | 130 |
| 9–13 | 240 |
| Boys 14–18 | 410 |
| Girls 14–18 | 360 |
| *Young Adults and Adults* | |
| Men 19–30 years | 400 |
| Men 31+ | 420 |
| Women 19–30 | 310 |
| Women 31+ | 320 |
| *Pregnant women* | |
| 18 years and under | 400 |
| 19–30 years | 350 |
| 31–50 | 360 |
| *Nursing women* | |
| 18 years and under | 360 |
| 19–30 years | 310 |
| 31–50 | 320 |

Although the new DRI is higher than the old RDA, many researchers believe they're still too low to prevent some health problems.

The research into the value of larger doses is now pretty solid. Many nutritionists and doctors now suggest 500 mg a day for adults. This amount could do a lot to help keep your blood pressure normal and prevent heart disease.

# Are You Deficient?

A lot of people don't get enough magnesium from their food to meet even the lowered DRI. By some estimates, in fact, nearly three-quarters of all Americans don't. Even so, very few healthy people are really deficient—you'd have to have very low amounts of magnesium for a long time to have any symptoms. If you're not basically healthy, though, you could become deficient, especially if you have any of these health problems:

➤ **You abuse alcohol.** Most alcohol abusers have poor diets that are too low in magnesium and other nutrients.

➤ **You have diabetes.** You may be excreting a lot of your magnesium in your urine— we'll talk about that some more later on in this chapter.

➤ **You have kidney disease.** Your kidneys may not be handling magnesium very well. Your doctor will prescribe medications that prevent magnesium deficiency. Do not take supplements!

➤ **You've been vomiting a lot or having severe diarrhea.** You lose a lot magnesium when this happens.

➤ **You use *diuretic drugs*.** Diuretics make you pass more urine, which lowers your magnesium level. This can become a real problem if you often use nonprescription diuretics ("water pills") without telling your doctor.

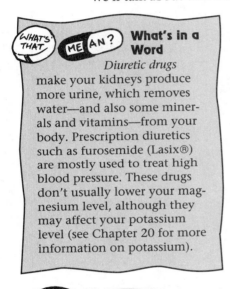

**What's in a Word**

*Diuretic drugs* make your kidneys produce more urine, which removes water—and also some minerals and vitamins—from your body. Prescription diuretics such as furosemide (Lasix®) are mostly used to treat high blood pressure. These drugs don't usually lower your magnesium level, although they may affect your potassium level (see Chapter 20 for more information on potassium).

**Warning!**
Nonprescription diuretics ("water pills") or herbal diuretics such as buchu or uva ursi ("dieter's tea") can make you pass too much urine and make your levels of magnesium and other important minerals such as potassium level drop too low.

A lot of people get some of their magnesium from the water they drink. In many areas, the water is "hard"—it has a lot of minerals such as calcium and magnesium in it. (A lot of bottled mineral waters also have magnesium, usually over 6 mg per quart.) People who live in areas where the water is "soft" and contains few minerals, or people who drink only distilled water, might be low on magnesium.

If you don't get enough magnesium, all your tissues are affected, but you'll feel it most in your heart, nerves, and kidneys. Generally, deficiency symptoms include nausea, loss of appetite, muscle weakness or tremors, and irritability. You might also have a rapid heartbeat. Severe magnesium deficiency can cause your heart to beat irregularly. Many nutritionists and doctors feel that breathing problems such as asthma are caused in part by magnesium deficiency. Extra magnesium can sometimes be very helpful for people with asthma. (We'll talk more about magnesium for heart problems and asthma later in this chapter.)

# Eating Your Magnesium

Magnesium is found in lots of foods. Good sources include nuts, beans, dark-green leafy vegetables (of course), whole grains, and seafood. Most people get a lot of their daily magnesium from milk, which has about 34 mg per cup. Soy foods such as miso and tofu (bean curd) are high in magnesium; soy milk actually has more magnesium than cow's milk. There isn't much magnesium in meat or foods that have been refined or processed a lot—just compare the 23 mg in a slice of whole wheat bread to the measly 5 mg in a slice of white bread.

Looking at the chart, you can see some delicious ways to get magnesium from your food. A peanut-butter sandwich on whole-wheat bread, for example, easily gives you nearly 100 mg.

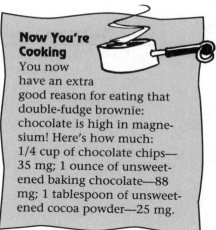

**Now You're Cooking**
You now have an extra good reason for eating that double-fudge brownie: chocolate is high in magnesium! Here's how much: 1/4 cup of chocolate chips— 35 mg; 1 ounce of unsweetened baking chocolate—88 mg; 1 tablespoon of unsweetened cocoa powder—25 mg.

## The Magnesium in Food

| Food | Amount | Magnesium in mg |
| --- | --- | --- |
| Almonds, dry roasted | 1 ounce | 84 |
| Banana | 1 medium | 33 |
| Black beans | 1 cup | 121 |
| Bread, whole wheat | 1 slice | 23 |
| Bread, white | 1 slice | 5 |
| Broccoli, cooked | 1/2 cup | 19 |
| Cashews, dry roasted | 1 ounce | 72 |
| Chick peas | 1 cup | 78 |
| Flounder | 3 ounces | 50 |
| Kidney beans | 1 cup | 80 |
| Lentils | 1 cup | 71 |
| Lima beans | 1 cup | 82 |
| Milk, low-fat | 8 ounces | 34 |
| Miso | 1/2 cup | 58 |
| Oatmeal, cooked | 1 cup | 56 |
| Okra | 1/2 cup | 46 |
| Peanut butter | 2 tablespoons | 51 |
| Peanuts | 1 ounce | 52 |
| Peas | 1/2 cup | 31 |
| Pinto beans, canned | 1 cup | 64 |
| Potato, baked with skin | 1 medium | 55 |

*continues*

### The Magnesium in Food   Continued

| Food | Amount | Magnesium in mg |
| --- | --- | --- |
| Shrimp | 3 ounces | 29 |
| Soy milk | 1 cup | 45 |
| Spinach, cooked | 1/2 cup | 79 |
| Swiss chard | 1/2 cup | 76 |
| Tofu | 1/2 cup | 118 |
| Walnuts | 1 ounce | 48 |
| Wheat germ | 1/4 cup | 69 |
| White beans | 1 cup | 113 |
| Yogurt | 8 ounces | 40 |

# Getting the Most from Magnesium

It's not that easy to get the RDA for magnesium just from your food—and it's even harder to get 500 mg a day that way. Even so, that's the best way to get your magnesium, along with all the other valuable vitamins and minerals also found in magnesium-rich foods.

### Food for Thought

Magnesium is the main ingredients in many antacids such as Maalox® and Mylanta®. Antacids are not the same as magnesium supplements. If you use antacids a lot, you'll probably get diarrhea. That leads us to the other use of magnesium: in larger amounts, it's a laxative in products such as milk of magnesia (magnesium hydroxide) and epsom salts. Use these laxatives only if your doctor recommends them, and not as a source of supplemental magnesium.

If you want to take a supplement, remember that your daily multi supplement probably has 10 to 50 mg of magnesium. Between your food and your multi, you won't need a large dose of supplemental magnesium to make up the difference. That's good, because large doses of magnesium—over 600 mg—can give you diarrhea.

The magnesium in supplements is always combined with some other harmless substance to make it stable. At the vitamin counter you'll find a lot of different choices, with names like magnesium orotate and magnesium gluconate. We suggest taking magnesium aspartate, magnesium glycinate, or magnesium citrate, because you absorb these the best. Avoid magnesium oxide—most people find it hard to tolerate. For the most benefit, take between 200 and 500 mg a day; don't go over 500 mg. Spread your magnesium out over the day and take the supplements with meals. If you get diarrhea from the supplements, cut back on your dose.

Your kidneys are very good at removing excess magnesium, so you're unlikely to have problems other than diarrhea from taking too much. Except for people with kidney problems, the excess will just pass out harmlessly in your urine.

**Warning!**
Do not take magnesium supplements or antacids containing magnesium if you also take the antibiotic drugs Cipro® or tetracycline! The magnesium will block the drugs from entering your bloodstream! If you take prescription diuretics, insulin, or digitalis, you may need more magnesium. Discuss magnesium supplements with your doctor before you try them!

| Thumbs Up/Thumbs Down | |
| --- | --- |
| **Magnesium works better with:** | **Magnesium is blocked by:** |
| Calcium | Alcohol |
| Potassium | Excess amounts of calcium |
| Thiamin | Fat-soluble vitamins (Vitamins A, E, K) |
| Vitamin C | |
| Vitamin D | |

# Magnesium and Your Heart

Low levels of magnesium seem to be related to some types of heart problems. Because magnesium helps your muscles relax, a shortage may cause a spasm in one of your coronary arteries. The spasm blocks the blood flow and can cause a heart attack. Some doctors think that a shortage of magnesium is behind many sudden heart attacks, especially in people who don't have a history of heart disease. In fact, intravenous magnesium is used in emergency rooms as a treatment for heart attacks.

**Food for Thought**

Tap water naturally has some minerals in it—on average, there's about 2 mg of magnesium in 8 ounces. If you live in an area with "hard" water—water that naturally has a lot of calcium and magnesium in it—you'll be getting more. In fact, the connection between high magnesium levels and lowered heart disease was made by comparing people from places with hard and "soft" water. The people who regularly drank hard water had a lot less heart disease.

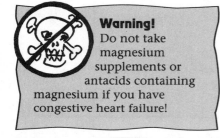

**Warning!**
Do not take magnesium supplements or antacids containing magnesium if you have congestive heart failure!

**What's in a Word**
*Cardiac arrhythmias* make your heart beat irregularly. Sometimes the arrhythmia makes you have an extra heartbeat or skip one; it could also make your heart beat too fast. Cardiac arrhythmias can be serious. See your doctor at once if you're having symptoms.

Magnesium may also protect against heart attacks caused by blood clots. Magnesium helps keeps the clots from forming by making your platelets (tiny blood cells that form clots) less "sticky." This makes them less likely to lump together into an artery-clogging clot.

Too little magnesium can also cause *cardiac arrhythmias*. When that happens, your heart beats irregularly. You might skip a beat or have an extra one, or your heart could beat too fast. If the problem is serious enough, your heartbeat doesn't quickly return to normal and you could die suddenly. Studies suggest that people with low levels of magnesium are more likely to die suddenly from heart rhythm problems.

# Magnesium Manages Blood Pressure

Magnesium helps your muscles relax. If you don't have enough magnesium, the walls of your blood vessels could tighten up, which raises your blood pressure. As it turns out, many people with high blood pressure don't eat enough magnesium. When they get more in their diet—up to 600 mg a day—their blood pressure drops. This doesn't work for everybody, though, so we can't say for sure that magnesium will make your high blood pressure go down. Even so, many doctors suggest that you try eating more magnesium-rich foods if you have high blood pressure. You could also try taking 400 mg a day in supplements, but talk to your doctor first.

Pregnant women sometimes get dangerously high blood pressure, especially in the last few months of the pregnancy. Magnesium may help prevent this problem. If you're pregnant, your doctor will probably prescribe a multi supplement that has magnesium in it. Don't take additional magnesium supplements unless your doctor recommends them.

# Help for Asthma

When you have an asthma attack, the muscles lining the airways in your lungs contract. This makes the airways get too narrow, so you have trouble breathing. Magnesium helps the muscles relax, so the airways open up and you can breathe more easily. In emergency rooms, intravenous magnesium is used to treat severe asthma attacks. Don't try to treat an attack on your own by swallowing magnesium supplements, though—it doesn't work and could be dangerous. Take your medicine instead.

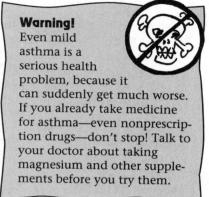

**Warning!**
Even mild asthma is a serious health problem, because it can suddenly get much worse. If you already take medicine for asthma—even nonprescription drugs—don't stop! Talk to your doctor about taking magnesium and other supplements before you try them.

If you have asthma, it might be because your diet is low in magnesium. Getting more through supplements and magnesium-rich foods—up to 1,000 mg a day—could help prevent attacks and make your attacks less severe. For the best results, spread the dose out over the day.

# Magnesium and Diabetes

High blood pressure is often a problem for people with diabetes—and people with diabetes often have low magnesium levels. Is there a connection? Some doctors think there is and recommend magnesium supplements for diabetic patients. Magnesium may also help diabetics control their blood sugar better and help prevent complications later on, like eye problems and heart disease. There's also some evidence that older people who are at risk for diabetes can prevent it by taking extra magnesium. If you have diabetes or are at risk for it, try to get as much magnesium as you can from your diet and consider taking between 200 and 300 mg a day in supplements. Talk to your doctor about taking supplements before you try them, especially if you have kidney problems because of your diabetes.

# Magnesium for Healthy Bones

We talked a lot about the importance of calcium for strong bones in the previous chapter. But calcium isn't the only mineral you need to keep your bones healthy—you also need enough magnesium. The magnesium helps keep your calcium levels in balance and makes sure you produce enough Vitamin D.

The general rule of thumb is that you need twice as much calcium as magnesium to prevent osteoporosis (bones that are thin, brittle, and break easily). Because women need more calcium as they get older, they also need more magnesium. According to the NIH, women aged 25 to 50 need 1,000 mg of calcium a day, so they also need to get 500 mg of magnesium. If you're a woman over age 50 and you're not taking estrogen, you probably need 1,500 mg of calcium and 750 mg of magnesium every day. This amount is hard to get through your diet alone—consider taking magnesium and calcium supplements.

# Magnesium and Migraines

People who get migraine headaches often have low magnesium levels. Does that mean that low magnesium causes migraines? Could be, although we're still not sure why. If you get migraines, try to get 500 mg of magnesium a day through your diet and by taking a magnesium supplement. This daily amount could reduce the number of attacks you get. It seems to work particularly well as a preventive for women who get migraines as part of their menstrual cycle.

One very interesting recent study showed that in about half the cases, intravenous magnesium stopped migraine headaches in their tracks. Unfortunately, once you have a migraine just swallowing magnesium supplements doesn't have the same effect.

# Other Problems Helped by Magnesium

There's a lot of controversy over whether magnesium helps some other health problems. We're not too sure about some of these—magnesium doesn't seem to do anything for prostate trouble, gallstones, body odor (we'll never understand how that one got started), or depression, for example, although some people claim it does. Let's look at two cases where the evidence shows that magnesium helps:

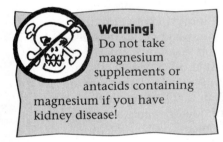

**Warning!**
Do not take magnesium supplements or antacids containing magnesium if you have kidney disease!

➤ **Premenstrual syndrome (PMS).** Some women swear that magnesium supplements relieve uncomfortable PMS symptoms, especially breast tenderness, headaches, and irritability. If you get severe PMS, try taking 300 to 500 mg a day for the two weeks leading up to your period. If you get severe cramps from your period, keep taking the magnesium during that time—it may help reduce cramping. Magnesium may help even more if you combine it with pyridoxine (refer to Chapter 8 for more information about this).

➤ **Preventing kidney stones.** Magnesium supplements seem to help keep calcium kidney stones from coming back. All you need is 100 to 300 mg a day. The magnesium seems to help more if you also take 10 mg a day of pyridoxine (Vitamin $B_6$). If you get kidney stones, talk to your doctor about magnesium supplements before you try them.

# The Least You Need to Know

➤ Magnesium is a mineral needed for over 300 different roles in your body.

➤ The adult RDA for magnesium is between 280 and 350 mg a day. Many researchers feel this is too low and suggest 500 mg a day.

➤ Foods high in magnesium include nuts, beans, dark-green leafy vegetables, and milk.

➤ Magnesium may help prevent heart rhythm problems and high blood pressure.

➤ Magnesium may be helpful for people with asthma and diabetes. It may also help prevent migraine headaches.

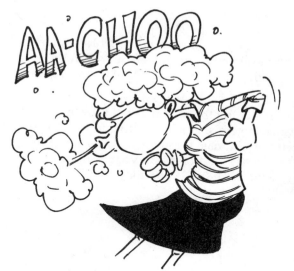

# Chapter 19

# Zinc: Immune System Booster

**In This Chapter**

➤ Why you need zinc

➤ Foods that are high in zinc

➤ How zinc helps colds

➤ How zinc helps prostate problems

➤ Why you need zinc for healthy skin, hair, and nails

Look up zinc in the encyclopedia and you'll learn all about this important industrial metal. You'll learn about how it's used to make pipes and galvanized metals that resist corrosion. You'll learn that 6.8 million metric tons of zinc are used every year. You might even learn that there are 338 zinc mines in the world. What you won't learn is that the same stuff that galvanizes metal is also incredibly important for your health.

Zinc is very important for your immune system. In fact, if you have a bad cold, taking extra zinc could get you back on your feet several days sooner. Zinc also helps you heal quickly from wounds, keeps your skin healthy, helps preserve your eyesight, and might even improve your memory. It's no surprise that today many doctors and nutritionists tell their patients to "think zinc!"

# Why You Need Zinc

Over 200 different enzymes in your body depend on zinc to work properly. Here's just one example: You need zinc to make the enzyme alcohol dehydrogenase, which breaks down alcohol. If you're deficient in zinc, your body can't process alcohol and you get very drunk on just a small amount.

You also need zinc to make many hormones, including the ones that tell your immune system what to do when you're under attack from germs. Zinc is essential for making the hormones that control growth and for the important male hormone testosterone. You have some zinc in every one of your body's cells, but most of it is in your skin, hair, nails, and eyes—and in your prostate gland if you're male. All told, your body contains just over 2.2 grams of zinc.

# The RDA for Zinc

Even though you use zinc in many important body processes, you don't need to eat much of it. Technically speaking, zinc is a trace element—a mineral you need in only very small amounts (we'll talk more about trace elements in Chapter 21). The adult RDA for zinc is 15 mg a day or less—an amount that most everybody easily gets from food. Check out the chart to see what your zinc need is.

| The RDA for Zinc | |
| --- | --- |
| Age/Sex | Zinc in mg |
| *Infants* | |
| 0–1 year | 5 |
| *Children* | |
| 1–10 years | 10 |
| *Adolescents and Adults* | |
| Males 11+ | 15 |
| Females 11+ | 12 |
| Pregnant women | 15 |
| Nursing women | 19 |

# Are You Deficient?

The first hint that zinc is an important nutrient came almost a century ago in Egypt, when doctors noticed that poor young boys who ate almost nothing but unleavened bread were very short and underdeveloped. It turned out that their diet had very little zinc. Once they got more zinc in their diet, they started growing normally again.

In our modern society, such a serious zinc deficiency is very rare. A slight deficiency in zinc isn't that uncommon. Surveys show that many women get only about half the RDA. You might be on the low side for zinc if:

➤ **You're a strict vegetarian or vegan.** Animal foods such as fish and meat are the best dietary sources of zinc. Fruits have virtually none. Children who don't eat animal foods are more at risk for zinc deficiency.

➤ **You eat a very high-fiber diet.** The fiber, especially fiber from whole grains, binds up the zinc in your diet and keeps you from absorbing it.

➤ **You're pregnant or breastfeeding.** You're passing a lot of your zinc on to your baby. If your diet is on the low side for zinc to begin with, you might be deficient. Talk to your doctor about supplements.

➤ **You're over age 50.** Your ability to absorb zinc from your food drops as you get older.

➤ **You abuse alcohol.** Alcohol abusers don't eat very well in general. Even moderate amounts of alcohol flush out the zinc stored in your liver and make you excrete the zinc stored in your liver.

Zinc deficiency has a number of symptoms: slowed growth in children, slow wound healing, frequent infections, skin irritations, hair loss, and loss of your sense of taste.

Generally speaking, you don't have to worry much about being deficient in this mineral. Anyone who eats a reasonably well-balanced diet will get plenty of zinc.

# Eating Your Zinc

The best food source of zinc by far is oysters. There are about 12 mg in a single raw oyster. Other foods that are good sources of zinc are lean meat, poultry, and organ meats. You only absorb about ten percent of the zinc you get from animal foods, and you absorb even less from the zinc in plant foods.

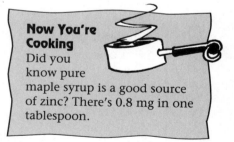

**Now You're Cooking**
Did you know pure maple syrup is a good source of zinc? There's 0.8 mg in one tablespoon.

There's a fair amount of zinc in beans, nuts, seeds, and whole grains, but your body can't use it very well. That's because these foods also have a lot of fiber. A substance called phytic acid in the fiber combines with zinc and keeps a lot of it from being absorbed. Fruits are low in zinc. For the best food sources of zinc, check the chart.

## The Zinc in Food

| Food | Amount | Zinc in mg |
|------|--------|-----------|
| Almonds, dry roasted | 1 ounce | 1.4 |
| Black beans | 1 cup | 1.9 |
| Beef, ground | 3 ounces | 4.6 |
| Beef liver | 3 ounces | 5.2 |
| Bread, whole wheat | 1 slice | 0.4 |
| Cashews, dry roasted | 1 ounce | 1.6 |
| Cheddar cheese | 1 ounce | 0.9 |
| Chicken, without skin | 3 ounces | 2.10 |
| Chickpeas | 1 cup | 2.5 |
| Egg | 1 large | 0.5 |
| Flounder | 3 ounces | 0.5 |
| Kidney beans | 1 cup | 1.9 |
| Lentils | 1 cup | 2.5 |
| Lima beans | 1 cup | 1.8 |
| Milk, 1% | 8 ounces | 1.0 |
| Oatmeal | 1 cup | 1.1 |
| Oysters, canned | 3 ounces | 77.3 |
| Oysters, raw | 6 medium | 76.4 |
| Oysters, smoked | 3 ounces | 103 |
| Peas, split | 1/2 cup | 0.9 |
| Peanut butter | 2 tablespoons | 0.9 |
| Peanuts | 1 ounce | 0.9 |
| Pecans | 1 ounce | 1.6 |
| Sunflower seeds | 1 ounce | 1.4 |
| Swiss cheese | 1 ounce | 1.1 |
| Turkey | 3 ounces | 1.7 |
| Walnuts | 1 ounce | 0.8 |
| Wheat germ | 1/4 cup | 3.6 |
| White beans | 1 cup | 2.5 |
| Yogurt | 8 ounces | 2.0 |

# Getting the Most from Zinc

You have a lot of choices at the vitamin counter when you're looking for a zinc supplement. What you want is a form that you can easily absorb, so we suggest zinc gluconate. Zinc picolinate, zinc citrate, or zinc monomethionate are also good options. Zinc sulfate is likely to upset your stomach— so skip it. Avoid zinc oxide—that form is really only useful in skin creams meant to block sunlight.

Most good multi supplements have the RDA for zinc. If you want to get more, try zinc supplements; they usually come in 10, 30, or 50 mg capsules. Zinc supplements in large amounts can block your absorption of calcium, copper, and iron. It's especially important to keep your copper and zinc levels in balance. If you regularly take extra zinc, be sure you're also getting some extra copper.

Take zinc supplements with meals to avoid stomach upsets. For best absorption, don't take zinc with a high-fiber meal. The fiber will reduce the amount you absorb.

Taking zinc in large doses (more than 150 mg per day) for a long period of time could lead to problems absorbing copper, lowered immunity, and lowered HDL cholesterol levels. Large doses of zinc could be toxic. It would be almost impossible to take enough zinc supplements to poison yourself—you'd throw it all up long before that.

**Warning!**
Do not take zinc if you are taking the antibiotic drug tetracycline. The zinc will keep the tetracycline from being absorbed into your bloodstream.

# Fighting Off Colds

The next time you catch a cold, zinc could help you get over it quicker. Your immune system needs zinc to work at top efficiency. In fact, your infection-fighting white blood cells contain a lot of the zinc in your body. Giving them a zinc boost when you have a cold seems to help them fight off the virus faster. It also seems to reduce cold symptoms such as a runny nose, coughing, and hoarseness.

For treating a cold with zinc, the best approach seems to be lozenges made of zinc gluconate with glycine. Put the lozenge in your mouth and let it dissolve slowly. Don't chew it or swallow it. Repeat every two hours or so for one or two days only. Adults shouldn't take more than 12 lozenges a day. Limit children to no more than six a day. You can buy zinc lozenges in any health-food store; many pharmacies now carry them as well. Most lozenges contain 22 or 23 mg—anything less won't help you very much. Just swallowing zinc supplements won't help your cold symptoms at all.

There are some drawbacks to zinc lozenges. Even though they're flavored to disguise their awful taste, they can leave a bad aftertaste in your mouth. If you take a lot of them they can affect your sense of taste and smell—your sense of taste and smell should return to normal a few days after you stop taking the extra zinc.

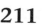

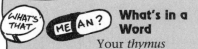

**What's in a Word**

Your *thymus gland* is a small but very important organ found in your neck just above your breastbone. It plays a very important role in your health by making some of the hormones that tell your immune system what to do. When you're born, your thymus is quite large. By the time you're a teenager, it's shrunk a lot, and by the time you're forty, it's shrunk even more. For a long time researchers thought that was normal, but recent studies show that zinc can revitalize your thymus and get it working again.

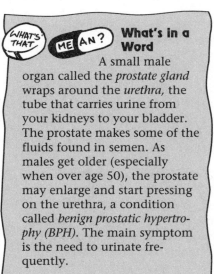

**What's in a Word**

A small male organ called the *prostate gland* wraps around the *urethra*, the tube that carries urine from your kidneys to your bladder. The prostate makes some of the fluids found in semen. As males get older (especially when over age 50), the prostate may enlarge and start pressing on the urethra, a condition called *benign prostatic hypertrophy (BPH)*. The main symptom is the need to urinate frequently.

Zinc may be a very useful immune system booster in general. It seems to give a real boost to your *thymus gland,* especially if you're over age 40. By then, your thymus may have naturally shrunk quite a bit, so it's not producing the hormones it used to—and those hormones stimulate your body to produce infection-fighting blood cells. Getting a little extra zinc—just 15 to 30 mg—every day may get your thymus moving again. That means your immune system will work better and fight off illness faster.

# Zinc Club for Men

Are the guys just kidding around when they tell you to eat oysters for a better sex life? Believe it or not, they're right. Oysters are by far the food highest in zinc—and you need plenty of zinc to make testosterone and other male hormones. You also need zinc to make healthy sperm and semen, so getting more zinc in your diet could help solve male infertility. In one study, men with low sperm counts took zinc supplements for six weeks. Their testosterone levels and sperm counts went up, and nearly half of them had pregnant wives before the study was over.

Zinc can also be very helpful for treating and possibly even preventing prostate problems. Your *prostate gland* is a small organ that wraps around the *urethra* at the neck of the bladder. As you get older, your prostate often naturally gets bigger, a condition called *benign prostatic hypertrophy (BPH)*. The enlarged gland squeezes the urethra and causes a need to go frequently (and also other urination problems). Sometimes the problems get so bad that medication or even surgery is needed.

A healthy prostate gland naturally has a lot of zinc in it, but men with BPH often have low zinc levels. Taking an extra 50 mg a day of zinc supplements seems to help some men with mild BPH by shrinking the prostate. It doesn't press as much against the urethra, and you can urinate more easily. It takes a while for the zinc to kick in—stay with the supplements for three to six months before you decide they're not working.

Finally, guys, despite rumors to the contrary, zinc doesn't stop balding or restore lost hair.

# Healthy Skin, Nails, and Hair

Zinc is really important for healthy skin. A shortage of zinc is often behind minor skin rashes and irritations that don't seem to have any real cause. These often clear up when patients start eating a diet higher in zinc or take zinc supplements. Zinc also sometimes helps people with psoriasis.

### Food for Thought

Teenagers might be able to ward off the dreaded zits with zinc. Many teenagers, especially boys aged 13 and 14, are low on zinc because there isn't enough in their diet. We know that a zinc deficiency causes skin problems. Are the two related? Many doctors think so and recommend more high-zinc foods for teens with severe acne. Prescription zinc ointments also seem to help prevent acne blemishes.

Sometimes a zinc shortage causes white spots on the fingernails or nails that break easily. Adding zinc to your diet could clear up the problem.

A form of zinc is used in some dandruff shampoos to control flaking. It's possible that you also absorb some of the zinc into your body through your scalp if you use one of these shampoos, but don't count on it. On the other hand, just eating more high-zinc foods or taking zinc supplements won't solve your dandruff problem.

# Zinc for Healing

Zinc is essential for healing wounds. Several studies have shown that patients recovering from surgery heal faster if they get enough zinc. The effect is dramatic if the patient was low on zinc to begin with; it didn't work as well on patients who had good zinc levels. If you're scheduled for an operation, talk to your doctor about taking zinc supplements for a few weeks before and after. It could make a difference in how quickly you recover.

# Think Zinc for Other Problems

Some zinc zanies recommend it for all sorts of health problems. Here are some ways zinc may make a difference:

➤ **Diabetes.** Some diabetics may be too low on zinc because they don't absorb it well and also excrete it quickly. Zinc supplements could help. Zinc might also help with two other problems diabetics often have: slow wound healing and frequent infections.

➤ **Macular degeneration.** This serious eye problem is the leading cause of blindness in the elderly. Your eyes naturally contain a lot of zinc—and a lot of it is concentrated in your retina, the part of your eye affected by macular degeneration. Zinc supplements could help prevent or slow down vision loss from macular degeneration.

➤ **Memory.** Can't remember where you left the car keys? Maybe you're not getting enough zinc. People who get the RDA do better on memory tests than those who don't.

Does zinc help Alzheimer's disease, rheumatoid arthritis, anorexia, or liver disease? Does it prevent cancer? Probably not, but we don't know for sure—the information in all cases is contradictory.

## The Least You Need to Know

➤ You need zinc to make over 200 different enzymes and many hormones, including testosterone.

➤ The adult RDA for zinc is 15 mg for men and 12 mg for women.

➤ Oysters are very high in zinc. Lean meats, beans, nuts, and seeds are good food sources.

➤ Zinc can help relieve cold symptoms and boost your immune system.

➤ Zinc can help male infertility and can relieve symptoms of benign prostatic hypertrophy.

➤ Zinc is important for healthy skin, hair, and nails and helps wounds heal faster.

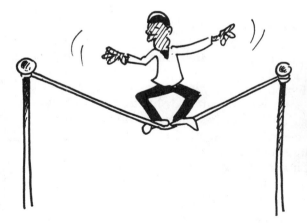

# Electrolytes: Keeping Your Body in Balance

## In This Chapter

➤ Why potassium, sodium, and chloride are vital to your health

➤ Why you need to keep your electrolytes in balance

➤ How sodium raises your blood pressure and how potassium lowers it

➤ How potassium can prevent strokes

Here's a chapter that should get you all charged up about an easy way to improve your health. We're talking about your electrolytes—the potassium, sodium, and chloride in your body. These minerals are electrically charged, so they can carry nutrients into and out of your cells. They also carry messages along your nerves and help control your heartbeat. Most important of all, your electrolytes have a lot to do with controlling your blood pressure.

Eat too much sodium and not enough potassium, and your blood pressure could shoot up to unhealthy levels. Cut back on the sodium and increase your potassium, though, and you'll be helping your blood pressure stay normal. The most electrifying thing of all is that you can do that easily, starting today, just by making some easy changes in your diet. And if you keep your blood pressure where it should be, other health problems, like heart disease and kidney trouble, may never get started.

# What's an Electrolyte?

*Electrolytes* are minerals that dissolve in water and carry electrical charges. In your body, potassium, sodium, and chloride are the electrolyte minerals. And since you're made mostly of water, these minerals are found everywhere in your body: inside your cells, in the spaces between cells, in your blood, in your lymph, and everywhere else. Each tiny particle of sodium and potassium in your body has a positive charge; each tiny particle of chloride has a negative one. Because electrolytes have electrical charges, they can move easily back and forth through your cell membranes. Why is that so important? Because as they move into a cell, they carry other nutrients with them and as they move out, they carry out waste products and excess water.

Potassium, sodium, and chloride are very closely linked—so closely that we really can't talk about them separately. Here's why: To keep your body in balance, your cells need to have a lot of potassium inside them and a lot of sodium in the fluids outside them. To keep the balance, sodium and potassium constantly move back and forth through your cell membranes.

You can see the link between sodium and potassium. Where does the chloride come in? Sodium combines easily with other elements. Here's a good example: Remember that familiar formula NaCl from science class? Na is the chemical symbol for sodium, while Cl means chloride. Put them together and you have sodium chloride, better known as ordinary table salt. You mostly need the sodium found in salt (table salt is about 40 percent sodium), but your body also needs the chloride. Among other things, you use it to make hydrochloric acid, the powerful digestive juice in your stomach.

> **WHAT'S THAT MEAN?**
>
> **What's in a Word**
>
> Minerals that dissolve in water and carry an electrical charge (positive or negative) are called *electrolytes*. The electrolytes in your body are potassium, sodium, and chloride.

> **WHAT'S THAT MEAN?**
>
> **What's in a Word**
>
> The chemical symbol for potassium is K, from the Latin word *kalium,* which means alkali, or a mineral salt. The chemical symbol for sodium is Na, from *natrium,* the Greek name for sodium. It's a lot easier to remember the chemical symbol for chloride—it's simply Cl. By the way, the chloride in your body isn't the same thing at all as the chlorine used to kill germs in drinking water and swimming pools.

# Why You Need Electrolytes

All three electrolytes—potassium, sodium, and chloride—keep the amount of water in your body in balance, carry impulses along your nerves, help make your muscles contract and relax, and keep your body from becoming too acidic or alkaline. You need electrolytes to carry glucose (blood sugar) and other nutrients into your cells and to carry waste products and extra water out again. Electrolytes also regulate your blood pressure and your heartbeat. In fact, sodium and potassium are so important for controlling your blood pressure that we'll talk about that more later on in this chapter.

# The RDAs for Electrolytes

Now that you know how important electrolytes are for keeping you alive, here's a surprise: There are no RDAs for them. Why? Every single living cell on earth—plant or animal—needs potassium, sodium, and chloride, which means that there's plenty of them in your food. Because the electrolytes are so easy to eat, nobody ever really gets deficient. By the logic of the RDAs, then, there's no reason to bother setting a minimum amount, since everybody gets whatever it is anyway. It makes sense—and as we'll explain later on in this chapter, too much sodium, not too little, is a much bigger health problem.

Even though there aren't any RDAs for potassium, sodium, and chloride, there are estimates of the minimum amounts you need to have. When you look at the chart, you'll see that the amounts are really pretty small.

| Estimated Minimum Requirements for Potassium, Sodium, and Chloride | | | |
|---|---|---|---|
| Age | Potassium in mg | Sodium in mg | Chloride in mg |
| *Infants* | | | |
| 0–0.5 year | 500 | 120 | 180 |
| 0.5–1 year | 700 | 200 | 300 |
| *Children and Adults* | | | |
| 1 year | 1,000 | 225 | 350 |
| 2–5 years | 1,400 | 300 | 500 |
| 6–9 | 1,600 | 400 | 600 |
| 10+ | 2,000 | 500 | 750 |

For the sake of comparison, figure there's about 3,000 mg of sodium in a teaspoon of salt. To stay healthy, you need to get less than a quarter of a teaspoon of salt every day. Many researchers think the sodium requirement is on the high side and that you can be perfectly healthy on only 200 mg (about one-fifteenth of a teaspoon) a day.

# Are You Deficient?

Ordinarily, you can't be deficient in electrolytes. You don't really need that much to begin with, and everyone gets plenty from their food.

The one exception is if you get sick with something that makes you vomit a lot or have severe diarrhea. In that case, you might quickly lose so many electrolytes (especially potassium) with the fluid that you run short. Unless you replace the fluids and electrolytes quickly this can be serious, especially in small children.

**217**

> ### Food for Thought
>
> If you have severe vomiting or diarrhea, you need to replace the electro-lytes and water you lose. Here's a good way to do it: In a large glass, com-bine 8 ounces of apple, orange, or any other fruit juice with half a teaspoon of honey and a pinch of ordinary table salt. In another glass, combine 8 ounces of plain water and a pinch of baking soda (sodium bicarbonate). Take a few sips from one glass, then a few sips from the other until you've drunk them both. The fruit juice contains the potassium you need, while the salt and baking soda provide sodium. The sugar from the juice and honey helps you absorb the electrolytes.

If you're low on potassium, you might get muscle cramps in your legs (this sometimes happens to athletes who sweat a lot in really hot weather). If you're low on potassium, you'll feel nauseous and very weak and listless. You'll start to feel better as soon as you get some more potassium into your system. In really severe cases, your heart could fail, but that's very unlikely for most people.

Sodium and chloride deficiencies are uncommon, since you get both elements from salt. Even when you sweat buckets, you still have plenty of salt in your body. It's much more important to replace the lost water.

## Potassium Pitfalls

Sodium, chloride, and potassium work together to keep the amount of water in your cells and around them (like in your blood) just what it ought to be. Sometimes the water balance gets a little out of whack. Extra hormones might make you hold on to too much water and get a little bloated. This often happens to women before and during their menstrual period. To relieve the discomfort, some women use nonprescription diuretic drugs ("water pills") and herbs such as buchu and uva ursi ("dieter's tea"). Diuretics reduce the amount of water in your body by making you produce more urine, but that can also make you excrete more electrolytes than you take in. You could accidentally make yourself sick, especially if you take too much or use them too often. Avoid using nonprescription diuretics—they may do more harm than good.

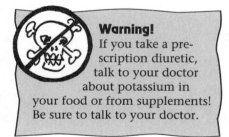

**Warning!**
If you take a pre-scription diuretic, talk to your doctor about potassium in your food or from supplements! Be sure to talk to your doctor.

If you have a heart condition, you might retain too much water because your heart isn't pumping very well. That can put a serious strain on it, so your doctor may prescribe a diuretic drug. Diuretics are also often prescribed to treat high blood pressure.

If your doctor prescribes a diuretic, it may be a "potassium-sparing" one such as triamterene (Dyrenium®) that doesn't affect your potassium levels. Other diuretics such as furosemide (Lasix®) *do* affect your potassium levels. If you need to take a diuretic that affects your potassium, your doctor may also tell you to eat potassium-rich foods or prescribe a potassium supplement.

## Other Prescription Drugs

Digoxin (Lanoxin®) is a digitalis—type drug that is often prescribed for people with heart failure and heart rhythm problems. If you also take a diuretic that lowers your potassium level, the combination of low potassium and digoxin could make your heart stop suddenly. On the other hand, if your potassium level gets too high, it could combine with the digoxin and make your heart rhythm get out of control. So, if you take any sort of digitalis-type drug for your heart, follow your doctor's instructions and be very careful about your potassium. Don't use salt substitutes, since they simply substitute potassium for sodium.

> **Warning!**
> If you take digoxin or any other digitalis-type heart medicine, talk to your doctor about potassium in your food or from supplements!

Another type of drug called an ACE inhibitor (Captopril® and Lotensin® are two well-known brands) is often prescribed to treat heart problems and high blood pressure. These drugs can make your potassium level go up. If you also take a potassium supplement or use a salt substitute, you could make your potassium level skyrocket—and that could make your heart beat irregularly or even stop. If you take an ACE inhibitor, follow your doctor's instructions and be very careful about your potassium. Don't use salt substitutes.

> **Warning!**
> If you take an ACE inhibitor drug for high blood pressure or your heart, talk to your doctor about potassium in your food or from supplements!

## Eating Your Electrolytes

Potassium is found in almost all foods, including fruits, vegetables, beans, meat, milk, and grains. Beans, fruits, and vegetables (especially potatoes) are the best natural sources. Some sodium and chloride are found in almost all foods.

We get plenty of both in the form of sodium chloride—the chemical name for plain old table salt. In fact, salt is so common in foods that we're not going to list any here. We'll stick to foods that are good sources of potassium.

> **Now You're Cooking**
> Molasses is a surprisingly good source of potassium. There's 293 mg in just one tablespoon of refined molasses, and 498 mg in the stronger-tasting blackstrap molasses.

## The Potassium in Food

| Food | Amount | Potassium in mg |
|---|---|---|
| Avocado | 1/2 medium | 550 |
| Banana | 1 medium | 451 |
| Beef, ground | 3 ounces | 205 |
| Black beans | 1 cup | 801 |
| Broccoli, cooked | 1/2 cup | 228 |
| Cantaloupe | 1 cup | 494 |
| Carrot, raw | 1 medium | 233 |
| Cauliflower, cooked | 1/2 cup | 200 |
| Chicken | 3 ounces | 195 |
| Chickpeas | 1 cup | 477 |
| Corn | 1/2 cup | 204 |
| Flounder | 3 ounces | 292 |
| Kidney beans | 1 cup | 713 |
| Kiwi | 1 medium | 252 |
| Lentils | 1 cup | 731 |
| Milk | 8 ounces | 381 |
| Okra | 1/2 cup | 257 |
| Orange | 1 medium | 250 |
| Orange juice | 8 ounces | 474 |
| Potato, baked with skin | 1 medium | 844 |
| Prune juice | 8 ounces | 706 |
| Spinach, cooked | 1/2 cup | 419 |
| Strawberries | 1 cup | 247 |
| Sweet potato | 1 medium | 397 |
| Tomato | 1 medium | 273 |
| Tomato juice | 6 ounces | 658 |
| Watermelon | 1 cup | 186 |
| Wheat germ | 1/4 cup | 259 |

# Getting the Most from Electrolytes

We don't recommend taking potassium supplements unless your doctor prescribes them for you. If you think you need extra potassium, the best way is to eat it. The nonprescription potassium supplements sold in health food stores contain only 99 mg (the FDA won't let them be bigger). That's about the amount of potassium in two big bites of a banana or a couple big swallows of orange juice—without the stomach upset potassium pills can cause. You easily excrete any excess potassium in your urine.

There's almost never any need for extra sodium or chloride. Most of us get plenty of salt from our food (or even too much) and don't need extra even in very hot weather or when we're sweating a lot. An exception might be someone running an ultramarathon in very hot weather and losing a lot of electrolytes from excess sweating.

# Shaking Up Salt

Everybody tells you to eat less salt, but it's hard to avoid. We sprinkle salt on our food as a seasoning and it is added to almost every processed food. Condiments like ketchup and soy sauce are loaded with salt. Baked goods made with sodium bicarbonate are full of sodium. And you can tell from their names that many food additives, like monosodium glutamate (MSG) and sodium nitrite, have a lot of sodium. In fact, salt is so common that the typical American diet contains between ten and fifteen times the RDA for sodium, or between 5,000 and 7,500 mg, or between almost two and four teaspoons of salt every day.

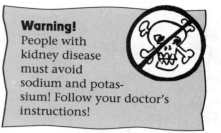

**Warning!**
People with kidney disease must avoid sodium and potassium! Follow your doctor's instructions!

**Quack, Quack**
If you sweat a lot from an athletic activity or hard work in hot weather—do you need those expensive sports drinks? No way! Drink a lot of plain water instead. It's important to replace the lost fluid. If you want to replace the lost potassium, have a piece of fruit or some OJ—there's over 500 mg in a cup.

Too much sodium and not enough potassium are the culprits behind many cases of high blood pressure (we'll talk more about that soon). For now, let's just say that almost all doctors and researchers agree: We eat too much salt. Cutting back on salt could reduce your chances of high blood pressure, stroke, kidney problems, and heart disease. It's an easy way to improve your health.

Step one is to just put the salt shaker away. We add salt to food to season it, not because we need it—our foods naturally have all the salt we need. If you stop adding salt, your food may taste a little bland at first, but after a few days you won't notice the difference.

The next step is to cut back on processed foods that are high in salt—lunch meats and snack foods would be good places to start. Other easy steps are choosing no-salt or low-salt foods. Try switching to unsalted butter, for example.

About half the extra salt we get comes from processed foods, but picking a low-sodium version can be a little confusing. Plenty of processed foods today claim to be low in sodium, but the labels all seem to say different things. Here's how the FDA says to sort out the claims:

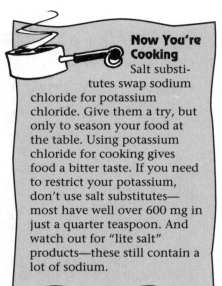

**Now You're Cooking**

Salt substitutes swap sodium chloride for potassium chloride. Give them a try, but only to season your food at the table. Using potassium chloride for cooking gives food a bitter taste. If you need to restrict your potassium, don't use salt substitutes—most have well over 600 mg in just a quarter teaspoon. And watch out for "lite salt" products—these still contain a lot of sodium.

➤ **Sodium-free or salt-free.** Less than 5 mg per serving.

➤ **Very low sodium.** 35 mg or less per serving.

➤ **Low sodium.** 140 mg or less per serving.

➤ **Light in sodium.** At least 50 percent less sodium per serving than the food ordinarily has.

➤ **Lightly salted.** At least 50 percent less sodium per serving than the food ordinarily has.

➤ **Reduced or less sodium.** At least 25 percent less sodium per serving than the food ordinarily has.

➤ **Unsalted, no salt added, without added salt.** No salt has been added during processing, even though salt is ordinarily added to that food.

There's one more requirement. If the label mentions only lowered salt or sodium, a line in the Nutrition Facts panel must say "Not a sodium-free food" or "Not for control of sodium in the diet." Still confused? We're not surprised. Here's a good way to choose: Look for the words "free" or "low" to get the least sodium.

# Electrifying News on High Blood Pressure

We know from many studies that people who eat a low potassium, high sodium diet are more likely to have high blood pressure. We know that if you already have high blood pressure, eating less sodium helps bring it down. We know that uncontrolled high blood pressure can lead to heart disease, kidney disease, and strokes. What we still don't know is exactly why sodium has such an impact on your blood pressure.

The balance between your potassium and sodium levels is important for keeping your blood pressure down. Many researchers believe that a good balance is roughly five parts potassium or even more to one part sodium. Unfortunately, our high-salt diets give many of us balances that are more like one part potassium to two parts sodium, or twice as much sodium as potassium. It's not surprising that one in four American adults—some 50 million people—has high blood pressure. Among adults over age 65, more than half have high blood pressure.

About 10 percent of the people who have high blood pressure are salt sensitive—sodium in their diet makes their blood pressure zoom up. These people should try very hard to reduce their sodium intake. Older people and African-Americans are most likely to be salt sensitive, but it makes sense for everyone to cut back. Studies show that overall, the average person who consumes less salt has lower blood pressure. In fact, a 1997 study in the prestigious British medical journal *The Lancet* suggests that older people who lower their salt intake also sharply lower their risk of stroke, even if they don't have high blood pressure.

Just cutting back on sodium isn't the whole solution. Many people with high blood pressure also benefit from *increasing* their potassium. When they do, they get a more natural balance in their electrolytes, and their blood pressure goes down. You don't need pills or supplements to get the benefits: just eating fewer salty foods and more foods rich in potassium will help. In many cases, lowering your sodium intake to under 2,000 mg a day and raising your potassium intake to over 3,500 mg a day has a very beneficial effect, especially for older people.

Proof that this works came in 1997 as part of the important Dietary Approaches to Stop Hypertension (DASH) study. Some people in the study ate a typical American diet; others ate a diet that was much lower in fat and much higher in fruits and vegetables—which are high in potassium. All the people in the study got about 3,000 mg a day of sodium but the people who ate the typical American diet got only 1,700 mg of potassium, while the people who ate lots more fruits and vegetables got about 4,700 mg of potassium. Guess whose blood pressure dropped? You're right. The typical Americans didn't improve at all, but the fruit and vegetable eaters saw their blood pressure drop substantially. And the higher their blood pressure was to begin with, the more it dropped.

What if you already take medicine for high blood pressure? Keep taking it as you cut back on sodium. Reducing your sodium almost always makes the drug work better. Cut back enough and make some lifestyle changes, and you might be able to take a smaller dose or maybe even stop taking medicine altogether. *Never* stop taking any medicine, but especially high blood pressure drugs, on your own. Always talk to your doctor first.

> **Warning!**
> Of course, less salt and more potassium won't help much if you don't also make lifestyle changes to help your blood pressure. Doctors recommend losing weight, quitting smoking, drinking less alcohol, and getting more exercise.

# Preventing Strokes with Potassium

Even if you don't have high blood pressure, potassium could help protect you against having a stroke. If your potassium intake is low, your odds of a stroke go up, no matter what other risk factors you may have, such a cigarette smoking or being overweight. According to one long-term study of older adults, just one daily serving of a potassium-rich food could cut your risk of a stroke by an amazing 40 percent. That's just one banana, glass of orange juice, or baked potato. And if you eat more than one serving a day, your odds against a stroke might improve even more.

# The Least You Need to Know

➤ Sodium, chloride, and potassium are electrolytes, minerals that have electrical charges and carry nutrients into and out of your cells.

➤ Electrolytes help regulate your blood pressure and heartbeat.

➤ There are no RDAs for potassium, sodium, and chloride. Most people get plenty of potassium from their food and too much sodium from salt (sodium chloride).

➤ Good food sources of potassium include beans, fruits, and vegetables.

➤ Too much sodium in your diet may raise your blood pressure to unhealthy levels, but potassium in your diet could help lower it.

➤ Potassium could help protect you against having a stroke.

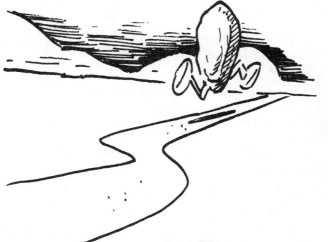

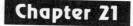

# The Trace Minerals: A Little Goes a Long Way

## In This Chapter

- ➤ What trace minerals are and why you need them
- ➤ The roles of iron, iodine, chromium, and selenium
- ➤ The roles of boron, copper, manganese, molybdenum, and other less important trace minerals
- ➤ Trace minerals you should avoid

True or false: Your body needs arsenic. Amazingly, the answer is true! Trace minerals—minerals you need in only tiny amounts—are full of surprises like that. Most of the trace minerals in your body do many important things, from carrying oxygen to building your bones to making the hormones and enzymes that tell your body what to do. You also have some trace minerals that don't seem to do anything useful at all.

The world of trace minerals is still being explored. We weren't even sure you needed boron, for example, until well into the 1980s. More roles for these tiny powerhouses are sure to be discovered as research continues.

# What's a Trace Mineral?

If you have less than a teaspoon of a mineral in your body, it's a *trace mineral*—one that you need, but only in very small amounts. In the human body, fifteen substances are considered necessary trace minerals (check out the chart for the whole list).

Although you need all the trace minerals, some are more important than others. Zinc, for example, is so important that we gave it its own chapter (see Chapter 19). Some of the other trace minerals, like nickel, are so minor and so easy to get from your food that there just isn't a lot to say about them. We'll concentrate on the trace minerals that could make a real difference to your health. Not every trace mineral has an RDA or even a Safe and Adequate Intake (SAI) amount. We just don't know about some of them, like nickel and boron.

| The Trace Minerals | | |
| --- | --- | --- |
| **Mineral** | **Function** | **RDA or SAI** |
| Boron | Builds healthy bones | None |
| Chromium | Controls blood sugar | 50–200 mcg |
| Cobalt | Needed for cobalamin (Vitamin $B_{12}$) | None |
| Copper | Needed for antioxidant enzymes, red blood cells, other enzymes | 1.5–3.0 mg |
| Fluoride | Protects against tooth decay, builds healthy bones | 1.5–4.0 mg |
| Iodine | Needed for thyroid hormones | 150 mcg |
| Iron | Needed for hemoglobin in red blood cells | 10–15 mg |
| Manganese | Needed for protein digestion, tissue formation | 2.5–5.0 mg |
| Molybdenum | Normal growth and development | 75–250 mcg |
| Nickel | Needed to make some enzymes and hormones | None |
| Selenium | Needed for antioxidant enzyme glutathione | 55–70 mcg |
| Silicon | Builds healthy bones | None |
| Tin | Unknown | None |
| Vanadium | Unknown | None |
| Zinc | Building a healthy immune system | 12–15 mg |

# Why You Need Trace Minerals

You might not need much of a trace mineral, but some are especially important when it comes to making the many different enzymes, hormones, and other chemical messengers your body uses every minute of every day. You need iodine to make thyroid hormones, which in turn control some very important parts of your metabolism, including your body weight. You need the trace mineral iron to carry oxygen in your blood and also to make other enzymes. Some trace minerals, such as selenium, are used to make the powerful natural antioxidants that protect you against free radicals. And some trace minerals work closely with vitamins to make them more active and long-lasting.

We still don't completely understand the roles of some other trace minerals, such as manganese. We know that you'll get health problems if you don't get the tiny amount you need, but we're still not sure why.

# RDAs and Safe and Adequate Intakes

In general, you need to be cautious about trace minerals. The toxic amount of a trace mineral often isn't that much higher than the safe amount. The adult RDA for selenium, for example, is between 55 and 70 mcg. The toxic amount is about 600 mcg, or less than ten times the RDA. Likewise, too much iron can be more harmful than too little.

Most people get plenty of all the trace minerals from their food and don't need to take supplements. If you feel you need more of a particular trace element, try to get it from your food whenever possible.

# Are You Deficient?

When was the last time you ever heard of anyone being deficient in copper? When was the last time you heard the word vanadium? As a rule, most people have all the trace minerals they need. With the exception of iron, you're not very likely to be deficient in any of them.

The bigger question is whether getting more of a trace mineral improves your health. Here too there just isn't a lot of solid evidence. In some cases—chromium, for example—it's possible that more is better. On the other hand, because we don't always know what too much might do, it's always best to be cautious and avoid super large doses of trace minerals.

# Eating Your Trace Minerals

Trace minerals are found in small amounts in a wide variety of foods. The amounts in your food generally come from the soil where the food is grown. Brazil nuts are high in

**Quack, Quack**

Some supplement pushers claim you need their super-duper (and expensive) mineral supplements because foods don't have enough minerals. Supposedly the soil they are grown in has been "depleted" of minerals by modern farming practices. These pushers are trying to confuse you by claiming that natural variations in soil minerals are caused by farmers—and that these variations have a bad effect on you. Don't be taken in.

selenium because the soil in the part of Brazil where they grow is high in selenium.

Trace minerals aren't evenly distributed around the world. To take selenium as an example again, parts of China have almost none—and some people there have a type of heart disease caused by severe selenium deficiency. Parts of the western United States, on the other hand, have very high selenium levels, and animals that graze on grass there sometimes get an overdose that causes illness and deformities.

Even if you eat a pretty unbalanced diet that's low in fresh fruits and vegetables, you're not very likely to be deficient in trace minerals. Some of them are inescapable. Iodine, for example, is added to almost all table salt—and as you know from reading Chapter 20, we all get more than enough salt every day. The water you drink gives you some of the trace minerals. Fluoride is often added to municipal water supplies, and chromium is found in "hard" water.

# Getting the Most from Trace Minerals

Most good daily multi supplements contain at least some of the trace minerals. The amounts vary—read the labels. A lot of multi supplements contain at least the RDA for iron. As we'll discuss a little further on, this may not be a good idea for some people. Again, read the label carefully.

Sometimes combination supplements contain one or two trace elements that are especially important. For example, calcium supplements sometimes come with magnesium and boron, because these two minerals are needed to build healthy bones. These supplements are on the expensive side. Do you really need the trace minerals as well? Probably not, especially if you also take a daily multi supplement.

There may be times when you want to take additional supplements of a particular trace mineral. Be very cautious here—take the smallest possible dose. Too much of a trace mineral could be as harmful as too little. Whenever possible, try to get your trace minerals from your food instead of pills.

# Singling Out Sulfur

Ok, we lied in the chapter title—sulfur isn't a trace mineral at all. About one-quarter of one percent of your body is made up of sulfur, so you have well over a teaspoon of the stuff in you. We're sticking it here because you need it and we don't know where else to put it.

Even though you need sulfur to make many amino acids and natural antioxidants (we'll talk more about this in Chapters 22 and 23) and the B vitamins thiamin, biotin, and pantothenic acid, there isn't much to say here. Sulfur is so common in your food that no one has ever been deficient in it, so no one has ever bothered to figure out an RDA or even a Safe and Adequate Intake for it. You also can't overdose on sulfur—you excrete any excess in your urine. Vitamin manufacturers don't generally make it into supplements, and reference books that give the breakdown of nutrients in food don't bother listing it. Good food sources of sulfur include eggs (sulfur is the awful smell in rotten eggs), clams, fish, lean beef, milk, and dairy products. Sulfur is also found in smaller amounts in all plant foods, especially cabbage, beans, garlic, onions, and wheat germ.

# Iron: Basic for Blood

Iron barely qualifies as a trace mineral, because you have just under a teaspoon of it in your body. You need it chiefly to carry oxygen in your blood. Every one of your red blood cells contains a protein called *hemoglobin*—and four atoms of iron are attached to every hemoglobin molecule. In your lungs, oxygen molecules attach to the iron atoms and are carried to your cells. When the oxygen reaches its destination, it's swapped for the waste carbon dioxide and carried back to your lungs. You get rid of it by exhaling.

How much iron you have determines how much oxygen gets to the rest of your body. Not enough iron, and you start making fewer red blood cells. Not enough red blood cells, and you become anemic— weak, tired, pale, short of breath.

Just how common is "iron-poor blood"? Not as common as all the advertising says, but common enough to be concerned. You could be low on iron for a long time before you become anemic. An important 1997 study found that one out of ten American women and small children were deficient in iron—or about 700,000 toddlers and 7.8 million women! Of those, about 240,000 toddlers and 3.3 million women were anemic. The results were so shocking that a national screening program for iron deficiency is being considered. Babies and toddlers need plenty of iron because they're growing so fast—and if they don't get it, they may fall behind in their mental development and never catch up. Teenaged girls need extra iron for growth, while women in general need extra iron to make up for the blood lost each month to menstruation. Pregnant and nursing women also need extra, because they're passing a lot of their iron on to their babies. Anyone, male or female, who is very athletic also needs extra.

**What's in a Word**
*Hemoglobin* is the oxygen-carrying protein that gives your red blood cells their color. Every molecule of hemoglobin has four atoms of iron in it.

**Warning!**
About 1.5 million Americans (mostly men) have a rare inherited condition called *hemochromatosis* that makes them build up too much iron. The extra iron can cause serious heart and liver problems. If you have this condition, you need to avoid iron.

# The RDA for Iron

The RDA for iron was lowered in 1989, once again showing that the RDAs are bare minimums and far from ideal—especially for women. Many doctors now suggest getting at least the RDA for men and closer to 20 mg a day for women. In general, that level or even a much larger dose—up to 75 mg a day—is quite safe.

| The RDA for Iron | |
| --- | --- |
| Age/Sex | Iron in mg |
| *Infants* | |
| 0–0.5 year | 6 |
| 0.5–1 year | 10 |
| *Children* | |
| 1–10 years | 10 |
| *Young Adults and Adults* | |
| Men 11–18 years | 12 |
| Men 19+ | 10 |
| Women 11–50 | 15 |
| Women 51+ | 10 |
| Pregnant women | 30 |
| Nursing women | 15 |

# Eating Your Iron

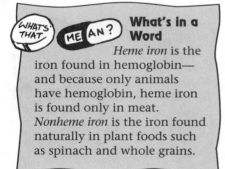

**What's in a Word**

*Heme iron* is the iron found in hemoglobin—and because only animals have hemoglobin, heme iron is found only in meat. *Nonheme iron* is the iron found naturally in plant foods such as spinach and whole grains.

The average American diet has about 6 mg of iron for every 1,000 calories you eat. That means you need to eat about 2,500 calories a day to get enough iron. Because women generally eat less than 2,000 calories a day, you need to be extra sure you're getting enough iron by choosing iron-rich foods.

Iron is found in many common foods. It falls into two categories: *heme iron,* found in meat, and *nonheme iron,* found in plant foods. You absorb heme iron from your food better than nonheme iron, but vegetarians don't need to worry—many delicious plant foods are high in iron. You can also increase the iron content of vegetable foods by using cast-iron cookware.

Rich sources of heme iron include organ meats, lean beef, chicken, oysters, and pork. Good sources of nonheme iron are whole grains, peas, beans, spinach, nuts, and blackstrap (unrefined) molasses. One of the best sources of iron is cream of wheat cereal—there's over 7 mg in six ounces. Many cold breakfast cereals such as bran flakes also have plenty of iron, both naturally and from added supplements. You're sure to find iron-rich foods you like in the chart.

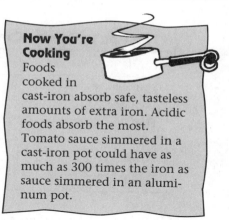

**Now You're Cooking**

Foods cooked in cast-iron absorb safe, tasteless amounts of extra iron. Acidic foods absorb the most. Tomato sauce simmered in a cast-iron pot could have as much as 300 times the iron as sauce simmered in an aluminum pot.

## The Iron in Foods

| Food | Amount | Iron in mg |
|---|---|---|
| Almonds, dry roasted | 1 ounce | 1.1 |
| Barley | 1 cup | 2.1 |
| Beef, ground | 3 ounces | 1.8 |
| Black beans | 1 cup | 3.6 |
| Bread, whole wheat | 1 slice | 0.9 |
| Broccoli, cooked | 1/2 cup | 0.6 |
| Brussels sprouts | 1/2 cup | 0.9 |
| Chicken | 3 ounces | 1.1 |
| Chick peas | 1 cup | 3.2 |
| Kale | 1/2 cup | 0.6 |
| Kidney beans | 1 cup | 3.2 |
| Lima beans | 1/2 cup | 1.8 |
| Liver, beef | 3 ounces | 5.8 |
| Liver, chicken | 3 ounces | 7.3 |
| Molasses, blackstrap | 1 tablespoon | 3.5 |
| Oysters, raw | 6 medium | 5.6 |
| Peanut butter | 2 tablespoons | 0.5 |
| Pecans | 1 ounce | 0.6 |
| Potato, baked | 1 medium | 2.7 |
| Prune juice | 8 ounces | 3.0 |
| Raisins, seedless | 2/3 cup | 2.1 |
| Spinach, cooked | 1/2 cup | 3.2 |

*continues*

### The Iron in Foods   Continued

| Food | Amount | Iron in mg |
|------|--------|-----------|
| Strawberries | 1 cup | 0.6 |
| Tomato | 1 medium | 0.5 |
| Tomato juice | 6 ounces | 1.1 |
| Walnuts | 1 ounce | 0.7 |
| Wheat germ | 1/4 cup | 1.8 |
| White beans | 1 cup | 6.6 |

## Getting the Most from Iron

If you're anemic, your doctor will prescribe an iron supplement. If you want to get more iron by taking an over-the-counter supplement, look for one containing carbonyl iron—you absorb this form best. Other good choices are ferrous sulfate or ferrous gluconate. Time-release or enteric-coated iron tablets are a waste of money, because they'll pass through your system before you absorb much iron from them.

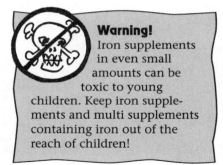

**Warning!**
Iron supplements in even small amounts can be toxic to young children. Keep iron supplements and multi supplements containing iron out of the reach of children!

Be careful with iron supplements—they can cause constipation or diarrhea. Don't exceed more than 30 mg a day. Take your iron supplements between meals. Some nutritionists recommend taking them with your Vitamin C supplements for better absorption.

A 1992 study of Finnish men suggested that high iron intake was related to heart disease. There's not a lot of other evidence for this, and so far it looks like getting the RDA or a bit more is perfectly safe for almost everyone.

## Iodine: Important for the Thyroid

You need iodine to make the *thyroid* hormones that regulate your body's metabolism. In fact, that's all iodine does for you, but it's a lot: Those thyroid hormones play a big role in your growth, cell reproduction, nerve functions, and how your cells use oxygen. One of the hormones, thyroxin, regulates how fast you use the energy from your food. If you don't have enough iodine, your thyroid swells up in an effort to make more hormones, a condition called *hypothyroidism.* The swelling is called a *goiter.*

# The RDA for Iodine

In total, you have between 20 and 30 mg of iodine in your body. The RDA is more than adequate to prevent a deficiency.

| The RDA for Iodine | |
| --- | --- |
| **Age/Sex** | **Iodine in mcg** |
| *Infants* | |
| 0–0.5 year | 40 |
| 0.5–1 year | 50 |
| *Children* | |
| 1–3 years | 70 |
| 4–6 | 90 |
| 7–10 | 120 |
| *Teens and Adults* | |
| 11+ | 150 |
| Pregnant women | 175 |
| Nursing women | 200 |

Until well into this century, iodine deficiency was a serious problem. People living in the Midwest and Great Lakes region, where the soil is very low in iodine, didn't get enough in their diets and often got goiters. Iodine deficiency during pregnancy causes a severe form of mental retardation called cretinism. To solve the iodine problem, in 1924 American salt producers began adding iodine to table salt at the rate of 400 mcg per teaspoon. Goiter and cretinism soon disappeared as public health problems and today iodine deficiency is very, very rare.

Iodine is added to a lot of daily multi supplements, but it's not really needed, because most people get more than enough from the salt in their food. Too much iodine (over 25 times the RDA) can also cause a goiter. More than 1,000 mg a day may also cause acne flare-ups in some people.

**What's in a Word**

Your *thyroid* is a small, butterfly-shaped gland found in your neck just below your Adam's apple. It produces hormones, including one called thyroxin that regulate your metabolism. A shortage of iodine can lead to *hypothyroidism,* or underactive thyroid. When that happens, your thyroid gland swells up and forms a lump called a *goiter* in your neck.

**Food for Thought**

Although iodine deficiency today is very rare, about six to seven million Americans, mostly women over age 40, have an underactive thyroid (hypothyroidism or myxedema) for other reasons. In most cases, there's no real reason for your thyroid to stop working well—it just does. Sometimes, again for no real reason, your own antibodies attack your thyroid and slowly destroy it, a condition called Hashimoto's disease. Symptoms include fatigue, cold hands and feet, constipation, dry skin, and hoarseness. Your doctor can easily do a blood test to see if your thyroid is working well. If it's underactive, you may need to take synthetic thyroid hormones.

# Chromium: Boon for Diabetics?

One of the hottest supplements today is chromium picolinate. Diabetics swear it helps them control their blood sugar better. Body builders swear it helps them build muscle faster. Some people claim it helps lower high cholesterol, while others claim it boost<u>s</u> your production of the anti-aging hormone DHEA.

Is chromium such a miracle mineral? Maybe, for some diabetics—but the other claims don't hold up as well.

Let's start with how much chromium you really need. Nobody knows. The Safe and Adequate range for adults is anywhere between 50 and 200 mcg. Why do you need it? In ways we still don't fully understand, chromium is involved with using fats, proteins, and carbohydrates. It's also needed to help the hormone insulin deliver glucose to your cells.

Because of the insulin connection, chromium is often touted as a way for diabetics to control their blood sugar. Chromium does seem to help some people with Type II, or adult-onset, diabetes, get glucose into their cells better. We suggest you skip chromium supplements and try to get between 50 and 200 mcg a day from your food. If you decide to try supplements, talk to your doctor first and keep a close eye on your blood sugar.

What about all those other things chromium is supposed to do? There's not a lot of evidence to back up the cholesterol or DHEA claims (see Chapter 27 on natural hormones for more on DHEA). The body builders may be disappointed too. The studies that showed chromium helps you lose fat and build muscle were badly flawed, and researchers haven't been able to reproduce them.

It's relatively easy to get at least 50 mcg of chromium a day from your food. Apples, broccoli, barley, corn, beef, eggs, nuts, mushrooms, oysters, rhubarb, tomatoes, and sweet potatoes are all good food sources. Most good daily multi supplements also have some chromium in them. If you decide to take a chromium supplement to help your diabetes, choose chromium glycinate or the patented type of trivalent chromium picolinate called Chromax-II GTF. (The GTF stands for glucose tolerance factor.) Skip supplements made with chromium chloride—you don't absorb this form very well.

# Selenium: An Essential Element

Your body's most abundant natural antioxidant is an enzyme called glutathione peroxidase. We'll talk a lot more about glutathione in Chapter 23, so for now we'll just mention that without selenium, you can't make glutathione. A recent major study has shown that selenium can be a powerful cancer-prevention supplement. People in the study took 200 mcg of selenium daily to see if their skin cancer rate would drop. It didn't—but their rates of colorectal, lung, and prostate cancer went down sharply.

Selenium may also help protect you against heart disease. It also helps your immune system work effectively and helps remove heavy metals such as lead from your body. Vitamin E works better and longer in your body when you have plenty of selenium. All that makes selenium pretty important for a mineral you need only in micrograms.

The RDA for selenium is quite low—you can easily get it from your food.

| The RDA for Selenium | |
| --- | --- |
| Age/Sex | Selenium in mcg |
| *Infants* | |
| 0–0.5 year | 10 |
| 0.5–1 year | 15 |
| *Children* | |
| 1–6 years | 20 |
| 7–10 | 30 |
| *Teens and Adults* | |
| Men 11–14 | 40 |
| Men 15–18 | 50 |
| Men 19+ | 70 |
| Women 11–14 | 45 |
| Women 15–18 | 50 |
| Women 19+ | 55 |
| Pregnant women | 65 |
| Nursing women | 75 |

Animal foods such as organ meats, seafood, lean meat, and chicken are all good sources of selenium. Whole grains such as oatmeal and brown rice are good plant sources of selenium, especially if they were grown in selenium-rich soil.

The benefits of selenium for cancer prevention and other health problems seem to kick in only at 200 mcg a day, though, so you may want to consider supplements. Selenium supplements come in two forms. Yeast-based supplements are made from yeast grown in a selenium-enriched medium. "Organic" selenium is bound to an amino acid in the form of selenomethionine. Avoid inorganic forms of this mineral such as sodium selenite or selenate—you don't absorb them very well. You need to be very cautious with selenium supplements. In amounts greater than 600 mcg a day, selenium can be toxic, although 200 mcg a day seems to be quite safe.

# Copper: Crucial for Your Circulation

Copper is involved in a lot of body processes, but its main functions are to help keep your heart and blood vessels healthy. You need copper to make an enzyme that keeps your arteries flexible—if you don't get enough, they could rupture. You also need copper to make the insulating sheath that covers your nerves. Copper works with iron to keep your red blood cells healthy. It's also very important for making the natural antioxidant superoxide dismutase (SOD) (we'll talk more about SOD in Chapter 23).

There's no RDA for copper, but you can check out the Safe and Adequate range in the chart. The average American diet gives you anywhere from 0.8 to 3.0 mg of copper every day.

| Safe and Adequate Range for Copper | |
| --- | --- |
| Age/Sex | Copper in mg |
| *Infants* | |
| 0–0.5 year | 0.4–0.6 |
| 0.5–1 year | 0.6–0.7 |
| *Children* | |
| 1–3 years | 0.7–1.0 |
| 4–6 | 1.0–1.5 |
| 7–10 | 1.0–2.0 |
| 11+ | 1.5–2.5 |
| *Adults* | |
| 18+ | 1.5–3.0 |

Hardly anyone is ever deficient in copper. There are some very rare inherited conditions such as Wilson's disease that make you store too much copper in your body, but on the whole, copper toxicity is also rare. You'd have to take in more than 10 mg a day to have any symptoms. The most common symptoms of copper overdose are nausea and vomiting.

Copper is found in a lot of common foods. There's over 2 mg of copper in a single oyster; other shellfish, such as lobster, are also good sources. Other good foods for copper include nuts, avocados, potatoes, organ meats, whole grains, and beans and peas. You may also be getting some from your drinking water if it goes through copper pipes. Copper is also found in most good daily multi supplements.

### Food for Thought

If you ever want to see sparks really fly, put a medical doctor and an alternative nutritionist together and ask them whether copper bracelets help arthritis. The doctor will flat out deny it and point to the lack of scientific evidence; the nutritionist will cite case after case where patients have been helped. So do the bracelets work? Who knows? If you have arthritis, try wearing one—it can't hurt and it might help.

It's important to keep your zinc and copper levels in balance, because the two minerals compete with each other to be absorbed into your body. Most nutritionists recommend a ratio of ten parts zinc to one part copper. In other words, if you're taking 30 mg of zinc, be sure to take 3 mg of copper as well—but don't take more than that.

# Fluoride: Fighting Tooth Decay

Here's a trace mineral we know you *don't* need. Even so, fluoride is very valuable for preventing tooth decay and even repairing decay in its earliest stages. Fluoridated drinking water reduces cavities in children by 20 to 40 percent and in adults by 15 to 35 percent—and the effect is even greater if you also use fluoridated toothpaste.

Fluoride helps build strong bones and keep them that way. There's some solid evidence that people who live in areas with fluoridated water have less osteoporosis. New drugs that combine calcium and fluoride for treating osteoporosis are now being investigated and show a lot of promise.

There's no RDA for fluoride, but today about 60 percent of the municipalities in the United States add it to their water supplies at the rate of one milligram per liter (which is another way of saying one part per million). That amount means the average adult will get between 1.5 and 4.0 mg a day just from drinking tap water.

The main reason water is fluoridated is that there really isn't any in food, with one exception: a cup of tea has about 0.3 mg. If you drink only bottled or filtered water or water from your own well, or if your community doesn't fluoridate its water, you and your family may not be getting the benefits of fluoride for your teeth and bones. Likewise, if you use "natural" toothpaste that doesn't have fluoride, you're not protecting your teeth fully.

There is no evidence at all that fluoride causes cancer, heart disease, kidney disease, Alzheimer's disease, or any other health problem.

# Manganese: Mystery Metal

Until 1972, when the first case came up, we didn't even know you could have a shortage of manganese. This mineral is still pretty mysterious. It seems to do a lot of the same things as magnesium, like help make your connective tissue, clot your blood, move glucose around your system, and digest your proteins. It may also be an antioxidant.

Most people take in anywhere between 2 and 9 mg of manganese a day. That seems to be enough, because manganese deficiency is extremely rare. There's no RDA, but we can tell you the Safe and Adequate range in the chart.

| Safe and Adequate Range for Manganese | |
|---|---|
| Age/Sex | Manganese in mg |
| *Infants* | |
| 0–0.5 year | 0.3–0.6 |
| 0.5–1 year | 0.6–1.0 |
| *Children* | |
| 1–3 years | 1.0–1.5 |
| 4–6 | 1.5–2.0 |
| 7–10 | 2.0–3.0 |
| *Teens and Adults* | |
| 11+ | 2.5–5.0 |

Foods that are high in manganese include tea, raisins, pineapple, spinach, broccoli, oranges, nuts, blueberries, beans, and whole grains.

Manganese can be very helpful for women with heavy menstrual flows. Eating more foods rich in manganese every day helps reduce the flow. Manganese is also an important mineral for building strong bones. If you don't get enough, you could be at greater risk for osteoporosis. Manganese also helps glucosamine to work better (see Chapter 22).

The best way to get more manganese is to eat more foods that contain it. Many daily multi supplements also contain manganese. Don't overdo, though—too much manganese can interfere with your iron absorption.

# Molybdenum: Making Enzymes

All of your tissues contain tiny amounts of molybdenum. It's needed to make several enzymes, particularly one called xanthine oxidase. You need this enzyme to grow and develop normally and to use iron in your body properly.

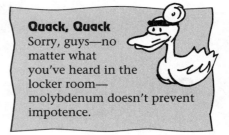

**Quack, Quack**
Sorry, guys—no matter what you've heard in the locker room—molybdenum doesn't prevent impotence.

The average adult gets between 45 and 500 mcg of molybdenum a day from food. As you can see from the chart, 45 mcg is a little less than ideal, but even so, molybdenum deficiency is almost impossible.

| Safe and Adequate Range for Molybdenum | |
| --- | --- |
| Age/Sex | Molybdenum in mcg |
| *Infants* | |
| 0–0.5 year | 15–30 |
| 0.5–1 year | 20–40 |
| *Children* | |
| 1–3 years | 25–50 |
| 4–6 | 30–75 |
| 7–10 | 50–150 |
| *Teens and Adults* | |
| 11+ | 75–250 |

The amount of molybdenum in your food depends on where it was grown. The soil in some parts of the country is much higher in molybdenum than others. In general, good food sources include whole grains, lean meat, organ meats, beans, dark-green leafy vegetables, and milk. Most people get plenty from their food and don't need extra, although molybdenum is often found in daily multi supplements.

**Food for Thought**

A careful study in one small region of China showed that people there had the world's highest rate of cancer of the esophagus—and also ate food grown in soil that was very low in molybdenum. The connection of cancer and low molybdenum seems clear, but so far there's no evidence that taking extra molybdenum prevents cancer.

# Other Trace Minerals

Did you know your body contains very tiny amounts of gold and silver? It does, but we have no idea why or what—if anything—would happen if you didn't have them. We do know why you have some other important trace minerals, though, so we'll run down the list and tell you the basics for each one.

➤ **Boron.** In the mid-1980s, researchers discovered that you need small amounts of boron to help you absorb calcium into your bones and keep it there. How much boron is still up in the air. There's no RDA or SAI yet, but many nutritionists today suggest getting 3 mg a day. That's not a problem, because most people get 2 to 5 mg a day from their food. Good dietary sources of boron are fruits, especially apples, pears, peaches, grapes, dates, and raisins. Nuts and beans are also high in boron.

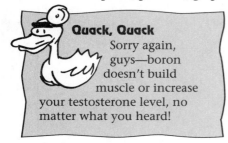

**Quack, Quack**
Sorry again, guys—boron doesn't build muscle or increase your testosterone level, no matter what you heard!

➤ **Cobalt.** Remember the chapter on cobalamin (Vitamin $B_{12}$)? You need cobalt to make this vitamin, which is essential for making red blood cells. In fact, that's *all* you need cobalt for. And because you don't need much cobalamin, you don't need much cobalt—a few micrograms is ample. If you're getting enough cobalamin from your food or supplements, you're getting plenty of cobalt.

➤ **Nickel.** We still don't know what nickel is doing there in your body, although it's probably involved with making some enzymes, hormones, and cell membranes. Too much nickel is associated with cancer, heart disease, and skin problems, but there's no known effects of too little nickel. Because you absorb very, very little nickel from your food, getting too much is almost impossible. Good food sources of nickel include chocolate, whole grains, nuts, beans, fruits, and vegetables.

➤ **Silicon.** You need silicon to make your bones, cartilage, and connective tissue. Nobody's ever been deficient in silicon because it's found in many foods, especially seafood, whole grains, root vegetables such as potatoes, and beans. Silicon supplements made from the plant horsetail are said to help your nails, hair, bones, and even arteries. Skip them—they're worthless.

➤ **Tin.** You've got this in your body, but we don't know what it does. This is one trace mineral you definitely don't have to think about.

➤ **Vanadium.** Recently a lot of vanadium products have come on the market, along with a lot of hype. Some of the ads even claim it "cures" diabetes. Don't believe it. Any possible benefit vanadium might have on your blood sugar is outweighed by its possible dangers even in moderate doses. There's no known need for vanadium in your body.

> **Quack, Quack**
> Germanium is a mineral used to make computer chips. Can it do anything for humans? Probably not, although some people claim, on almost no evidence, that it boosts your immune system. This is one of the more expensive ways to waste your money—the capsules run about a dollar apiece.

# Minerals You Should Miss

There are some minerals that are OK in trace amounts but definitely not OK beyond that. Here's the rundown:

➤ **Aluminum.** Too much aluminum can cause nerve and brain damage. The average person doesn't need to worry much about this, but if you're a heavy user of aluminum-based antacids you could have a problem.

➤ **Arsenic.** Believe or not, you actually need this in very, very small amounts. Most people get about 140 mcg a day from their food. Doses larger than 250 mcg a day are toxic.

➤ **Cadmium.** Your body doesn't have any known use for cadmium, so it's never developed a way to get rid of it. Unfortunately, cadmium is found in cigarette smoke and air pollution, so you could accumulate a toxic amount over many years. If you don't already have enough good reasons to stop smoking, cadmium is another.

> **Quack, Quack**
> A few years back researchers found aluminum in the brains of people with Alzheimer's disease. This gave rise to the rumor that food cooked in aluminum pots and pans could cause Alzheimer's. Not so: aluminum cookware is perfectly safe.

➤ **Lead.** This stuff is really bad for you, even though your body normally has a tiny amount of it. Even small amounts of extra lead can cause nerve damage, anemia, mental impairment, and muscle weakness. Recent research also ties lead exposure to high blood pressure. Most cases of lead poisoning occur from exposure to lead-based paint and air pollution. Young children are especially at risk.

➤ **Mercury.** This is another mineral that you have naturally in very small amounts. In larger amounts, though, it can do real damage and should be avoided. Mercury is used in a lot of industrial processes, so it can end up in air and water pollution. Fish such as tuna and swordfish that swim in mercury-contaminated water and eat smaller fish also contaminated with mercury may accumulate high levels of it. If you then eat the fish, you'll also get the mercury that's in it. Experts suggest eating these fish no more than once a week—less if you're pregnant or breastfeeding. What about the mercury in your silver dental fillings? We're not sure if this is really dangerous or not—talk to your dentist.

How can you avoid all these dangerous minerals? To a degree, you can't in our industrial society. There are some simple steps you can take, though: have lead paint removed, stop smoking, and avoid contaminated food, water, and air.

## The Least You Need to Know

➤ Your body needs very small amounts of some minerals.

➤ In almost all cases, you can get enough of the trace minerals from your food.

➤ Iron deficiency is fairly common, especially among toddlers and women. The RDA for iron is 12 to 15 mg.

➤ Other important trace minerals are iodine, chromium, and selenium.

➤ The trace minerals boron, cobalt, copper, manganese, and molybdenum are needed in very small amounts for good health.

# Part 4
# Exploring Other Supplements

There's a wide and wonderful world of supplements beyond vitamins and minerals. It's so wide and wonderful, in fact, that it's easy to get lost in it. We're here to help you stay on the right road. To do that, we have to leave out most herbal products—there are so many useful ones that it would take a whole other book (or maybe two) to write about them. Instead, in this section we'll concentrate on other supplements, like amino acids, essential fatty acids, natural hormones, and flavonoids. These are safe, easy-to-take supplements that can help you with your everyday good health.

New research and new products come along all the time in this fast-changing area. Not all of them deliver what they promise. We've tried to clear up the confusion so you can set a straight course toward better health.

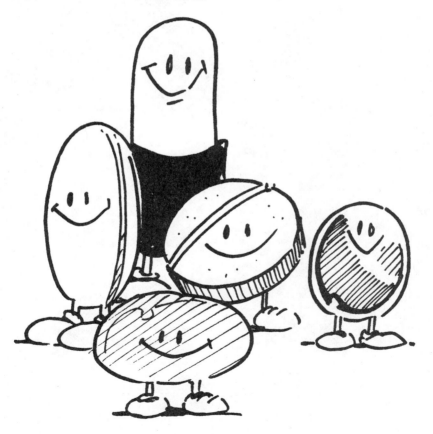

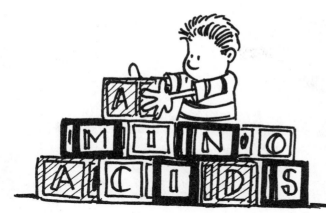

# Chapter 22

# Amino Acids: The Building Blocks of Life

## In This Chapter

➤ What amino acids are

➤ Why amino acids are essential to life

➤ How your body uses amino acids to make hormones, enzymes, and antioxidants

➤ How individual amino acids can help health problems

Your body is a very busy place. Every second of every day, all around the clock, year after year, you make thousands of different enzymes, hormones, antioxidants, and chemical messengers. Every day millions of new cells replace old cells. Your taste buds, for example, only last a day or so, while you replace your entire skin every 30 days. Every day you make *millions* of red blood cells to replace the ones that wear out as they pound through your blood vessels.

The building blocks of everything that happens in your body are just twenty-two amino acids. All cells are made from them, and your body is regulated by them. Where do the amino acids come from? From the protein in the foods you eat, because proteins are nothing more than long chains of amino acids.

# Why You Need Amino Acids

Pretty much all of you that's not bones and teeth is made up of *protein*. All that protein is made up of different combinations of *amino acids*. And all those amino acids are made just from atoms of hydrogen, oxygen, nitrogen, and carbon, with a little sulfur thrown in here and there.

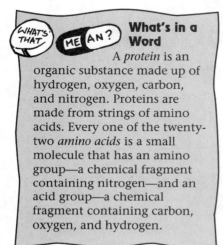

**What's in a Word**

A *protein* is an organic substance made up of hydrogen, oxygen, carbon, and nitrogen. Proteins are made from strings of amino acids. Every one of the twenty-two *amino acids* is a small molecule that has an amino group—a chemical fragment containing nitrogen—and an acid group—a chemical fragment containing carbon, oxygen, and hydrogen.

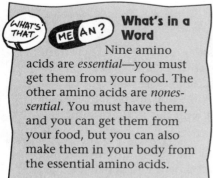

**What's in a Word**

Nine amino acids are *essential*—you must get them from your food. The other amino acids are *nonessential*. You must have them, and you can get them from your food, but you can also make them in your body from the essential amino acids.

Amino acids are the building blocks of protein. The human body needs twenty-two different amino acids to make up the 50,000-plus proteins that make you, just as we can make all the words in the English language from just 26 letters.

The amino acids fall into two basic categories: *essential* and *nonessential*. Essential amino acids are the nine aminos you must get from your diet—like vitamins, you have to have them and, unlike vitamins, you can't get them any other way. (The amino acids arginine, histidine, and cysteine are essential for growing babies but not for adults.)

Nonessential amino acids are the amino acids you can make in your body by combining two or more of the essential amino acids. Nonessential doesn't mean unnecessary. You don't have to get these aminos from your food (although they are found in foods), but you still need to have them. That means your food has to contain enough of the essential amino acids to build them.

Your body contains many other amino acids, such as carnitine and taurine, that don't fall into the essential/nonessential categories. We know that some of these aminos play important roles in your body. There are others that we still don't fully understand, but researchers are working on them. We believe there may be some exciting new developments in this area in the next few years.

Amino acids may have complicated names, like phenylalanine, or confusingly similar names, like glutamine, glycine, and glutamic acid. To make them easier to remember, we've listed them all in a chart. We're going to be talking about the different aminos by name, so refer back to the chart if you get mixed up.

| The Amino Acids | |
|---|---|
| **Essential Amino Acids** | **Nonessential Amino Acids** |
| Histidine | Alanine |
| Isoleucine | Arginine (essential for babies) |
| Leucine | Asparagine |
| Lysine | Aspartic acid |
| Methionine | Carnitine (essential for babies) |
| Phenylalanine | Cysteine |
| Threonine | Glutamic acid |
| Tryptophan | Glutamine |
| Valine | Glycine |
| | Proline |
| | Serine |
| | Taurine (essential for babies) |
| | Tyrosine |

# 50,000 Proteins from Just 22 Aminos

You need all twenty-two amino acids to make the bigger protein molecules that keep you alive. Amazingly, those twenty-two aminos can be assembled into so many different three-dimensional combinations that your body can make over 50,000 different proteins. That includes all the proteins that make up your tissues and form all the many enzymes, hormones, neurotransmitters, and other chemical messengers that keep your body working.

The instructions for making all those proteins are encoded in your genetic material—the DNA in the nucleus of every one of your cells. In a very complicated sequence of events, your DNA tells your cells to put together specific amino acids, anywhere from two or three to a thousand or so, to make whatever protein happens to be needed at that moment. Amazingly, some cells in your body can produce as many as 10,000 different proteins! When exactly the right aminos are linked together in exactly the right order, they coil and fold up into exactly the shape of that protein and

**Quack, Quack**
Some people claim that taking supplements containing nucleic acids (DNA and RNA) can help "revitalize" you. Others sell hair and skin products made with nucleic acids, claiming that they somehow restore a youthful appearance. We can always hope, of course, but these products are worthless.

no other. That protein, folded into its particular shape, fits like a key into a lock with other proteins as it carries out its specific job in your body. When the job is done, other proteins come along and recycle it; breaking it back down so that its amino acids can be used again in another combination. The intricate complexity of your body is truly awesome!

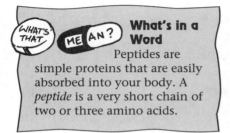

**What's in a Word**
Peptides are simple proteins that are easily absorbed into your body. A *peptide* is a very short chain of two or three amino acids.

When two or three amino acids combine into a short chain, they form a very simple protein called a *peptide*. You make a lot of different peptides. We're just starting to understand how many and how important they are. Most of your neurotransmitters, the chemical substances that send messages to and from your brain and help regulate your body, are peptides. They have complicated names only a biochemist could remember, like bradykinin, leucine, enkephalin, and substance P.

# The RDA for Amino Acids

Figuring out the RDA for amino acids gets complicated, because you really need to know two things: How much protein you need, and then how much of that protein should be made up of each of the nine essential amino acids. Bear with us as we work it out.

First, the protein. How much do you really need? Probably a lot less than you're getting. The RDA for protein is figured using a very complicated formula, but it basically comes down to this: You need 0.36 grams of protein for every pound of body weight. So, if you're that mythical 130-pound woman, you need about 47 grams of protein (130 × 0.36) every day.

To put your protein needs in a different way, you need to get about 10 to 15 percent of your daily calories from protein. A gram of protein has about 4 calories, so our imaginary 130-pound woman gets about 188 calories a day from protein.

Let's get real with these numbers. There's about 28 grams in an ounce. A quarter-pound hamburger has about 14 grams of protein; a baked chicken leg has about 30 grams. In an average American diet, you reach your daily protein quickly. In fact, you probably go way over it every day.

Now let's look at the amino acids. Animal proteins, such as meat, eggs, and milk, contain all nine of the essential amino acids, along with some of the nonessential ones. Nutritionists call these "high-quality" or "complete" proteins. The protein in eggs is such high quality that eggs are used as the standard to measure other proteins by (see the chart for the breakdown). So, the proportions of the essential amino acids in an egg set the standard for how much of each essential amino acid you need. Looking at the egg chart, you can see that you need relatively little tryptophan, for example, compared to leucine.

| Amino Acids in an Egg | |
|---|---|
| **Amino Acid** | **Amount in mg** |
| Arginine | 377 |
| Cysteine | 146 |
| Histidine | 149 |
| Isoleucine | 343 |
| Leucine | 537 |
| Lysine | 452 |
| Methionine | 196 |
| Phenylalanine | 334 |
| Threonine | 302 |
| Tryptophan | 76 |
| Tyrosine | 257 |
| Valine | 383 |

Now let's combine what we know about protein and what we know about amino acids. We know you need 0.36 mg of protein for every pound of your body weight. We know that protein needs to contain the different essential amino acids in roughly the same proportions as those found in an egg. Based on that, we can then figure out how much of each essential amino you need to get every day. The breakout is shown in the chart in terms of milligrams per each pound of your body weight. Checking the chart, you can see that a 130-pound woman needs to get 1,040 mg (130 × 8), or almost exactly 1 gram, of leucine every day. To put that in perspective, there's close to 2 grams of leucine in a quarter-pound hamburger.

| Adult Requirements for Essential Amino Acids | |
|---|---|
| **Amino Acid** | **Requirements in mg/lb** |
| Histidine | 5–7 |
| Isoleucine | 6 |
| Leucine | 8 |
| Lysine | 7 |
| Methionine | 8 |
| Phenylalanine | 8 |
| Threonine | 4 |
| Tryptophan | 2 |
| Valine | 6 |

# Eating Your Aminos

Very few people in our modern society get less than the RDA for protein. Most get more—vegetarians get about 50 to 100 grams a day, and meat eaters get a lot more. Protein deficiency—and therefore amino acid deficiency—is almost unheard of. You'd have to be on a very weird and restrictive diet, or have a serious health problem, to be too low in protein.

It is important to get the right balance of amino acids, though. If you're a strict vegetarian or vegan, you need to be sure you're getting enough variety in your food to give you plenty of all the essential aminos. Plant foods don't contain as much protein as animal foods, and they usually don't have enough of all the essential amino acids. Corn, for example, is very low in tryptophan and cysteine.

Most people get plenty of high-quality protein in their diet and don't need to worry about getting enough amino acids. You don't need to take amino acid supplements if you're in good health and eat a well-balanced diet.

Sometimes, though, you might want to be sure of having enough of the amino building blocks for a particular protein. For example, you need to have plenty of cysteine, glycine, and glutamic acid to make the antioxidant glutathione. If you need extra glutathione to fend off extra free radicals—because you have an infection, for example—you might need some extra amino building blocks. (Glutathione is so important to your health that we'll talk more about it in chapter 24 on super antioxidants.) In that case, check out your health-food store for *free-form* amino acid supplements. Read the label carefully. If it doesn't say free form, the aminos you want are probably in there only as part of a protein chain made up of a combination of amino acids. Your digestive system will have to break down the chain in order to release the amino acids. Free aminos are already in their simplest form, so they're absorbed into your body right away.

Watch out for amino acid formulas that claim to contain all the essential and nonessential amino acids. Read the labels carefully. Some of these formulas are really just protein powders with some added free amino acids. They're high in calories because they're designed for weight gain and building body mass.

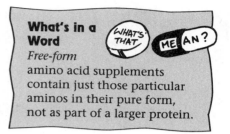

**What's in a Word**
*Free-form* amino acid supplements contain just those particular aminos in their pure form, not as part of a larger protein.

Most people take their amino supplements by swallowing them in convenient capsules. If you'd rather take the powder form, just put a spoonful on your tongue and wash it down with a few swallows of a cold liquid. Aminos don't dissolve, so you'll have trouble stirring them into a drink.

Never add free form amino acids to hot foods or use them in cooking. The heat changes their structure and makes them ineffective.

# Amino Alert!

Some health problems can be made worse by amino acids. If you have kidney disease, you need to be very careful about how much protein you eat. Adding extra amino acids to your diet could cause problems, so be sure to discuss them with your doctor or nutritionist first.

In large doses, lysine can interfere with insulin production, so don't take supplements of this amino acid if you have diabetes or blood sugar problems. (We'll talk about lysine for treating herpes a little later in this chapter.)

There are some rare genetic conditions that are worsened by amino acids. People with phenylketonuria (PKU), for instance, can't make the enzyme that converts the essential amino acid phenylalanine to the nonessential amino acid tyrosine. These people have to avoid phenylalanine in all forms—including aspartame, the artificial sweetener better known as Nutra-Sweet®.

**Warning!**
If you take a monoamine oxidase (MAO) inhibitor drug such as Nardil® or Marplan® to treat depression and anxiety, be sure to avoid foods and amino acid supplements containing phenylalanine, tryptophan, and especially tyrosine.

**Warning!**
Some dieters try liquid protein diets as a fast way to lose weight. We strongly recommend against these because of possible heart failure. The FDA agrees and says they shouldn't be used even under your doctor's supervision.

# Arginine for Immunity

Arginine may be helpful for stimulating your immune system, healing wounds, and slowing the growth of cancer. One reason may be that arginine stimulates your thymus, the small gland in your upper chest that produces an important kind of infection fighting white blood cell.

Arginine, along with methionine and glycine, forms the building blocks of creatine, a protein that is needed for making energy in your muscles and for muscle growth. Based on the logic that if you eat more of the building blocks you'll make more of the protein, some bodybuilders and athletes take supplements of all three. Straight creatine supplements are now also very popular. Do these work? They don't work any better than just eating a well-balanced diet.

What about avoiding foods high in arginine, such as nuts, whole grains, and chocolate, if you have herpes? We'll talk more about that a little later on when we get to lysine.

# Carnitine for Cardiac Cases

Carnitine is an amino acid you make in your body from the essential aminos lysine and methionine. In foods, carnitine is found in meat, especially beef, pork, and lamb. There's virtually none in plant foods, so vegetarians should be sure they're getting enough foods that contain lysine and methionine, the building blocks for carnitine.

Your heart contains more carnitine than any other part of your body. It's there to help the mitochondria (the tiny power plants) in your heart cells produce energy. How? It helps by carrying fatty acids into the mitochondria, where they're converted to energy. Some researchers believe that taking supplemental carnitine may help people with heart problems by making their hearts work more efficiently. Extra carnitine can sometimes be very helpful for people with angina or heart failure. If you have a heart condition, discuss carnitine with your doctor before you try it. (And read Chapter 26 on Coenzyme $Q_{10}$.)

Recent research suggests that carnitine may help people with chronic fatigue syndrome (CFS), a mysterious illness that causes extreme tiredness, depression, loss of concentration, muscle pain, and other symptoms. In one study, 28 patients were given 3 grams of carnitine a day. All the patients showed clear improvements in their well-being and mental outlook, and only one had any side effects. The researchers think carnitine works by improving energy production.

Because carnitine is involved in moving fatty acids around your body, it seems reasonable to think that it may also help lower your cholesterol. Carnitine is sometimes helpful for lowering blood triglycerides and LDL ("bad") cholesterol and raising HDL ("good") cholesterol. If you have high cholesterol, discuss carnitine with your doctor before you try it.

Today many claims are being made for carnitine. Some people say it improves athletic performance and endurance, helps Alzheimer's disease, improves memory, and treats depression. At this point, the research for athletes doesn't prove much, although it may help people who do endurance sports like triathlons. The research on Alzheimer's and depression in the elderly is much more solid. Carnitine, in the form of acetyl-L-carnitine, is often helpful to these people, with no real side effects. It may be worth trying, but be warned: It's expensive. The going price of a 500 mg capsule is over a dollar and the suggested dosage is four capsules a day for people with Alzheimer's and similar problems.

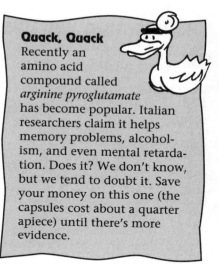

**Quack, Quack**
Recently an amino acid compound called *arginine pyroglutamate* has become popular. Italian researchers claim it helps memory problems, alcoholism, and even mental retardation. Does it? We don't know, but we tend to doubt it. Save your money on this one (the capsules cost about a quarter apiece) until there's more evidence.

# Cysteine for Pollution Protection

In Chapter 9 on folic acid, we talked about an amino acid called homocysteine and how too much of it can damage your heart. You naturally make homocysteine when you use cysteine, but that's no reason to avoid cysteine—this nonessential amino acid is very important to your health. Cysteine is one of the few amino acids to contain sulfur, so you need plenty of it to make glutathione, your body's most abundant natural antioxidant. We'll talk more about glutathione and cysteine in Chapter 24, so for now we'll discuss the role of cysteine in removing toxins from your body.

You're exposed every day to all sorts of toxins in the air you breathe and the foods you eat. All those toxins end up in your liver, where cysteine and glutathione corral them and escort them out of your body. In fact, cysteine is so good at protecting your liver that it's used in emergency rooms to treat overdoses of acetaminophen (Tylenol®), which can cause serious liver damage.

A good way to keep your cysteine level high is to eat foods that contain cysteine or methionine, the essential amino acid your body needs to make cysteine. Good choices are eggs, meat, dairy products, and whole grains. If you want to try supplements, we suggest taking N-acetyl-L-cysteine (NAC), which is made naturally from cysteine. For reasons not fully understood, NAC is absorbed better than cysteine supplements.

# Glutamine for the Gut

What's the difference between glutamine and glutamic acid? Not much, the two are very closely related, and your body converts them back and forth very easily. These amino acids are used to make many different neurotransmitters. Glutamine is particularly important for your brain and nerves.

Glutamic acid and glutamine are very abundant in foods. Some of the glutamine from your food is absorbed directly into the cells of your small intestine to nourish them, while the rest is absorbed into your bloodstream for use in other parts of your body. Some doctors and nutritionists believe that glutamine supplements may be very helpful for people with intestine problems like ileitis and Crohn's disease. Talk to your doctor before you try glutamine supplements.

# Lysine: Help for Herpes?

Some researchers believe that the balance of arginine and lysine in your body plays a role in treating the painful genital blisters and cold sores caused by the herpes virus. *Herpes* is the name of a group of viruses. *Herpes simplex* type 1 (HSV-1) is the virus that causes cold sores. Herpes simplex type 2 (HSV-2) is the virus that causes genital herpes. *Herpes zoster* is a related virus that causes chicken pox and shingles.

The thinking is that the virus "feeds" on arginine and is "blocked" by lysine. There really isn't a lot of solid evidence one way or the other for this, but many people with herpes swear that lysine works to stop an outbreak. Since not much else helps, it's certainly worth trying. Arginine-rich foods to avoid include chocolate, nuts, seeds, beer, coconut, grains such as oats, whole wheat, peanuts, soybeans and soy products, and wheat germ. Lysine-rich foods to load up on include fish, lean meats, chicken, soy products, milk, and cheese. You can also buy lysine supplements. Many patients say that taking 2,000 to 3,000 mg of lysine at the first sign of an attack helps ward it off or keep it from being as bad.

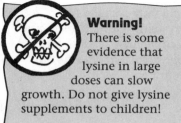

# Methionine and Taurine

Methionine and taurine, along with cysteine, are sulfur-containing amino acids. Methionine is an essential amino acid you have to get from animal foods such as eggs, fish, milk, and meat in your diet. Taurine is an amino acid that some researchers now believe should be listed in the nonessential category.

You make cysteine in your body only from methionine. You make taurine from methionine and cysteine and also get it from animal foods. Methionine may play a role in keeping your cholesterol down, but there's not enough evidence to make taking supplements worthwhile. Some researchers believe that taurine can help heart problems such as heart failure and arrhythmias. We're starting to realize that taurine is more important than we thought, but it's still too soon to recommend supplements—especially because they may have a depressing effect on your nervous system.

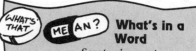

### What's in a Word

*Serotonin* carries impulses in the parts of your brain that control your mood and emotions. If you have plenty of serotonin to carry the impulses, you feel calm and confident. If you're short on serotonin, you might feel depressed, tense, angry, or anxious. You might also crave sugary carbohydrates and overeat. Too much serotonin, however, can be harmful to your heart—that's why some prescription drugs such as phenfluramine (Redux®) that raise your serotonin level were recalled by the FDA.

### Food for Thought

Recently a form of methionine called SAM (S-adenosylmethionine) has become available as a supplement. SAM levels tend to be low in clinically depressed people and in the elderly. Taking SAM supplements can be helpful for relieving severe depression. They may also help older people with memory problems or Alzheimer's disease. SAM seems to work best if you take 400 mg three or four times a day and are sure to get enough of all the B vitamins every day. If you have bipolar disorder (manic depression), take SAM only if your doctor recommends it.

# Tryptophan for Natural Sleep

You need the essential amino acid tryptophan to make serotonin and melatonin, both important body chemicals that help control your mood and sleep patterns. (We'll talk more about melatonin in Chapter 27 on natural hormones.) *Serotonin* is a neurotransmitter—a substance you make to carry nerve impulses across the tiny gaps between nerves.

Your body makes neurotransmitters from amino acids almost instantly, just when they're needed, and then breaks them down again very quickly to reuse the building blocks.

If you don't have enough tryptophan, you won't be able to make enough serotonin and melatonin, and you may start to feel depressed and have trouble sleeping. If you've been traveling through time zones, your melatonin levels may be off from jet lag and tryptophan could help get them back in sync again.

If you want to get more tryptophan as a way to help insomnia, one simple way is to eat it. Good sources of tryptophan include turkey, peanuts, avocados, oranges, bananas, cottage cheese, fish, lean meat, and milk. A lot of unsweetened breakfast cereals, like bran flakes, are also high in tryptophan. If you've been having insomnia, try having a snack of one of these foods—a turkey sandwich or a bowl of shredded wheat with milk—an hour before bedtime. It works surprisingly well for a lot of people.

# Phenylalanine, Tyrosine, and Migraines

Two amino acids, phenylalanine and tyrosine, are said to help depression, mostly because both are important for making the brain chemicals epinephrine, norepinephrine, and dopamine. In theory, if you're low on phenylalanine you can't make tyrosine, and if you're low on either of these amino acids, you can't make enough of the brain chemicals. The upshot could be that you get depressed. The evidence for this chain of events is on the thin side, so we can't say for sure that taking supplements of these aminos will help.

**Food for Thought**

The migraine drug sumatriptan (Imitrex®) works by mimicking serotonin, a neurotransmitter your body makes from tryptophan. The drug makes the small blood vessels in your brain contract, which relieves the migraine pain. Sumatriptan pills work for about 60 percent of the people who take them; the injected form works 80 percent of the time. If you suffer from migraines, talk to your doctor about a prescription for sumatriptan.

There are some good reasons not to take them. Large doses of either amino or both together could raise your blood pressure. Don't use these supplements if you have high blood pressure. If you take an MAO inhibiting drug such as Nardil® or Marplan® for depression, don't take these aminos—they could raise your blood pressure dangerously high. In fact, you should avoid foods high in phenylalanine and tyrosine, such as nuts, seeds, cheese, lima beans, avocados, bananas, and non-fat dried milk.

Both phenylalanine and tyrosine form tyramine, a substance that can trigger migraine headaches. If you get migraines, you should probably avoid supplements of these two amino acids and foods that are naturally high in tyramine. We list the worst offenders in the chart, but in general alcohol, many fruits, and all aged, dried, pickled, preserved, fermented, cured, or cultured foods are out.

| Foods High in Tyramine | |
| --- | --- |
| Aged cheeses | Pineapple |
| Avocados | Prunes |
| Bananas | Raisins |
| Beer | Seeds such as sesame seeds or pumpkin seeds |
| Beans | Sauerkraut |
| Chocolate | Soy sauce |
| Nuts, including peanuts | Wine |
| Organ meats | Yogurt |
| Pickled herring | |

# Glucosamine: Real Help for Arthritis

Glucosamine isn't exactly an amino acid. It's sometimes called an amino acid sugar, because it's made from glucose and an amine (one molecule of nitrogen and two of hydrogen). However you want to define it, glucosamine turns out to be very helpful for the treatment of arthritis.

Here's how we think it works. You make glucosamine in your body and use it to make cartilage in your joints. As you get older, you lose your ability to make glucosamine (we don't know why) and your *cartilage* starts to break down. You then get stiffness and pain—arthritis—in the joint. If you take supplemental glucosamine, it seems to stimulate your body into repairing the cartilage, which relieves the arthritis symptoms.

Glucosamine doesn't always work for everyone, and it can take a few weeks to start kicking in, but many arthritis sufferers call it a wonder drug. Their pain and stiffness improve markedly, and they can sometimes cut back on or even stop the powerful drugs they've been taking for pain and swelling. Best of all, glucosamine has no real side effects and you can't overdose, although some people may get very mild stomach upsets from it.

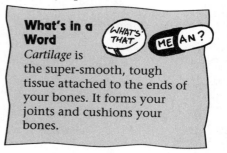

**What's in a Word**
*Cartilage* is the super-smooth, tough tissue attached to the ends of your bones. It forms your joints and cushions your bones.

No foods contain glucosamine, so if you want to try it you'll have to take supplements made from chitin, the processed shells of shrimp, crabs, and lobsters. We strongly recommend glucosamine sulfate over other forms, since the sulfur is important for building cartilage. The usual dose is 500 mg two or three times a day, preferably with meals to avoid digestive upsets or heartburn. Glucosamine is even more effective if you're getting enough Vitamin C and manganese (see Chapter 13 for Vitamin C and Chapter 21 for trace minerals).

What about all those cartilage products that are supposed to help arthritis? They contain chondroitin sulfate, which is just a cruder form of glucosamine sulfate. They do work for some people. If they don't for you, try glucosamine.

**Food for Thought**

Glucosamine works so well for arthritis that many manufacturers now offer it. It's best to take a good product that contains glucosamine sulfate, but glucosamine hydrochloride or N-acetyl glucosamine (NAG) work well for many people. To be sure you're getting a good product, choose a reliable manufacturer such as Solgar, Enzymatic Therapy, or Twin Labs.

# The Least You Need to Know

➤ Amino acids are the building blocks of protein.

➤ Most people get all the amino acids they need from the protein in their food. Protein deficiency is very rare.

➤ You need all twenty-two amino acids to make the 50,000-plus proteins you need for life.

➤ Amino acids make the many enzymes, hormones, neurotransmitters, and other chemical messengers that regulate your body.

➤ Some individual amino acids can help health problems, including heart disease, insomnia, and herpes.

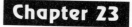

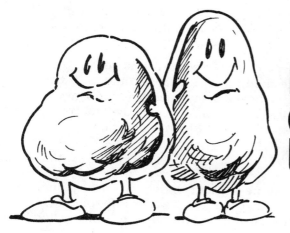

# Chapter 23

# Essential Fatty Acids: When Is Fat Good?

## In This Chapter

➤ What the essential fatty acids are and why you need them

➤ Foods that are high in essential fatty acids

➤ How essential fatty acids can help your heart

➤ How essential fatty acids can help other health problems

Here's what we're *not* going to do in this chapter: We're not going to tell you how bad red meat is for you. We're not going to warn you about the dangers of high cholesterol. We're not even going to lecture you about going on a low-fat diet. If you ever read a newspaper, open a magazine, or watch television, you don't need us—you know already.

We're going to talk about the good fats—the ones you have to have for good health. Really, it's true: There are some fats you simply can't live without. Not only that, these same fats could help you live longer and better by keeping your heart healthy and possibly preventing cancer. All that, just from swapping that steak or burger for some shrimp or fish a few times a week. And once you feel the benefits of doing that, maybe you'll start thinking about that low-fat diet.

# What's So Essential about Fat?

All that anti-fat information out there could make you think that all fat, no matter what, is just plain bad for you. As always, the truth is lot more complicated. Bear with us as we explain a little about fats in general.

You definitely do need some fat in your diet and in your body. The fat you eat is a source of quick energy and you have to have some fat in your diet to absorb and use Vitamins A, D, E, and K. You need fat to make your cell walls and many important hormones, enzymes, neurotransmitters, and other chemical messengers in your body. And you need some stored fat in your body to keep you warm and to cushion your organs.

# Good Fat versus Bad Fat

You need some fat for good health, but there are different kinds of fats. Which ones are best? The answer gets a little complicated, so hang in there as we get into some definitions. (If you don't want to read all this, just skip down to the last line of this section.)

➤ **Fat.** A fat is an organic substance made from molecules of hydrogen, carbon, and a little oxygen. Fat doesn't dissolve in water.

➤ **Triglycerides.** Almost all the fat in our foods comes from triglycerides. These are fats made from a backbone of glycerol (carbon atoms linked together) and three (that's where the *tri-* comes from) fatty acids. Your body stores fat in the form of triglycerides.

➤ **Fatty acids.** A fatty acid molecule is made from a chain of carbon atoms bound to hydrogen atoms. At the tail end of the chain is a carbon atom attached to two oxygen atoms—that's what makes the fat an acid. There are different kinds of fatty acids (and we'll talk about them later in this chapter), but for now you need to remember that the chains of carbon and hydrogen atoms vary in length. They're usually from 12 to 24 carbon atoms long.

➤ **Saturated fats.** If every carbon atom in the fatty acid is matched up with a hydrogen atom, the fat is saturated—it can't hold any more hydrogen. Saturated fats are bad fats, since they've been shown to raise your cholesterol. They're usually solid at room temperature, like butter and lard, and come from animals—meat, poultry, and whole-milk dairy foods. Some vegetable oils, such as palm oil and coconut oil, are also saturated.

➤ **Monounsaturated fats.** In monounsaturated fats, there's a missing hydrogen atom. An extra carbon atom takes its place. Monounsaturated fats are good fats, since they can help lower your cholesterol. Good examples of monounsaturated fats include olive oil, canola oil, and peanut oil.

➤ **Polyunsaturated fats.** These fat molecules have several missing hydrogen atoms, so they have several extra carbon atoms in their place. Polyunsaturated fats are also good for you, since they can help prevent heart disease. Good examples are corn oil, safflower seed oil, sunflower seed oil, and fish oil.

➤ **Trans-fatty acid.** If you add extra hydrogen to an unsaturated fat such as corn oil, it changes from a liquid to a soft solid—like margarine, for example. The process is called hydrogenation. Trans-fatty acids, or trans fats for short, aren't good for you. They behave a lot like saturated fats in your body and can raise your cholesterol.

Here's what it all comes down to: mono and poly fats—good; saturated and trans fats—bad.

# The Good Fats

Let's get back to those fatty acids. You have twenty different fatty acids in your body, but they're all made from just two: *linoleic acid* and *linolenic acid*. These two fatty acids are *essential*. You must get them from your food because your body can't make them. (Some experts feel only linoleic acid is essential, since you can make some linolenic acid from it.) Like amino acids for proteins, essential fatty acids are the building blocks for all the other fats in your body (although you also get the other fats from foods). Essential fatty acids are also the building blocks for your cell membranes and for many of the important hormones and other chemical messengers that tell your body what to do.

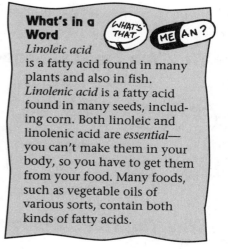

**What's in a Word**
*Linoleic acid* is a fatty acid found in many plants and also in fish. *Linolenic acid* is a fatty acid found in many seeds, including corn. Both linoleic and linolenic acid are *essential*—you can't make them in your body, so you have to get them from your food. Many foods, such as vegetable oils of various sorts, contain both kinds of fatty acids.

# Omega-3 and Omega-6

Researchers divide the fatty acids into four separate groups, depending on where their double carbon bonds fall relative to the acid tail of the chain. The tail end is called the omega end (from the last letter of the Greek alphabet). If we start counting from the omega end of linoleic acid, the first double carbon bond we come to is at the sixth carbon atom. So, another name for linoleic acid is *omega-6;* the fatty acids made from linoleic acid are in the omega-6 family. The double carbon bond for linolenic acid comes at the third atom, so linolenic acid is also called *omega-3,* and the fatty acids made from it are in the omega-3 family.

Omega-3 and omega-6 essential fatty acids are especially important for making *prostaglandins* in

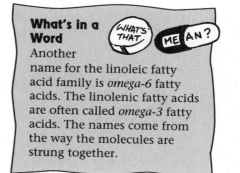

**What's in a Word**
Another name for the linoleic fatty acid family is *omega-6* fatty acids. The linolenic fatty acids are often called *omega-3* fatty acids. The names come from the way the molecules are strung together.

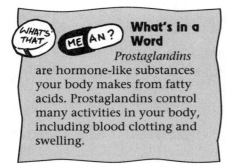

your body. Prostaglandins are hormone-like substances made from fatty acids. They regulate many activities in your body, including inflammation, pain, and swelling. They also play a role in controlling your blood pressure, your heart, your kidneys, and your digestive system. Prostaglandins are important for allergic reactions, blood clotting, and making other hormones.

Prostaglandins are a double-edged sword: some cause swelling and others relieve it. You use omega-3 fatty acids to make some kinds of prostaglandins and omega-6 fatty acids to make others. By changing the amounts of omega-6 and omega-3 fatty acids in your body, you may be able to change your prostaglandin levels.

## Why You Need Omega-6

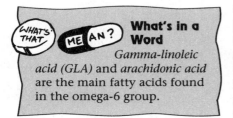

Omega-6 fatty acids (linoleic acid) are the most common polyunsaturated fatty acids in food. The omega-6 family actually has three members: *gamma-linoleic acid (GLA)*, *arachidonic acid*, and dihomo-linoleic acid. Of the three, GLA is probably the most useful for helping health problems. Arachidonic acid, on the other hand, is needed to make some prostaglandins that cause unpleasant symptoms, like swelling.

## Why You Need Omega-3

Omega-3 fatty acids (linolenic acid) are found in the leaves and seeds of many plants, in egg yolks, and in cold water ocean fish. The omega-3 family has three related members:

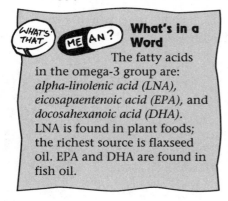

*alpha-linolenic acid (LNA), eicosapentenoic acid (EPA)*, and *docosahexanoic acid (DHA)*. LNA is found in plant foods, especially nuts, soybeans, canola oil, and flaxseed oil. EPA and DHA are found in fish oil.

Fish oil has been shown to have a lot of very good effects on your health. It can lower your triglyceride and cholesterol levels, reduce your high blood pressure, prevent blood clots, and help some digestive problems. It may even prevent cancer. In fact, fish oil is so helpful for some medical problems that we'll discuss it separately later in this chapter.

# Getting the Most from Essential Fatty Acids

Most people get their omega-3 and omega-6 essential fatty acids from their diet. Omega-6 fatty acids are found in all foods that have polyunsaturated fats in them. Especially good sources are cooking oils such as corn oil, safflower oil, sunflower oil, and soybean oil. Nuts and seeds, such as walnuts, peanuts, almonds, and sunflower seeds, are also good sources. The tiny seeds of the borage, black currant, and evening primrose plants are very rich sources of omega-6 fatty acids in the form of GLA, so they're often used to make supplements.

Omega-3's in the form of EPA and DHA are found in all fish and seafood—the oilier the fish, the more it has. As you can see from the chart, cold-water fish such as salmon, bluefish, herring, and tuna are excellent sources. So are cod, flounder, mackerel, and shrimp. Canola oil, soybean oil, and walnut oil are also good sources of omega-3 fatty acids. Another good way to get omega-3's is by taking flaxseed oil. Your body converts the LNA in the oil into EPA and DHA.

# Fish Oil Supplements

If you don't like to eat fish or want to get larger amounts of fish oil than you can get from eating fish, you can try fish oil supplements. In large amounts, fish oil capsules can give you gas, diarrhea, and heartburn. If you take a lot of them, you get fish breath and a fish body odor. (You'll be very popular with the neighborhood cats, but not with anybody else!) You can avoid the fish breath problem by taking slow-release capsules, but these are more expensive.

Read the label carefully when you buy fish oil supplements. The amounts of EPA and DHA are less than the size of the supplement. For example, a 1,000 mg capsule might have only 180 mg of EPA and 120 mg of DHA, or 300 mg of combined omega-3's. To get 1 gram of EPA/DHA, you'd have to take four capsules. We recommend MaxEPA® as a reliable brand. Store your fish oil capsules in a cool, dark place—the refrigerator is ideal. Spread your dose out over the day.

> **Now You're Cooking**
> To get the most from the essential fatty acids in cooking oils, purchase oils made using modified expeller presses (read the label)—this method keeps the oil from being oxidized during processing. Store the oil in the refrigerator.

> **Warning!**
> Fish oil naturally has no Vitamin E. This vitamin is usually added to fish oil supplements to help keep the oil from oxidizing. If you take fish oil supplements, be sure to take extra Vitamin E—up to 200 IU a day—to keep the oil from oxidizing inside you.

### Food for Thought

Cod liver oil is a moderately good source of omega-3 fatty acids, but it has some drawbacks (aside from its awful taste). One tablespoon of cod liver oil has 123 calories, over 4,000 RE of Vitamin A, and 34 IU of Vitamin D. You need to be careful about getting too much of these fat-soluble vitamins, so we don't recommend cod liver oil for getting your omega-3's. Get your A's and D's from other sources. To get more omega-3's, eat more fish and take EPA or DHA supplements.

### The Omega-3's in Fish

| Fish | Omega-3 in grams |
|------|------------------|
| Bass | 0.6 |
| Bluefish | 1.2 |
| Catfish | 0.6 |
| Crab, Alaska king | 0.6 |
| Flounder | 0.3 |
| Herring | 1.1–1.7 |
| Mackerel | 2.2–2.6 |
| Mullet | 1.1 |
| Salmon, canned Chinook | 3.0 |
| Salmon, pink | 1.0–1.9 |
| Salmon, sockeye | 1.3 |
| Sardines | 2.9 |
| Shrimp | 0.3–0.4 |
| Swordfish | 0.2 |
| Trout | 1.1–2.0 |
| Tuna, canned | 1.5–1.7 |

*Note: Amounts are for 3.5-ounce (100 grams) servings.*

If you're a vegetarian or don't like the side effects of fish oil, you can get your omega-3's from flaxseed oil (also sometimes called linseed oil). Enzymes in your body convert the linolenic acid in the flaxseed oil into EPA and DHA—the fatty acids that are best for your heart.

| The Omega-3's in Vegetable Oils | |
|---|---|
| Oil | Omega-3 in mg |
| Canola oil | 111 |
| Flaxseed oil | 533 |
| Soybean oil | 68 |
| Walnut oil | 104 |
| Wheat germ oil | 69 |

*Note: Amounts are for 1 gram (1,000 mg).*

There's no RDA for essential fatty acids, and true deficiencies are rare. Even so, some nutritionists believe that today we eat so many saturated and trans fats that many of us don't get enough essential fatty acids for optimal health. The essential fatty acids we do eat tend to be unbalanced. We eat too many omega-6's, mostly from the corn and sunflower seed oils used in many processed foods, and not enough omega-3's. This imbalance, some researchers believe, causes many health problems by getting your prostaglandins and other body chemicals out of whack. Our recommendation? Cut back on omega-6 foods and try to get at least 1,000 mg (1 gram) of omega-3's every day. Checking the chart, you can see you can easily get that much from just one small serving of canned tuna, sardines, or salmon.

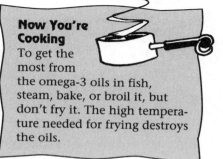

**Now You're Cooking**
To get the most from the omega-3 oils in fish, steam, bake, or broil it, but don't fry it. The high temperature needed for frying destroys the oils.

# Nothing Fishy About It: Omega-3 Helps Your Heart

In the 1930s, Danish researchers studied the Eskimos of Greenland. They found that the Eskimos ate very large amounts of fatty fish and seal meat (seals eat nothing but fish), yet they almost never got heart disease. The researchers decided that the omega-3 fatty acids EPA and DHA kept the Eskimos' hearts healthy. Can they do the same for you?

Several long-term studies have shown that men who eat fish several times a week have less heart disease than men who don't eat fish regularly. The most convincing is the DART (Diet and Reinfarction Trial) study of 1989, which looked at men who had already had heart attacks. The men who were told to eat lots of fish had 29 percent fewer second heart attacks than those who continued with their pre-heart attack diets. Some other studies, though, haven't really shown any difference in the overall heart disease rate. In 1995, for example, the ongoing Physicians' Health Study showed that there was no association between the amount of fish oil the men in the study ate and their chances of having a heart attack.

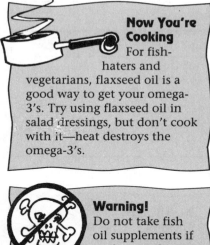

**Now You're Cooking** For fish-haters and vegetarians, flaxseed oil is a good way to get your omega-3's. Try using flaxseed oil in salad dressings, but don't cook with it—heat destroys the omega-3's.

**Warning!** Do not take fish oil supplements if you have a clotting disorder or take blood-thinning drugs such as warfarin!

When it comes to another heart problem, the benefits of fish oil are clearer. We're pretty sure that fish oil supplements can help prevent sudden death from heart rhythm problems. In one important study, there were eight sudden deaths in the control group that didn't take fish oil supplements and none in the group that did—even though the fish oil group didn't lose any weight or improve their cholesterol levels.

Fish oil supplements may also reduce heart attacks by preventing blood clots from blocking the arteries leading to your heart. The fish oil makes your platelets—the tiny cells in your blood that form blood clots—less "sticky," so they're less likely to lump together and form a clot. "Thinner" blood also helps prevent strokes.

If you take fish oil on a regular basis, you may thin your blood to the point where it takes you a little longer to stop bleeding. This sounds scary, but actually fish oil doesn't thin your blood any more than a daily aspirin tablet does—and many doctors recommend aspirin for patients with heart problems. On the other hand, if you have any sort of bleeding problem or are taking a blood-thinning drug such as coumadin or warfarin, skip the fish oil supplements. If you want to try fish oil supplements for your heart, discuss them with your doctor first. You'll probably need to take at least three grams a day.

# Fish Oil and Fat Levels

Taking fish oil supplements can lower your triglyceride level if it's too high. One drawback is that fish oil supplements might lower your overall triglycerides but raise your LDL ("bad") cholesterol. There's a way around this problem. Combining fish oil with garlic supplements seems to lower your triglycerides *and* lower your LDL cholesterol. You need a lot of both for the treatment to work: about 5 to 15 grams of fish oil and 1 gram of garlic (we'll talk more about garlic in Chapter 25). Large amounts of fish oil (over 5 grams a day) can cause your blood to become dangerously "thin" and make you bleed too easily. If you want to take big doses of fish oil, talk to your doctor first and get your blood checked often.

A lot of studies show that fish oil lowers your cholesterol level. It does, but *only* if you also lower the amount of saturated fat you eat. If you take fish oil capsules but continue with a high fat diet, your cholesterol won't go down. In fact, it might even raise your LDL level which you definitely don't want.

Some researchers believe that the GLA in evening primrose oil can reduce your LDL cholesterol. You need to take a fair amount—up to three grams a day.

# Helping High Blood Pressure

Fish oil lowers your blood pressure, but not by much and only if it's pretty high to begin with. The effect isn't really worth the trouble. There are better, natural ways to lower your blood pressure (check back to the chapters on calcium and magnesium, for instance).

# Fish Oil and Diabetes

If you have diabetes, be extremely cautious about fish oil supplements. They could raise your blood sugar and lower your insulin production. If you want to try fish oil as a way to lower your triglycerides, talk to your doctor first. Use small amounts (no more than 1,000 mg a day) and keep a very close eye on your blood sugar.

GLA, an omega-6 fatty acid, is sometimes helpful for nerve damage cause by diabetes (diabetic neuropathy). The doses needed are low—less than 500 mg a day. If you want to try this, talk to your doctor first—and also read about lipoic acid in Chapter 24.

# Calming Crohn's Disease

Fish oil supplements can be very helpful for keeping Crohn's disease, a chronic inflammation of the colon, under control. In one recent study, patients who took fish oil supplements were able to keep their symptoms from coming back much longer than patients who didn't. They did just as well on the fish oil as patients who were taking a powerful drug and they didn't have the drug's side effects. The patients in the study took a slow-release form of fish oil capsules that kept them from getting unpleasant side effects like gas and fishy breath.

# Helping Rheumatoid Arthritis

Rheumatoid arthritis is a serious and very painful disease that causes inflammation and stiffness of your joints. It's not the same as the ordinary sort of wear-and-tear arthritis some of us get. Some of the pain and swelling of rheumatoid arthritis comes from "bad" prostaglandins that are made from arachidonic acid—which is an omega-6 fatty acid. For some patients, omega-3 oils seem to help counteract the "bad" prostaglandins and relieve the symptoms. The doses needed are fairly high, in the range of 3 grams of fish oil or flaxseed oil a day. Since rheumatoid arthritis is usually treated with powerful anti-inflammatory drugs that can have nasty side effects, omega-3 oils are certainly worth a try. Be sure to discuss them with your doctor before you try them.

# Fish Oil Fights Cancer

Fish oil may play an important role in preventing cancer and slowing tumor growth. So far the studies are all on animals, but they're encouraging. The fish oil may have an effect on the cancer cell membranes by keeping the nutrients the cancer needs to grow from entering the cells. Another possible explanation is that the fish oil blocks the formation of some prostaglandins and hormones that nourish the cancer. Research is continuing in this very interesting area.

Substances called lignans in flaxseed oil may help prevent breast cancer. They seem to work by keeping estrogen, the female hormone, from helping the cancer get started and grow. (This is such an important area of research that we'll discuss it separately in chapter 27 on hormones.)

# GLA: The Promise of Evening Primrose Oil

The GLA in evening primrose oil may be helpful for relieving PMS symptoms, especially breast tenderness and swelling. It seems to work best if you take 500 to 1,000 mg every day (not just in the days before your period), along with 50 mg of pyridoxine. (For more on how pyridoxine helps PMS, check back to chapter 8.)

Many people claim that taking GLA supplements helps their skin, hair, and nails look better. Supplements seem to work best if you have dry skin or hair—it probably won't do much for you if your skin or hair are normal or oily. Brittle nails seem to improve if you take GLA supplements. GLA also often helps people with mild eczema.

# Other Good Fats

Omega-6's and omega-3's aren't the only good fats. There's also the omega-9 or oleic acid group, for example. Oleic acid is found in olive oil, peanut oil, avocados, and nuts. These monounsaturated fats seem to play a role in keeping your heart healthy and preventing cancer. We don't have space here to go into the many advantages of the Mediterranean diet (lots of olive oil, grains, fresh fruits and vegetables, and fish), but we urge you to look into it. Instead, we'll concentrate here on the health benefits of some specific fat-related supplements.

## The Weight Loss Pill

A fatty acid called conjugated linoleic acid (CLA) is being touted as a weight loss pill. It's said to magically burn off body fat and build up muscle. Does this sort of hype sound familiar? All sorts of silly supplements make those claims. Is there any more truth to them for CLA? Of course not—save your money.

## Helping Senility

Phosphatidylserine is a fatty substance found in your cell membranes. It's involved in keeping the cell membranes, especially the ones in your brain, stable. Because of that, phosphatidylserine (PS) supplements made from soy oil may be helpful for some Alzheimer's disease patients and older people with memory problems. This is a promising line of research that may be worth exploring, but discuss PS supplements with your doctor before you try them.

Some people claim that PS improves concentration, memory, and mental focus for everyone, not just the elderly. If you've reached that middle-aged point in life where you can't remember where you put your reading glasses, you might want to try it.

## Building Brain Cells

A lot of the interest in fish oil supplements has been on treating heart problems. Until recently, nobody paid much attention to how the DHA (docosahexenoic acid) in fish oil can help build your brain cells.

### Food for Thought

Your brain is actually 60 percent fat—and DHA is the most abundant fat in your brain. (Remember this fact the next time someone calls you a fathead!) It's also the most abundant fat in breast milk, since babies need it to nourish their growing brains. DHA seems to be important mostly for connecting brain cells to each other and making sure the signals get through right. Since you have ten *billion* nerve cells in your brain (roughly the same number of cells as stars in our galaxy, the Milky Way) you can see how important DHA is.

Your body makes some DHA naturally, but we get most of it from eating fish, eggs, red meat, and organ meats. If you've been cutting back on meat and eggs, if you're a strict vegetarian, or if you're a nursing mother, you might not be getting enough. In the long run, that could lead to memory problems or early senility. Supplements that contain only DHA derived from fish oil or algae are now available.

## The Least You Need to Know

➤ You need essential fatty acids to make your cell membranes.

➤ Essential fatty acids are also needed to make many body chemicals, including hormones and prostaglandins.

➤ Good sources of essential fatty acids in food oils are flaxseed oil, canola oil, soybean oil, walnut oil, corn oil, safflower oil, and wheat germ oil.

➤ Fish, especially cold-water fish such as salmon, tuna, and sardines, are good food sources of essential fatty acids.

➤ Fish oil supplements can help prevent heart attacks, lower cholesterol, and treat some intestinal problems.

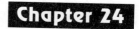

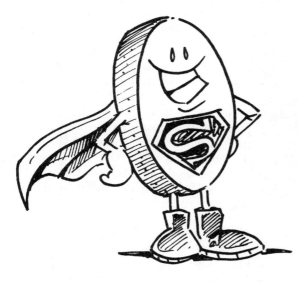

# Super Antioxidants

➤ Why you need glutathione
➤ Foods that are high in glutathione
➤ The antioxidant powers of cysteine and selenium
➤ What lipoic acid can do for you

Antioxidants, antioxidants, antioxidants. By now you've gotten the message: You need plenty of antioxidants to corral those damaging free radicals before they can wreck your body. The best antioxidant of all is the one you make naturally in your body: an amazing substance called glutathione. Lots of this super antioxidant is everywhere in your body.

But glutathione does more than just mop up free radicals like a very thirsty sponge. It also rounds up all sorts of dangerous toxic wastes in your body and whisks them quickly away, before they can do any harm. The best news of all about glutathione? You can easily get more of it into your system just through the foods you eat.

## The Crucial Role of Glutathione

Every second of every day, your body makes damaging free radicals. And every second of every day, your body makes a powerful substance called glutathione (abbreviated GSH)

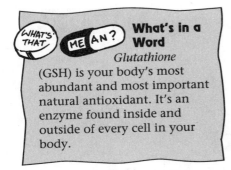

that grabs hold of those free radicals and smothers them. Glutathione also picks up any toxic substances (from air pollution, say) that have found their way into your body and escorts them out.

What is this amazing stuff? *Glutathione* is a tripeptide—a small protein made from just three amino acids. Molecules of cysteine, glycine, and glutamic acid combine in your cells to make glutathione. Of the three aminos needed to make glutathione, cysteine is the most important, because cysteine contains sulfur, which is also needed to make glutathione. You also need the trace mineral selenium to make glutathione. Your body generally has plenty of glycine and glutamic acid (or its close cousin glutamine), but sometimes the cysteine and selenium are in short supply. When that happens, you could end up without enough glutathione to defend your body.

# Are You Deficient?

Your glutathione level naturally drops as you get older. That's bad, because this lowers your defenses against free radicals and toxins and leaves you open to disease. The higher your glutathione level, the less likely you are to get heart disease, diabetes, high blood pressure, and a whole range of other problems. Glutathione protects your eyes against free radicals and helps prevent cataracts and other blinding eye conditions. Most important of all, glutathione boosts your immune system and helps it work at top efficiency—and that keeps you healthy no matter what your age.

You might be low on glutathione for a lot of reasons aside from just getting older. We could write a whole book about why (in fact, we did—it's called *Glutathione: The Ultimate Antioxidant*), but for now let's just give a few good reasons:

➤ You're sick with a bad cold or flu or have an injury of some sort. You're making a lot of extra free radicals that need to be squelched, and your immune system needs glutathione to make white blood cells, so you're using up glutathione faster than you can make it.

➤ You're exposed to a lot of toxins. Glutathione finds toxic wastes in your body and carts them off. If you're exposed to a lot of toxins every day—air pollution, exhaust fumes, or dry-cleaning chemicals, for example—your glutathione is very, very busy. You're using so much of it to eliminate toxins that there's not a lot left to fight free radicals.

➤ You have a chronic disease such as asthma or rheumatoid arthritis. You need extra glutathione to boost your immune system and fend off the extra free radicals your disease creates—and a shortage of glutathione makes your symptoms worse by letting free radicals attack. This gets very circular. It's even possible that a shortage of glutathione is why you're sick to begin with.

You can easily see why it's so important to be sure you have enough glutathione in your system.

# Boosting Your Glutathione Level

It's easy to raise your glutathione level—some glutathione is found in almost all fruits and vegetables. We've listed some of the best sources in the chart. Cooking destroys a lot of the glutathione, so eat these foods raw or just lightly steamed.

Some vegetables contain substances that naturally make your body make more glutathione. The best choices here are broccoli, cabbage, Brussels sprouts, cauliflower, kale, and parsley. Recent research shows that fish oil also makes you produce more glutathione (see Chapter 23 for more information about fish oil).

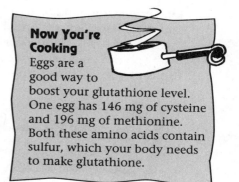

**Now You're Cooking**
Eggs are a good way to boost your glutathione level. One egg has 146 mg of cysteine and 196 mg of methionine. Both these amino acids contain sulfur, which your body needs to make glutathione.

## Foods High in Glutathione

| Food | Glutathione in mg |
| --- | --- |
| Acorn squash | 14 |
| Asparagus | 26 |
| Avocado | 31 |
| Broccoli | 8 |
| Cantaloupe | 9 |
| Grapefruit | 15 |
| Okra | 7 |
| Orange | 11 |
| Peach | 7 |
| Potato | 13 |
| Spinach | 5 |
| Strawberries | 12 |
| Tomato | 11 |
| Watermelon | 28 |
| Zucchini | 7 |

*Note: Amounts are for 3.5-ounce (100 grams) servings.*

You can also take glutathione supplements. This doesn't always work well for everyone. Remember, glutathione is a tripeptide, a small protein made from three amino acids. Some of the glutathione you swallow in a supplement gets broken down into its amino acids by your digestive juices, and some gets absorbed straight into your body through your small intestine. If you're low on glutathione to begin with, you'll probably absorb a lot. For maximum protection against free radicals and toxins, we suggest getting at least 100 mg a day of glutathione. This could be hard to get from your food alone, so you might want to take supplements. Glutathione supplements are extremely safe—even taking several grams at a time is harmless. Take your glutathione supplements with meals to absorb the most from them.

### Food for Thought

If you want to try glutathione supplements, we recommend either GSH 250 Master Glutathione Formula or Glutaplex (both made by Douglas Labs). Both formulas contain glutathione, NAC, lipoic acid, selenium, riboflavin, glutamine, and glycine. GSH 250 is stronger—take it if you really need an antioxidant boost. If you regularly eat lots of fresh fruits and vegetables, the smaller amounts in Glutaplex may be all you need.

## Supplements to Boost Glutathione

### Quack, Quack

Glutathione is only one of several powerful antioxidants you make. Superoxide dismutase (SOD) and catalase are two others. SOD is an enzyme that demolishes the superoxide radical; catalase is an enzyme needed to capture hydroxyl radicals. Some manufacturers sell SOD and catalase supplements, but these supplements are worthless: Your digestive juices destroy them as soon as you swallow them. If you want to try SOD supplements, choose the enteric-coated version from Solgar.

If you don't want to take glutathione supplements, you can eat foods high in cysteine or take cysteine supplements instead. You have to have plenty of cysteine to make glutathione, because cysteine has that all-important sulfur molecule in it. By taking supplements, you make sure you've got enough. We recommend cysteine supplements in the form of *N-acetyl cysteine* (NAC). This form is easily absorbed by your body.

Most people have plenty of the other two aminos—glycine and glutamic acid—needed to make glutathione. Even so, taking extra glutamine (your body converts glutamine to glutamic acid very easily) helps raise your glutathione level. This seems to work not because you're short on the glutamine building block but because glutamine stimulates your liver to make more glutathione. Glutamine is found in almost all foods. The best sources are lean meats, eggs, wheat germ, and whole grains.

If you want to take extra glutamine, we recommend the less expensive powder form over tablets. The powder is tasteless and odorless and dissolves easily in water. Drink it down or sprinkle it on cold foods such as your breakfast cereal. Don't mix it with acidic liquids like orange juice or put it on something hot—you'll destroy the glutamine.

The usual dose for extra glutamine is anywhere from 1,000 mg to 5,000 mg.

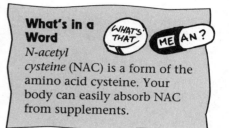

**What's in a Word**

*N-acetyl cysteine* (NAC) is a form of the amino acid cysteine. Your body can easily absorb NAC from supplements.

**Food for Thought**

NAC supplements can do more than just boost your glutathione level. Raising the level of cysteine in your blood seems to stimulate your immune system and make you produce more infection-fighting T4 white blood cells.

Riboflavin (Vitamin B$_2$) helps your body combine amino acids into proteins, so be sure you're getting enough. The RDA for riboflavin is just under 2 mg a day. If you want to boost your glutathione level, though, you'll need more. We suggest 25 to 50 mg a day—a dose that's perfectly safe. Vitamin C also helps boost your glutathione level. We suggest taking 500 mg a day.

You also need to be sure you've got enough selenium in your system. That's because you need selenium to make one of the vital enzymes needed to make glutathione in your cells. We suggest getting 25 mcg a day. (Refer to Chapter 21 on trace minerals to learn more about why you need tiny amounts of this mineral.)

Finally, lipoic acid helps you make glutathione and use it more efficiently. Lipoic acid is so important that we're going to discuss it separately.

# Lipoic Acid: The Vitamin That's Not a Vitamin

When researchers in the 1950s isolated *lipoic acid*, they thought at first they had found a new vitamin. Lipoic acid is essential for helping your mitochondria—the tiny power plants in your cells—turn glucose into energy. The researchers thought you got your lipoic acid from your food, especially animal foods. If you have to have something, and you can only get it from your food, it's a vitamin, right? After some more study the researchers found that your body makes the very small amounts of lipoic acid you need for producing energy.

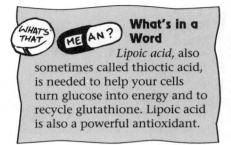

**What's in a Word**

*Lipoic acid*, also sometimes called thioctic acid, is needed to help your cells turn glucose into energy and to recycle glutathione. Lipoic acid is also a powerful antioxidant.

That's not the end of the story, though. In the late 1980s, researchers found that lipoic acid is also a very powerful antioxidant—one that's both water-soluble and fat-soluble. They also realized that you use lipoic acid as part of the complicated process that recycles your glutathione so it can capture more free radicals. Because almost all the lipoic acid you make naturally is busy being used in your mitochondria, there's not a lot left over for your glutathione—and there's none left over to act as an antioxidant.

Lipoic acid helps boost your glutathione level by helping you recycle it better. But because you naturally don't have a whole lot of lipoic acid, you can only recycle so much glutathione and no more—unless you take lipoic acid supplements. The usual dose is fairly small, just 200 mg a day.

Lipoic acid supplements can also give you extra free radical protection throughout your body. This could help prevent a lot of health problems, including atherosclerosis and cataracts. Lipoic acid could also be useful for people with liver disease.

## Helping Diabetic Neuropathy

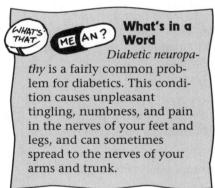

**What's in a Word**

*Diabetic neuropathy* is a fairly common problem for diabetics. This condition causes unpleasant tingling, numbness, and pain in the nerves of your feet and legs, and can sometimes spread to the nerves of your arms and trunk.

People with diabetes sometimes get a painful nerve condition called *diabetic neuropathy*. We still don't know exactly what causes the problem, but lipoic acid can often help. The doses needed are fairly high. In Europe, where doctors can prescribe lipoic acid, the usual dose is 600 to 1,200 mg a day. It has been widely used in Germany for over 25 years for treating diabetic neuropathy.

If you have diabetes and want to try lipoic acid, be sure to talk to your doctor first. The lipoic acid may also improve your blood sugar level, so you'll have to watch the level carefully and adjust your medication if needed.

## The Least You Need to Know

➤ Glutathione is your body's most abundant natural antioxidant.

➤ You can boost your glutathione level by eating foods high in glutathione and by taking glutathione supplements.

➤ You also can raise your glutathione level by taking supplements of cysteine, selenium, and glutamine—the building blocks for glutathione.

➤ Lipoic acid is another powerful antioxidant you make in very small amounts. Lipoic acid supplements can help raise your glutathione level.

➤ Lipoic acid can be very helpful for diabetic neuropathy, a painful nerve condition.

# Chapter 25

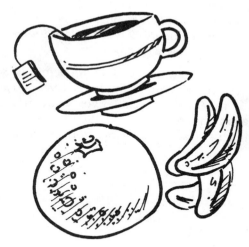

# Flavonoids for Humanoids

## In This Chapter

➤ What flavonoids are

➤ Foods that are high in flavonoids

➤ How flavonoids mop up free radicals

➤ Flavonoids protect you against cancer and heart disease

➤ Protecting your eyes with flavonoids

Everywhere you go, people are telling you to eat lots of fresh fruits and vegetables. Why? It's not just that these foods are crammed with vitamins and minerals. It's not just that they're low in calories, low in fat, and high in fiber. It's because they're packed with flavonoids—the stuff that gives them their color and taste. And it's the flavonoids, as much if not more than the other stuff, that makes fruits and vegetables so good for you.

There are so many flavonoids and they're so good for you that we're still trying to figure them all out. So far, we've managed to identify some really important ones, like alpha carotene, but there's plenty more we haven't pinned down yet. We know they're in there, though, and that you should get as many of them as possible. How? By following the advice everyone's giving you: Eat lots of fresh fruits and vegetables—five to nine servings a day.

# What Are Flavonoids?

Flavonoids—also called bioflavonoids—give fruits and vegetables their bright colors. These chemically complicated substances make oranges orange, red peppers red, and blueberries blue. But flavonoids do more than just give color and flavor to plant foods—they also give powerful antioxidant protection to the people who eat them.

Flavonoids are part of a much larger family of plant substances called phytochemicals. So far, scientists have discovered over 4,000 different phytochemicals in plants. Over 600 are flavonoids or carotenoids, and of those, about 50 to 60 stay active after you've eaten them and are valuable for your health. Most flavonoids are great antioxidants. Others may be helpful for their ability to relieve swelling, pain, and allergic reactions. Some may even help you fight off viruses.

## Food for Thought

Flavonoids were discovered in the late 1930s by Albert Szent-Györgi, discoverer of Vitamin C. He gave a friend a crude sample of Vitamin C made from lemons to help his bleeding gums. The bleeding stopped temporarily. Later, Szent-Györgi gave him a purer form of Vitamin C—and it didn't work. In purifying it, he had removed the flavonoids. When his friend used just the "impurities," the bleeding stopped completely. Szent-Györgi looked more closely at what he had taken out. He called it Vitamin P for vascular permeability (a fancy way to say blood vessels that bleed easily). Vitamin P turned out not to be absolutely essential in your diet—so technically it's not a vitamin.

## Now You're Cooking

Flavonoids in fruits and vegetables aren't hurt much by cooking. In fact, cooking breaks down tough cell walls in vegetables and makes flavonoids easier to absorb. Don't peel fruits and vegetables—many flavonoids are in the skin. Boil or steam fresh vegetables lightly or use frozen vegetables. Canned produce has very little left in the way of flavonoids, vitamins, minerals, or taste.

There's a lot we still don't know about flavonoids. When you get right down to it, our lack of knowledge is the best reason of all to be sure you eat plenty of fresh fruits and vegetables every day. Somewhere in that big mix of flavonoids are the ones that keep you healthy—and that's not even counting the vitamins, minerals, and fiber in fruits and veggies.

There are so many different flavonoids that it's hard to sort them all out. One reason is that plant foods have lots of different flavonoids in them. Broccoli, for example, is a good source not just of cancer-fighting indoles but also of the antioxidants quercetin and lutein—and also of Vitamin C, calcium, potassium, folic acid, chromium, and boron. Oranges have over 40 different flavonoids, including almost all the ones we'll talk about in this chapter.

On top of all that, flavonoids are what make many medicinal herbs work—but describing all that would take a whole other book. In this chapter we'll stick to explaining the major flavonoid groups.

# Carotenoids: Orange You Glad You Know

Carrots, sweet potatoes, squash, and other orange and red foods get their color from substances called *carotenoids*. The carotenoids are such a large and important family that we need to break them down into two main branches. Orange and red foods contain large amounts of *carotenes*. Carotenoids are also found in green leafy vegetables such as broccoli, kale, spinach, and Brussels sprouts.

All the carotenoids are fat-soluble. To get the most carotenoids from these foods, eat them with a little dietary fat. Supplements containing mixed carotenoids usually contain mostly beta carotene along with alpha carotene, lutein, lycopene, and other carotenoids in varying combinations. These supplements are often made from a type of algae called *Dunaliella salina*. They're a good insurance policy if you don't eat many fruits and vegetables.

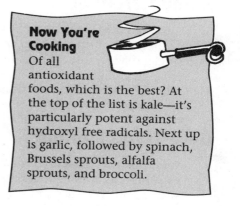

**Now You're Cooking**
Of all antioxidant foods, which is the best? At the top of the list is kale—it's particularly potent against hydroxyl free radicals. Next up is garlic, followed by spinach, Brussels sprouts, alfalfa sprouts, and broccoli.

Carotenoids are orange- or red-colored substances found in many fruits and vegetables. Carotenoids are divided into two groups. Carotenes contain only carbon and hydrogen atoms. They're found in carrots, squash, and many other orange- or red-colored foods. Your body can convert alpha and beta carotene into Vitamin A; the carotenes are also very powerful antioxidants. Xanthophylls contain carbon, hydrogen, and oxygen atoms. These carotenoids are found in many dark-green leafy vegetables and in egg yolks. They're also orange or yellow (*xantho* means yellow in Greek), but the color is covered up by the green chlorophyll in these foods. Xanthophylls are great antioxidants, but they have no Vitamin A activity.

**Food for Thought**

The no-calorie fat substitute Olestra® promises us guilt-free potato chips. It may be promising more cancer as well. Why? Because Olestra passes through your body without being digested, it carries away fat-soluble nutrients, including vitamins A, D, E, and K. To make up for the loss, the manufacturer has agreed to add these vitamins to Olestra. But Olestra also carries away cancer-fighting carotenoids—and there are no plans to add them to Olestra. By some estimates, three servings a week of a snack food containing Olestra would lower your carotenoid level by 10 percent. Over the whole United States population, that could lead to over 30,000 extra cancer deaths every year.

# The Carotenes

No, these aren't adolescent carrots. They're flavonoids found in many orange- and red-colored fruits and vegetables. The most important member of the carotene family is beta carotene. Because you convert some of the beta carotene you eat into Vitamin A, we talked a lot about it in Chapter 3, so check back there to find out more. In this section, we'll focus on three other very important carotenes: alpha carotene, beta-cryptoxanthin, and lycopene.

## Alpha Carotene

Although beta carotene is the most abundant carotene in foods, its close cousin alpha carotene is a much stronger antioxidant, especially for quenching those destructive singlet oxygen free radicals. Alpha carotene is found in all the same foods as beta carotene, including carrots, sweet potatoes, cantaloupe, broccoli, kiwi, spinach, mangos, and squash. As a rough rule of thumb, the amount of alpha carotene in a food is about 10 to 20 percent of the amount of beta carotene.

## Beta-Cryptoxanthin

Sounds like a character from a horror movie about zombies, doesn't it? Actually, cryptoxanthin is a carotene found in oranges, mangoes, papayas, cantaloupes, peaches, prunes, and squash. You may not realize it, but you eat some every time you eat butter, because cryptoxanthin is also used to color butter. It's a very good quencher of singlet oxygen free radicals.

## Lycopene

Pizza lovers, rejoice! Lycopene is a cancer-fighting anti-oxidant found in large amounts in tomatoes—it's what makes them red. (Watermelon and pink grapefruit have lycopene too, but in much smaller amounts.) Lycopene is the most abundant carotene in your body. Surprisingly, most people have levels that are far higher than their beta carotene levels. A major study in 1995 showed that men who eat lots of tomato-based foods are much less likely to get prostate cancer. In general, lycopene seems to protect against cancer of the digestive tract, including colon cancer, and against lung cancer. New research suggests that lycopene may also help ward off heart disease. In 1997, a major European study showed that men who eat the most lycopene are only half as likely to have a heart attack as the men who eat the least. We're sure there will be plenty of research on this very promising flavonoid in the coming years.

> **Now You're Cooking**
> You absorb lycopene well only if you eat it with dietary fat—like the olive oil in tomato sauce or the cheese on your pizza. Cooked tomatoes are better, because cooking breaks down the cell walls and releases the lycopene. To get the most lycopene from fresh tomatoes, eat them with an oil-based salad dressing.

Any sort of tomato-based food gives you lycopene—check out the chart for some good choices.

| The Lycopene in Food | |
| --- | --- |
| **Food** | **Lycopene per ounce (in mg)** |
| Canned tomatoes | 3 |
| Fresh tomatoes | 3 |
| Ketchup | 5 |
| Pink grapefruit | 1 |
| Spaghetti sauce | 5 |
| Tomato juice | 3 |
| Tomato sauce | 5 |
| Tomato soup | 3 |
| Watermelon | 1 |

**Food for Thought**

In the 1830s and 1840s, Dr. Miles' Compound Extract of Tomato was a popular remedy for just about everything. The firm's slogan was "Tomato Pills Cure Your Ills." Dr. Miles and his many competitors were on to something, even if they didn't know what it was—the vitamins, minerals, and lycopene in tomatoes are indeed good for you, although we can't say they cure anything. And even if they didn't help, tomato pills didn't hurt—which is more than can be said for many of the standard medical treatments of the time.

# The Xanthophylls

Xanthophylls are carotenoids that are mostly found in dark-green leafy vegetables. They aren't converted in your body into Vitamin A. In general, all xanthophylls are valuable antioxidants. The xanthophylls lutein and zeaxanthin also protect your eyes against free radical damage.

## Lutein and Zeaxanthin

Your macula—the part of your retina you use for acute vision—is crammed with lutein and zeaxanthin. They help protect the delicate cells of your macula from the harmful effects of ultraviolet light in sunshine. A major study at Harvard Medical School showed that older people who ate the most high-carotenoid foods had the lowest rates of age-related macular degeneration—which is one of the major causes of blindness in the elderly. Lutein and zeaxanthin probably work because their yellow color blocks light from the ultraviolet (blue) end of the spectrum. Both lutein and zeaxanthin are also effective antioxidants. All dark-green, leafy vegetables are good sources of these xanthophylls; spinach and collard greens are especially good choices. The lutein and zeaxanthin used in supplements are often made from the petals of marigolds!

## Capsanthin

This antioxidant xanthophyll is found in red peppers—the redder the better. Redder doesn't mean hotter, though. Capsanthin is found in hot peppers, of course, but capsanthin supplements are made from paprika, which is made from sweet red peppers.

## Have a Nice Cup of Tea

When you brew yourself a nice cup of tea, you're actually brewing a potent antioxidant mix. Tea has two substances in the catechin family—epigallocatechin gallate and epicatechin gallate—that are the most potent antioxidants of all the flavonoids. That makes tea into more than just a relaxing hot drink—it protects against heart disease, stroke, and cancer. Catechins help make your platelets, the tiny cells in your blood that make it clot, less "sticky." When your platelets are less sticky, they're less likely to clot, which means you're less likely to have a heart attack or stroke from a clot in an artery. In one recent study, Dutch men who drank four cups of tea a day had a much lower risk of stroke than those who didn't—whether or not they also took vitamins. The catechins in tea also act as powerful antioxidants that can keep cancer from getting started. Tea also has antibacterial action: It kills the bacteria that cause cavities and gum disease. Japanese men who drink a lot of green tea (nine or more cups a day) have lower cholesterol levels.

The benefits of tea are found mostly in green tea, the kind used in China and Japan, because green tea has the most catechins. Green tea is made by steaming and then drying the fresh tea leaves. The steaming removes an enzyme that oxidizes the catechins and makes them less potent. Oolong tea (the kind served in Chinese restaurants) and black tea (the kind used in typical tea bags) aren't

> **Now You're Cooking**
>
> To brew tea, bring cold water to a rapid boil. Pour hot water into the teapot to warm it, then empty. Use one rounded teaspoon of loose tea (or one tea bag) for each cup; add one more for the pot. Pour in boiling water, cover the pot, and let tea steep (three to five minutes). Stir gently and pour. Use a strainer if you used loose tea.

steamed. Instead, they're exposed to the air for a few hours and then allowed to ferment. The process oxidizes the catechins and makes them less potent. Even so, these teas are nearly as potent as green tea. One cup of green tea has about 375 mg of catechins; a cup of black tea has 210 mg.

You need to drink at least five cups of mild-tasting green tea a day to get any real benefit. If you don't want to drink that much, try supplements containing green tea extract. One capsule is roughly the same as five cups of tea.

### Food for Thought

After water, tea is the world's most popular beverage. About 75 percent of the world's tea production is black tea; well over two million tons are made every year. Most of the rest is green tea; about 560,000 tons are made every year. Of the 47 *billion* cups of tea Americans drink every year, about 37 billion are iced.

One cup of brewed tea has about 40 mg of caffeine; a cup of instant tea has about 35 mg. As a caffeine comparison, one cup of brewed coffee has about 110 mg of caffeine; a cup of instant coffee has about 60 mg. The caffeine in tea is all released in the first minute of brewing.

# Quercetin: The Flavonoid from Onions

The flavonoid quercetin is very active—it's the important ingredient in a lot of medicinal plants. Quercetin helps reduce inflammation and swelling, block allergies, kills viruses, and acts as an antioxidant. It may even help diabetics control their blood sugar and avoid eye problems.

Quercetin is found in many different plant foods, but ordinary onions are the richest source. Their high quercetin content explains why onions are widely used in folk medicine as a treatment for allergies and asthma—the quercetin slows or prevents allergic reactions and relaxes swollen bronchial tubes. Quercetin also blocks your production of an enzyme that changes glucose into a damaging sugar alcohol. If you have diabetes, high sugar alcohol levels can cause cataracts, diabetic neuropathy, and other complications. Eating onions can help keep your blood sugar closer to normal, which will help you avoid some of the health problems diabetes can cause.

Quercetin can help prevent cancer by blocking the growth of cancer cells. In a major Chinese study, people who ate the most onions had the least stomach cancer. A lot of the research on this is still in the test-tube stage, though, so we can't really be sure about how quercetin helps cancer in people.

**Food for Thought**

Onions contain many other phytochemicals, including allylic sulfides that help lower your LDL ("bad") cholesterol level. Onions also help lower your blood pressure, prevent blood clots and improve your circulation. It's no surprise that many doctors today tell their heart patients to eat an onion every day. To get rid of onion breath, chew on a sprig of fresh parsley. If you prefer taking a quercetin supplement, the usual dose is between 200 and 400 mg three times a day. For best absorption, take the capsules about 20 minutes before meals.

There are over 500 plants in the big *Allium* family, including onions, scallions, chives, leeks, shallots, and garlic. The highest quercetin levels are in red onions, yellow onions, and shallots. Quercetin isn't absorbed all that well in your digestive tract. You absorb more from cooked onions than raw ones. (You'll also have better breath.)

# Garlic: It's Good for You

Garlic is a member of the extended onion family, but it stands out from all the others because of one phytochemical: allicin. This sulfur-containing compound is what gives garlic its pungent smell and taste. In folk medicine, garlic is used for everything from athlete's foot to influenza (to say nothing of its ability to ward off vampires). There's some truth to garlic's antibiotic activity, but recent research has concentrated on garlic as an antioxidant, a way to lower cholesterol, and a way to prevent cancer.

Garlic is one of the most potent antioxidant foods around—it's especially good for capturing peroxyl free radicals. The antioxidant effect of garlic could be why people who eat a lot of it tend to be healthier in general.

Until very recently, researchers believed garlic really did help cholesterol. They had good reasons: Several solid studies backed them up. Garlic supporters argue that the patients in the study just weren't taking enough. Whether or not that's the case, a study in 1997 in Israel gave new support to garlic as a weapon against high cholesterol and atherosclerosis. For now, all we can say is that garlic may be helpful and probably won't hurt.

The news on the cancer front is better. A sulfur compound found in aged garlic has been shown to slow down the growth of prostate cancer cells—but so far, only in the test tube. Garlic shows great promise as a preventive measure and as a treatment for prostate cancer, but so far we don't know enough to recommend an amount to take.

What about garlic for heart problems? A chemical in garlic called ajoene (*ajo* is Spanish for garlic) seems to thin your blood and prevent your platelets from forming clots that can lead to a heart attack. Ajoene (methyl allyl trisulfide) may also help dissolve clots once they form. Other garlic compounds may help your heart by lowering your blood pressure.

The benefits of garlic come from eating one to three fresh cloves every day. Not too many people like to eat that much garlic, though—and not too many people like to be around people who do. Raw garlic, cooked garlic, and even garlic powder from the spice shelf all give you the benefits of garlic. To avoid stomach upsets and garlic breath, though, try garlic supplements. These fall into two categories: dried garlic pills (the most popular brand is Kwai®, imported from Germany) or aged garlic in pills or liquid form (the most popular brand is Kyolic®, imported from Japan). Dried garlic (Kwai) has allicin; aged garlic (Kyolic) doesn't. On the other hand, aged garlic offers more protection against cancer. Because nobody really knows which compounds in garlic are the most important, it's hard to say which type of supplement is better. You need to take four 1,000 mg powdered garlic tablets, four gelcaps of aged garlic, or one teaspoon of liquid aged garlic to get the equivalent of two to three fresh garlic cloves.

## Anthocyanins for Healthy Eyes

Did you ever notice that not too many foods are blue? If more of them were, we might all have sharper eyesight. That's because blue fruits such as blueberries, blue grapes, and plums are high in a group of flavonoids called anthocyanins. The anthocyanins are very effective free-radical fighters, especially in the tiny blood vessels of your eyes. They're valuable for preventing eye problems, especially those affecting your retina, such as macular degeneration.

Just eating a lot of blueberries probably won't help protect your eyes, though. Supplements made from bilberries (a Scandinavian plant very similar to blueberries) are available. The standard capsules contain 25 percent anthocyanins. To get any real benefit from them, you'll need to take between four and eight 60 mg capsules a day.

## Resveratrol: Red Wine Rescuer

The French ignore all the things we Americans do to stay healthy.

They eat foods high in fat and calories. They smoke cigarettes. They wouldn't dream of going to the gym to work out. They also live longer and have less heart disease than anyone else in westernized society. What's going on here?

It's what scientists call the French paradox. What seems to save the French from their bad habits is what some might consider another bad habit: They drink a lot of red wine. And red wine is high in healthful flavonoids, including catechins and anthocyanins. As we've already explained, these flavonoids are great antioxidants that help protect your heart. Resveratrol, another substance in red wine, lowers your cholesterol and helps prevent artery-clogging blood clots. Resveratrol has an extra benefit: It blocks tumor growth and may even help precancerous cells return to normal.

A study in 1992 found that people who ate nuts several times a week cut their risk of heart disease—even though nuts are very high in fat. In 1997, researchers discovered that peanuts contain lots of resveratrol—about 73 micrograms in an ounce. By comparison, a five-ounce glass of red wine contains over 800 micrograms of resveratrol.

Many doctors recommend a glass or two of red wine with your evening meal. Not only does the alcohol help you relax, it's how the flavonoids in red wine get into your system—they're soluble in alcohol but not water (although we still don't know if you absorb much resveratrol that way). If you don't want to drink alcohol, try eating plenty of red or purple grapes or drinking purple grape juice. The flavonoids are concentrated in the purple or red grape skins. You have to drink three times as much grape juice to get the same benefit as one glass of wine, though. You could try one of the new red wine supplements instead. These capsules contain the flavonoids in powder form, without the alcohol.

## Unexpected Health from Unlikely Plants

Many, many plant foods contain valuable flavonoids. So do parts of plants we don't normally eat. And so do some plants that we don't think of as food at all. Here's a run-down of some of the flavonoids now available in supplements.

➤ **OPCs.** Oligomeric proanthocyanidins (you can see why we prefer the abbreviation) are flavonoids found in many plants and in red wine. Supplements are made from grape seeds or pine bark. (The commercial mixture from pine bark is called pycnogenol.) OPCs are very active free-radical scavengers, especially for trapping hydroxyl free radicals. Enthusiasts also claims that OPCs help problems caused by poor circulation, such as easy bruising, varicose veins, hemorrhoids, and intermittent claudication. Do they? Yes—OPCs and pycnogenol can be very helpful, especially for varicose veins. Try them and see if they work for you. The usual dose for general antioxidant protection is 50 mg a day. For circulation problems, the dose is between 150 and 300 mg daily.

➤ **Citrus flavonoids.** Several flavonoids found in citrus fruits, including hesperidin, quercetin, rutin, and naring in, are helpful for improving circulation in your tiny blood vessels. They work a lot like OPCs. If you want to take supplements, look for a brand that lists the amounts of rutin and hesperidin on the label—brands that don't, aren't as reliable. The usual dose for circulatory problems is between 2,000 and 6,000 mg a day.

➤ **Rutin.** This flavonoid is found in citrus fruits and also in red wine, berries, and buckwheat. As we've already discussed, rutin is useful for circulatory problems. New research suggests it can also help protect the DNA in your genes. Exposure to free

**Warning!**
Flavonoids in grapefruit juice, including quercetin, kaempferol, and naringin, can cause dangerous drug interactions. They seem to block one of your liver enzymes and keep it from breaking down certain drugs, so the drugs build up to dan-gerous levels in your bloodstream. Don't drink grapefruit juice if you take felodipine (Plendil®) or nifedipine (Adalat® or Procardia®) to treat high blood pressure or angina or terfenadine (Seldane®) to treat allergies.

radicals, pollution, and toxins can damage your DNA and make it send out garbled messages. You make enzymes that continually check out your DNA and make repairs when they come across any damage. In lab animals, rutin revs up the repair enzymes and reduces DNA damage. Humans aren't lab rats, so it's too soon to say if this will work in people.

# Ginkgo Biloba and Your Brain

One of the best-selling herbs on the market today is an extract made from the leaves of the ginkgo biloba tree. What makes this stuff so popular? Flavonoids. The flavonoids in ginkgo are safe, very powerful antioxidants that can boost your memory and mental alertness. Ginkgo can also be very helpful for *cerebral insufficiency*, or poor blood flow to your brain, and for poor circulation in your feet, legs, and hands. Ginkgo can also help some cases of male impotence by improving circulation to the penis.

Ginkgo's powerful antioxidant action is particularly good for squelching free radical attacks on your cell membranes. In fact, some researchers think ginkgo can actually reverse free radical damage to brain cell membranes.

In Europe, doctors are allowed to prescribe ginkgo—and they do. It's one of the most widely prescribed medicines in Germany, for example. In the United States, ginkgo is sold over the counter in pharmacies and health food stores. The standard version (sometimes labeled EGb) is a capsule or liquid that contains 24 percent ginkgoflavoneglycosides and 6 percent terpene lactones (those are just the scientific terms for the active flavonoids in ginkgo). Don't buy anything else.

The usual dose for cerebral insufficiency is 40 mg three times a day. This would also be a good dose for other circulatory problems. A lot of people take 40 to 80 mg a day as a preventive measure to keep their mental function high. Does this work? We can't remember!

In 1997, a serious study of ginkgo biloba as a treatment for Alzheimer's disease appeared in the *Journal of the American Medical Association*. The study showed that ginkgo biloba in the form of EGb slowed the progression of the disease in about a third of the patients. The dosage in the study was 40 mg three times a day over a year-long period—an

**What's in a Word**

*Cerebral insufficiency* is a general term for problems caused by poor blood circulation to your brain. It's most common in older people, where it often causes symptoms of senility such as memory loss, poor concentration, confusion, anxiety, and depression.

**Now You're Cooking**

We don't recommend tea made from crushed ginkgo leaves—you won't get very much of the active ingredients. To get the most from ginkgo, buy the EGb in capsules or as an extract.

amount that had no side effects and worked almost as well as the prescription drug tacrine. The researchers think that the antioxidant powers of gingko are probably responsible for the improvement. The results of the study are very encouraging—we feel that more research will lead to better uses of ginkgo biloba as an effective treatment for this devastating disease.

Ginkgo can be helpful for situations where you want to be mentally alert—before a big exam or interview, for example. If you want to try this, take just 40 mg an hour or so in advance.

Ginkgo is very, very safe and is unlikely to cause any side effects. It works by improving the blood flow through the tiny blood vessels of your brain, so you get more oxygen and other nutrients. As it improves circulation to your brain, though, you might get some dizziness or even a mild headache. To be on the safe side, start with smaller doses and gradually build up the amount over several weeks. It can take six weeks or even longer before you start to notice any improvement from taking ginkgo. Stick with it.

# The Least You Need to Know

➤ Flavonoids are the substances that give color and flavor to plant foods.

➤ To get the most flavonoids, eat a variety of fresh fruits and vegetables every day.

➤ Most flavonoids are powerful antioxidants. Many are also helpful for preventing or treating specific health problems such as asthma or eye problems.

➤ Carotenoids, including beta carotene and lycopene, are powerful antioxidants. Lycopene may help prevent prostate and lung cancer.

➤ Other important flavonoids include quercetin, found in onions, and catechins, found in tea.

➤ Garlic contains many flavonoids and other valuable substances, as do red wine, blueberries, citrus fruits, grape seeds, and the herb ginkgo biloba.

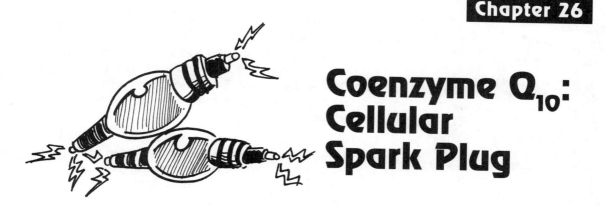

# Chapter 26

# Coenzyme Q$_{10}$: Cellular Spark Plug

## In This Chapter

➤ What coenzyme Q$_{10}$ (ubiquinone) is

➤ How coenzyme Q$_{10}$ makes energy in your cells

➤ Foods that are high in coenzyme Q$_{10}$

➤ How coenzyme Q$_{10}$ can help people with heart failure

➤ How coenzyme Q$_{10}$ can lower your blood pressure

What makes you tick? At the most basic level—inside your cells—it's something called coenzyme Q$_{10}$. You need this special stuff to release energy in your cells. Without it, you come to a stop.

Coenzyme Q$_{10}$ acts a lot like the spark plugs in your car engine. Spark plugs convert gasoline to energy inside the pistons of the engine. The energy drives the pistons, which drive the car. Coenzyme Q$_{10}$ in your cells works the same way. If one of your spark plugs isn't working right, your car engine stops running well. If all the spark plugs aren't working, your car sputters to a stop, even if the gas tank is full. Something very similar happens in your body if you run low on coenzyme Q$_{10}$—you can't produce enough energy to keep your body running.

# Co Q What?

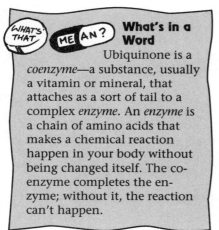

**What's in a Word**

*Quinones* are brightly colored organic substances found in all living plants and animals that need oxygen to survive. *Ubiquinone* is one name for a quinone that is found in all human cells. Its name comes from the prefix *ubi-*, meaning everywhere, combined with quinone.

**What's in a Word**

Ubiquinone is a *coenzyme*—a substance, usually a vitamin or mineral, that attaches as a sort of tail to a complex *enzyme*. An *enzyme* is a chain of amino acids that makes a chemical reaction happen in your body without being changed itself. The coenzyme completes the enzyme; without it, the reaction can't happen.

Back in 1957, researchers found something in beef hearts that seemed to be basic for making energy in living cells. They analyzed it and found it was a *quinone*, one of a group of substances that are found in all living plants and animals that use oxygen. Early researchers called the substance *ubiquinone,* meaning a quinone that was found everywhere.

The basic structure of quinone differs slightly among living things. In humans, the quinone has 10 units in a side chain of molecules. In the 1960s, researchers discovered that ubiquinone in humans is a very important *coenzyme*, so they started calling it coenzyme $Q_{10}$, or $CoQ_{10}$ for short.

$CoQ_{10}$ works in the mitochondria of your cells. These mini power plants provide the energy that runs your body. In a very complex process, $CoQ_{10}$ shuttles tiny, electrically charged particles back and forth in the mitochondria among the three essential enzymes that are needed to generate energy. Without $CoQ_{10}$, the whole process grinds to a halt.

Starting in the 1970s, coenzyme $Q_{10}$ research really took off in Japan. It was approved there as a treatment for heart failure in 1974. Today, it is one of the five most widely prescribed drugs in Japan. It's also widely prescribed in Italy, Sweden, Denmark, and Canada. In the United States, though, no drug company makes coenzyme $Q_{10}$ and it is not considered a drug. Instead, it's a food supplement that you can buy in any health food store. All coenzyme $Q_{10}$ supplements are imported from Japan.

# $CoQ_{10}$ for Cardiac Cases

So far, the most exciting news about coenzyme $Q_{10}$ is that it can be extremely helpful for some types of heart disease. In a number of serious studies, coenzyme $Q_{10}$ has been shown to be especially good for people with *heart failure.*

The biggest benefit seems to come from the way $CoQ_{10}$ improves energy flow in your mitochondria. Your heart muscle has the most mitochondria of any muscle in your body, and it also has—or should have—the highest level of coenzyme $Q_{10}$. People with heart failure, though, frequently have low coenzyme $Q_{10}$ levels, which is probably why they often improve when they start taking $CoQ_{10}$. Their hearts start to pump harder and circulate their blood better.

Coenzyme $Q_{10}$ has no side effects and doesn't cause any bad drug interactions. Best of all, studies show that heart failure patients who take coenzyme $Q_{10}$ feel better overall and have to spend less time in the hospital.

In early studies of $CoQ_{10}$, heart patients were given just 30 mg a day and showed some improvement. Today the usual dose for heart disease is anywhere from 100 to 300 mg a day. Because you can't overdose on coenzyme $Q_{10}$, these doses are quite safe.

If you have heart failure or any other sort of heart disease and want to try coenzyme $Q_{10}$, you *must* talk to your doctor first. The sooner you start taking $CoQ_{10}$ after your heart disease has been diagnosed, the better it will work, but it will still take several weeks to start helping. You *must* continue to take your medication—coenzyme $Q_{10}$ should be taken along with, not instead of, any drugs your doctor prescribes. A few months after you start taking coenzyme $Q_{10}$, your symptoms may get a lot better. You may even want to take less of your prescription medicines. *Never* try to change your heart drugs on your own—you *must* talk to your doctor.

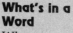

**What's in a Word**

When your heart is damaged or weak and can't pump blood to the rest of your body very well, you have *heart failure*. Symptoms of heart failure include extreme tiredness, breathlessness, and swelling in the ankles and legs. Drugs such as digitalis, diuretics, and blood thinners are often used to treat heart failure.

$CoQ_{10}$ may give you another heart benefit as well. It seems to reduce the "stickiness" of your platelets, the tiny cells that form blood clots. If your platelets are less likely to clump together to form an artery-blocking clot, you're less likely to have a heart attack. This is a promising new area of research, but it's far too soon to recommend $CoQ_{10}$ as a blood thinner or as a way to prevent heart attacks. That's because some studies show that coenzyme $Q_{10}$ might interact with blood-thinning drugs and make them less effective.

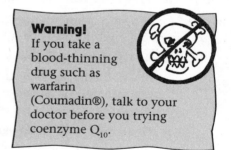

**Warning!**
If you take a blood-thinning drug such as warfarin (Coumadin®), talk to your doctor before you trying coenzyme $Q_{10}$.

# Lowering Your Blood Pressure

Coenzyme $Q_{10}$ could help lower your blood pressure, especially if it's high because of a heart problem. It works like this: $CoQ_{10}$ helps your heart work better, and when your heart pumps more efficiently, your blood pressure goes down. Coenzyme $Q_{10}$ may also help if your blood pressure is high for no particular reason (essential hypertension). Somewhat less than half of the people with essential hypertension are low on coenzyme $Q_{10}$. If you're one of them, taking supplements may help. Ask your doctor about having a blood test to check your $CoQ_{10}$ level. (For more information about your blood pressure, look in Chapter 2 for basic information; also check Chapter 17 on calcium and Chapter 18 on magnesium.)

If you want to try coenzyme $Q_{10}$ for your blood pressure, talk to your doctor first. $CoQ_{10}$ takes a while to start helping. You'll have to take about 200 mg a day for several months before you see a drop. In the meantime, you *must* keep taking your high blood medicine—*coenzyme $Q_{10}$ should be taken along with, not instead of, any drugs your doctor prescribes*. After you start taking $CoQ_{10}$, your blood pressure may drop and you may need less of your prescription drugs. *Never* try to change your high blood pressure medicine on your own—you *must* talk to your doctor.

# Cholesterol and CoQ$_{10}$

Those artery-clogging cholesterol deposits are made in part when the LDL ("bad") cholesterol in your blood reacts with oxygen. Coenzyme $Q_{10}$ may help keep your cholesterol from oxidizing, which in turn keeps it from plugging up your arteries. Some researchers claim it works even better than Vitamin E or carotenes, but there haven't been enough studies yet to prove this.

If you have high cholesterol, your doctor may prescribe a drug such as lovastatin (Mevacor®) to bring it down. These drugs work well, but they may also block your production of coenzyme $Q_{10}$, because some of the processes blocked by the drug are the same steps needed to make coenzyme $Q_{10}$. If you need to take medicine to lower your cholesterol, talk to your doctor about taking coenzyme $Q_{10}$ supplements as well.

# Other Benefits of Coenzyme Q$_{10}$

A lot of health claims are made for coenzyme $Q_{10}$. Some are nonsense—$CoQ_{10}$ probably won't do anything for male infertility—but some claims have real value.

➤ **Improving immunity.** Your coenzyme $Q_{10}$ level drops when you've got a serious illness. Taking supplements might give your immune system a jolt and help you produce more infection-fighting antibodies, but it takes at least a month of daily supplements for the effect to kick in.

➤ **Diabetes.** $CoQ_{10}$ could benefit diabetics by helping to prevent many complications, such as heart disease. It also may help keep blood sugar levels down. This is an area that needs a lot more research before we can recommend it. If you have diabetes and want to take $CoQ_{10}$ supplements, talk to your doctor first.

➤ **Gum disease (gingivitis).** Many people with gum disease (gingivitis) have low $CoQ_{10}$ levels. Good dental care, along with taking extra $CoQ_{10}$, could help clear up the problem faster.

➤ **Improved athletic performance.** Because coenzyme $Q_{10}$ is so important for producing energy in your body, a lot of serious athletes are interested in it. There's some evidence that coenzyme $Q_{10}$ is a safe, natural way to improve endurance. The better shape you're in, the better it works, although it seems to help even ordinary couch potatoes.

➤ **Improved energy.** Taking coenzyme $Q_{10}$ can help improve your overall energy level. This is good for anyone who works long hours, and it's very good for the elderly, people recovering from cancer treatment, and people with chronic fatigue syndrome.

➤ **Treating cancer.** Some experimental work suggests coenzyme $Q_{10}$ in high doses could slow or even stop tumor growth. A lot more work remains to be done, though, before this becomes a useful treatment for cancer.

Among researchers today there's a lot of interest in $CoQ_{10}$. We think many of the claims for it will be validated by serious research over the next few years.

## Food for Thought

Every day you hear about "natural" remedies for health problems—remedies your doctor says don't work or aren't proven. Should you try them, even though they're not part of mainstream medicine? We can't say. We can tell you to carefully consider the source. Advertisements, word-of-mouth recommendations, or the advice of a part-time clerk at the vitamin counter aren't good enough. The information you get this way is often distorted or just plain wrong. Before you start taking vitamins, minerals, and other supplements to treat a health problem, seek qualified help from a nutritionally oriented physician or other professional who can give you rational advice based on solid scientific evidence.

# Getting Your Coenzyme Q₁₀

About half the coenzyme $Q_{10}$ in your body comes from the foods you eat; almost all the rest is made in your liver. Many foods have at least some coenzyme $Q_{10}$ in them, so the average person eats about 5 mg a day. Good sources of coenzyme $Q_{10}$ in food include oily, cold-water fish such as tuna, mackerel, and sardines. Organ meats, beef, and vegetable oils such as soy or canola oil are also good sources. Wheat germ, rice bran, and soy foods such as tofu all have some coenzyme $Q_{10}$.

You have to eat a lot of these foods to get any real amount of coenzyme $Q_{10}$. To get 30 mg of $CoQ_{10}$ in one sitting, for instance, you'd have to eat a whole pound of sardines or more than two pounds of peanuts. The process of making coenzyme $Q_{10}$ in your body is very complicated—it takes at least 15 steps and needs plenty of Vitamin C, Vitamin E, selenium, and the B vitamins.

All things considered, we suggest raising your $CoQ_{10}$ level by taking supplements. These are fairly inexpensive—a 30 mg capsule costs about a quarter. You have a choice of sublingual (under the tongue) lozenges, chewable tablets, tablets, and oil-based gelcaps.

We recommend the gelcaps. They're easy to swallow and give you the small amount of fat you need to absorb the $CoQ_{10}$ better.

Coenzyme $Q_{10}$ supplements are extremely safe. They don't cause any drug interactions or side effects and you can't overdose on them. Bear in mind, though, that they won't do anything for you if your coenzyme $Q_{10}$ level is normal—the supplements only help if your level is low.

## The Least You Need to Know

➤ Coenzyme $Q_{10}$ is a vitamin-like substance essential for making energy in your cells.

➤ You get some coenzyme $Q_{10}$ in your food and make the rest in your body.

➤ Coenzyme $Q_{10}$ supplements are sold in drug stores and health food stores. They are very safe and unlikely to interact with other drugs.

➤ Coenzyme $Q_{10}$ can be very helpful for treating heart failure.

➤ Coenzyme $Q_{10}$ can help lower your blood pressure.

# Chapter 27

# Help from Natural Hormones

## In This Chapter

➤ How hormones help regulate your body

➤ Your diet can help your hormones

➤ How melatonin can helps jet lag and insomnia

➤ How natural hormones can help women avoid menopause problems and breast cancer, and help men avoid prostate cancer

➤ Natural hormones can lower your cholesterol

Women have them. Men have them. Teenagers *really* have them. What are they? Hormones—chemical messengers that control and coordinate what goes on in your body. Hormones regulate your blood pressure and heartbeat. They control your growth, your sleep cycle, your blood sugar, your sexuality, and lots of other things in your body. They even play a role in your emotions. And when your hormones get out of whack, a lot of things can start to go wrong.

The good news is that sometimes you can help your hormones get back in sync safely and easily. Insomnia and jet lag, for instance, are really helped a lot by natural hormones—there's no need for dangerous sleeping drugs. And just changing your diet to include small amounts of soy foods every day can help solve some of the problems of menopause.

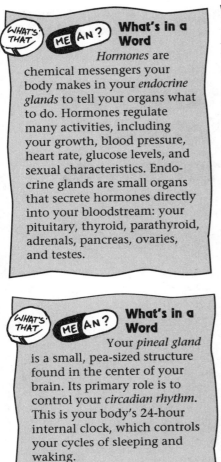

**What's in a Word**

*Hormones* are chemical messengers your body makes in your *endocrine glands* to tell your organs what to do. Hormones regulate many activities, including your growth, blood pressure, heart rate, glucose levels, and sexual characteristics. Endocrine glands are small organs that secrete hormones directly into your bloodstream: your pituitary, thyroid, parathyroid, adrenals, pancreas, ovaries, and testes.

**What's in a Word**

Your *pineal gland* is a small, pea-sized structure found in the center of your brain. Its primary role is to control your *circadian rhythm*. This is your body's 24-hour internal clock, which controls your cycles of sleeping and waking.

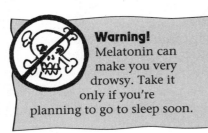

**Warning!**
Melatonin can make you very drowsy. Take it only if you're planning to go to sleep soon.

# What's a Hormone?

*Hormones* are the chemical messengers your body makes in your *endocrine glands*—your thyroid or pancreas, for example. Hormones coordinate what goes on in your body, making all your tissues and organs work together smoothly. Your endocrine system and the hormones it makes are marvelously complex—far too complex to explain in detail here. Diabetes or an underactive thyroid, for example, are hormone problems that you need to work with your doctor to treat. In this chapter, we'll focus on insomnia, jet lag, and menopause symptoms—hormone-related problems you can do a lot to help through diet and supplements.

# Melatonin: From A to Zzzz

Melatonin is a hormone made by your *pineal gland* (a small gland inside your brain). Your pineal gland controls your sleep/wake cycle and your body's internal clock—what scientists call your *circadian rhythm*. Melatonin's main function is to help you fall asleep, but today all sorts of other claims are made for it. Can melatonin cure insomnia, prevent jet lag, block cancer, restore immune function, improve your sex life, and even retard aging? Let's look more closely at what melatonin can really do.

## Melatonin for a Good Night's Rest

Melatonin does help you sleep. When your eyes notice it's getting dark, that information gets sent to your pineal gland, which then starts to make melatonin, which makes you drowsy. That's why melatonin is sometimes called "the hormone of darkness." Most people begin making melatonin at sunset, reach a peak at around two in the morning, and then gradually taper off toward sunrise. Until you're about 40, you make plenty of melatonin. After that, you make less and less as you get older, which may be one reason many elderly people don't sleep well.

Taking melatonin supplements on a regular basis a few hours before bedtime does help many people with frequent sleep problems get to sleep faster and stay asleep longer. If you only have occasional nights where you just can't seem to get to sleep, melatonin probably won't do much for you, especially if you're under age 40. On the other hand, because it's not addictive and has no side or morning-after effects (unlike most over-the-counter sleep medicines), it's worth a try. The dosage for getting to sleep varies hugely from person to person. Some people need just 100 mcg, while others take several milligrams. For most people, 100 to 400 mcg taken two to four hours before bedtime works very well.

## Relieving Jet Lag

For many tired travelers, melatonin is helpful for dealing with jet lag—the fatigue and insomnia that come from passing quickly through several time zones. Travel through time zones throws off your circadian rhythm. So do shift work and night jobs. Melatonin can help reset your internal clock to nighttime at your destination, which helps you get to sleep.

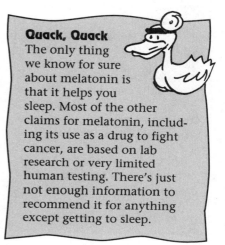

**Quack, Quack**
The only thing we know for sure about melatonin is that it helps you sleep. Most of the other claims for melatonin, including its use as a drug to fight cancer, are based on lab research or very limited human testing. There's just not enough information to recommend it for anything except getting to sleep.

To deal with jet lag, take a 3 mg dose of melatonin the first night you're at your destination. Be sure you have nothing else to do but nod off at that point, because the melatonin could make you very sleepy. You should sleep well and wake up feeling pretty close to normal. If you have trouble getting to sleep the next few nights, keep using the melatonin. Don't use it for more than five days in a row—by then you should be adjusted to your new time zone. If you're adjusting to a change in shifts or a switch to night work, follow the same schedule.

## Maximizing Your Melatonin

Important as melatonin is, your body produces it only in very small amounts—you make no more than about 300 mcg in a night. Taking larger doses of melatonin supplements doesn't seem to do any harm, though. Even in doses as large as 6 grams, melatonin isn't toxic. If you're pregnant or nursing, skip the melatonin—we don't know if you pass it on to your baby or not, or what happens if you do. And don't give melatonin to kids—they already make plenty of it. We recommend synthetic (also called pharmacy-grade) melatonin. "Natural" melatonin is made from the pineal glands of slaughtered cows and could contain dangerous viruses and impurities. If you don't want to take melatonin supplements, try eating foods that are high in the amino acid tryptophan, like turkey. Your body uses tryptophan to make melatonin. (For more information about tryptophan, see Chapter 22 on amino acids.)

## It's Soy Good for You

Soybean foods such as soy milk, tofu, and miso may be the best foods around for protecting women against breast cancer and relieving the symptoms of menopause. They may also help protect men against prostate cancer—and they help keep everyone's cholesterol down.

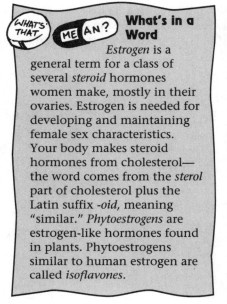

**What's in a Word**

*Estrogen* is a general term for a class of several *steroid* hormones women make, mostly in their ovaries. Estrogen is needed for developing and maintaining female sex characteristics. Your body makes steroid hormones from cholesterol—the word comes from the *sterol* part of cholesterol plus the Latin suffix *-oid*, meaning "similar." *Phytoestrogens* are estrogen-like hormones found in plants. Phytoestrogens similar to human estrogen are called *isoflavones*.

Soybeans are very high in *phytoestrogens*, hormone-like compounds found in plant foods. They're also high in *isoflavones*, phytoestrogens that are chemically close to the human female hormone *estrogen*. Two soy isoflavones, *genistein* and *daidzein*, can help prevent breast cancer.

Here's why. Estrogen is a *steroid* hormone—in other words, it's a hormone your body makes in your adrenal glands and your ovaries from cholesterol. Your breasts, ovaries, and uterus all have special receptors for estrogen. But too much estrogen can trigger breast cancer. And once the cancer starts, estrogen can make it grow faster.

What if you could block the estrogen receptors? That would slow the cancer down or even stop it—and that's exactly what successful cancer-fighting drugs such as tamoxifen do. What if you could block the receptors *before* the cancer starts? That's exactly what soy isoflavones, especially genistein, can do. Genistein and daidzein act like very weak estrogen—just strong enough to beat your real estrogen to the receptors, but not strong enough to trigger cancer.

Although we think of estrogen as the main female hormone, men make it in small amounts as well. Estrogen may play a role in triggering prostate cancer.

Soy foods have lots of other valuable anticancer substances as well. Soy foods are good sources of natural chemicals, such as protease inhibitors, saponins, phytosterols, and phytates, which block cancer cells and keep them from developing.

**Food for Thought**

Breast cancer is the second most common form of cancer in the western world, but it is much less common in Asia. In the United States, nearly 200 out of every 100,000 women will get breast cancer. In Japan, only 52 will—a rate about four times lower. Japanese women seem to get their cancer protection from the soy foods they eat. Among Japanese men, prostate cancer is also much less common. Here too, the cancer protection seems to come from soy foods.

Soy foods can also help menopause symptoms, especially hot flashes. Nearly half of all American women have this annoying problem for a year or so as they go through the early stages of menopause, but only about 10 percent of Japanese women get them. Again, soy foods seem to make the difference. The average Japanese woman eats a pound of tofu (bean curd) a week.

Today Premarin®, a drug that replaces estrogen in menopausal women, is one of the most widely prescribed drugs in America. Premarin can be very valuable for many women, especially in the first years after menopause. If you don't replace the estrogen your body has naturally stopped making, you're more likely to develop heart disease and osteoporosis. On the other hand, if you keep taking estrogen, you raise your chances of getting cancer, especially breast cancer. The decision to go ahead with estrogen replacement therapy is a serious one. You and your doctor need to weigh the pros and cons very carefully. As you do, discuss the safe alternative of genistein and daidzein supplements with your doctor. (And also read the section on preventing osteoporosis in Chapter 17 on calcium.)

Soy foods may also be helpful for lowering cholesterol levels—for women and men. A number of studies show that soy foods not only lower your LDL ("bad") cholesterol, they raise your HDL ("good") cholesterol. Also, the soy isoflavones may help keep the LDL cholesterol from oxidizing and forming artery-clogging deposits.

# Eating Your Soy

You can get the natural benefits of genistein, daidzein, and all the other good stuff in soy just by eating more soybean foods. The best choices are tofu (bean curd), soy milk, miso (fermented soybean paste used in soups), tempeh (a chewy cake made from fermented soybeans), and textured soy protein (TSP—also called textured vegetable protein or TVP). Fermented soy foods have the most genistein. Soy sauce and tamari don't have much in the way of isoflavones, though, even though they're also fermented.

Tofu is so popular today that you can find it in just about any supermarket—check the produce section. It's just as nutritious as meat, but when you eat tofu you get the soy isoflavones along with far fewer calories, almost no saturated fat, and a goodly dose of calcium. Soy milk is also easy to find in supermarkets. You can use the unflavored kind just like regular milk. The flavored versions are tasty and low in fat and calories.

Soy burgers, soy hot dogs, soy cheese, and soy ice-cream, which all taste a lot like the real thing, are also very popular now. They're low in calories and fat, but these foods are highly processed and have a lot of additional ingredients, so they don't have much in the way of isoflavones left. Soybean oil, which is the primary ingredient in vegetable cooking oil, doesn't have many isoflavones either.

You may have to visit your health-food store to find miso, tempeh, and textured soy protein. While you're there, look for other interesting soy foods, like roasted soybeans (fun for snacks), soy flour (follow the package instructions), dried soy beans (soak them for a *long* time and use them like any

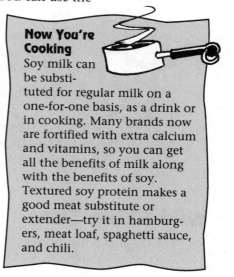

**Now You're Cooking**

Soy milk can be substituted for regular milk on a one-for-one basis, as a drink or in cooking. Many brands now are fortified with extra calcium and vitamins, so you can get all the benefits of milk along with the benefits of soy. Textured soy protein makes a good meat substitute or extender—try it in hamburgers, meat loaf, spaghetti sauce, and chili.

bean), and natto, a food made from fermented whole soybeans (use it as a side dish or condiment). Check out ethnic Asian and vegetarian cookbooks to find great soy recipes.

**Now You're Cooking**
Soy protein powder, available at your health food store, is another way to get the benefits of soy in your diet. Mix the powder with juice or use it in shakes and smoothies. As little as 30 to 40 grams a day—roughly three to four tablespoons—may be enough to help your hot flashes.

How much soy do you need to eat to relieve menopause problems and get cancer protection? Most researchers believe that anywhere from 20 to 50 mg of soy isoflavones every day will help, depending on how severe your symptoms are. There's about 30 to 40 mg of isoflavones (about 80 percent of it genistein) in a typical serving of soy food. What's a typical serving? Half a cup of tofu or tempeh, one cup of soy milk, or a quarter cup of textured soy protein. Based on that, you don't really need to eat large servings of soy foods—just 12 ounces of soy milk a day could be enough to cool off your hot flashes. You'll get the isoflavones along with lots of other useful nutrients, like protein, calcium, boron, lecithin, folic acid, and omega-3 fatty acids—and you'll get additional protection against artery-clogging cholesterol.

You can't always arrange to have soy foods in your daily diet—or maybe you just can't stand the taste of the stuff. In that case, you can buy nonprescription supplements that contain genistein and daidzein. They can be very helpful as an alternative to prescription hormones for relieving menopause symptoms, particularly hot flashes and vaginal dryness. Generally, the supplements come in 12 mg tablets or capsules. The usual dose is two or three daily. To be sure of getting a good product with enough active isoflavones, choose supplements from a reliable manufacturer such as Solgar, Twinlab, or Carlson.

If you're already taking Premarin or any other hormone replacement pills and you think you'd rather eat more soy foods or try genistein supplements instead, talk to your doctor first. You'll have to taper off the pills—don't just stop taking them.

**Food for Thought**
Americans eat so little soy that the amounts can't even be tracked, although we grow half of the world's soybeans. The annual American soybean crop comes to about 50 million metric tons and is worth over $12 billion. Almost all the soybeans grown in the United States are used for animal feed or vegetable oil or are exported.

# Wild About Yams

The original birth control pills were made from a substance called diosgenin, first discovered in Mexican wild yam roots. Diosgenin is very similar to the female hormone *progesterone.* Although using a tincture or cream made from wild yam is *not* an effective birth control method, wild yam can be helpful for relieving PMS and some menopause symptoms. That's because it has some of the same effects as progesterone.

Many researchers believe that PMS symptoms are caused by an imbalance between your estrogen and your progesterone levels. You make lots of estrogen in the time between your menstrual period and your next ovulation. From ovulation to your next period, you make lots of progesterone. The two hormones should balance each other out, but for many women, they don't. Their estrogen, for reasons we don't fully understand, is dominant. The two hormones get out of sync, and the result is PMS.

As you go through menopause, you may stop making progesterone before you stop making estrogen. Once again, your hormones are out of sync and there's nothing to block the estrogen. This time the result is hot flashes, vaginal dryness, the start of osteoporosis—and an increased risk of breast cancer and heart disease.

As we discussed earlier about estrogen, there are many pros and cons to taking progesterone supplements. If you decide against hormone replacement therapy, you could try wild yam tincture or cream as a natural way to replace your progesterone. The usual dose for the tincture is 25 drops a day, taken in a glass of water or juice. Wild yam cream seems to be more helpful, though. By law, the creams have no more than 5 mg of diosgenin, which your body converts to progesterone, per ounce. Most women rub half a teaspoon or less into the skin of the inner thigh or lower abdomen twice a day. The diosgenin is absorbed into your bloodstream through your skin.

> **Quack, Quack**
> Despite the rumors, sweet potatoes contain no progesterone or estrogen, so you won't get any natural hormones by eating them. The confusion arises because we use the words yam and sweet potatoes interchangeably to mean the sweet, orange-colored tuber traditionally served at Thanksgiving. Scientifically, though, yams are the tuberous roots of a tropical vine in the *Dioscorea* family. Mexican wild yam (*Dioscorea villosa*) is far too bitter to eat—and it's not an effective form of birth control.

> **What's in a Word**
> *Progesterone* is a female hormone made in the ovaries. Women make a lot more progesterone when they ovulate about halfway through their menstrual cycle. If the egg isn't fertilized, their progesterone level quickly drops off.

# DHEA: Eternal Youth?

You have two adrenal glands, each about the size of a grape. Your adrenals sit on top of your kidneys and produce a number of different steroid hormones. The hormone they make the most is *dehydroepiandrosterone,* or *DHEA* for short. Your body converts DHEA into other steroid hormones, including small amounts of testosterone and estrogen, as you need them. As you get older, your production of DHEA naturally drops off. Studies suggest that people with high DHEA levels live longer and have less heart disease and cancer. Other studies hint that DHEA helps prevent Alzheimer's disease, autoimmune diseases such as lupus, osteoporosis, and other problems. The ads for DHEA supplements promise that it builds muscle, burns fat, stimulates your sex drive, and, of course, slows aging.

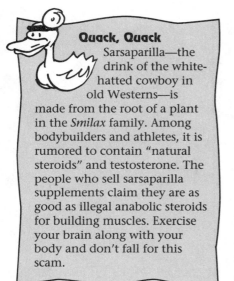

**Quack, Quack**
Sarsaparilla—the drink of the white-hatted cowboy in old Westerns—is made from the root of a plant in the *Smilax* family. Among bodybuilders and athletes, it is rumored to contain "natural steroids" and testosterone. The people who sell sarsaparilla supplements claim they are as good as illegal anabolic steroids for building muscles. Exercise your brain along with your body and don't fall for this scam.

If you think this all sounds too good to be true, you're right. Most of the studies are based on work done in the test tube, on animals, or in very limited human trials. There's no real evidence that DHEA does anything good for you—and it may be harmful. It could speed up the growth of tumors, especially those that feed on estrogen or testosterone. A man who has prostate cancer, which grows faster in the presence of testosterone, clearly shouldn't take DHEA. But what about the many older men who have prostate cancer in such an early stage that it's still undetectable? For many of these men, the cancer will never develop into a problem or need treatment—but if they take DHEA, they might stimulate the cancer into growing. Women who take DHEA risk raising their testosterone level (yes, all women naturally make small amounts of this hormone). And women who have naturally high testosterone levels are six times more likely to get breast cancer. Women should definitely not take any chances here—stay away from DHEA.

We believe you should take DHEA supplements only if your doctor has found that your level is very low and recommends them. Your DHEA level can be checked easily with a convenient blood test.

## The Least You Need to Know

➤ Hormones are chemical messengers your body makes in your endocrine glands, including your pineal gland, adrenal glands, and sex organs.

➤ Hormones regulate your body and control many functions.

➤ The hormone melatonin controls your body's internal clock. Melatonin supplements can help you cope with insomnia from jet lag or shift changes.

➤ Menopausal women stop making the female hormone estrogen. Soy foods such as tofu (bean curd) contain genistein and daidzein, plant estrogens that can help replace the missing hormone.

➤ Eating soy foods every day may help protect women against breast cancer.

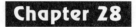

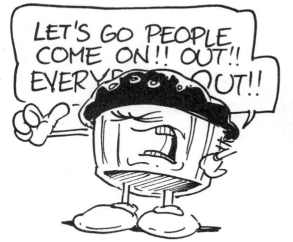

# Chapter 28

# Fiber: Moving Things Along

**In This Chapter**

➤ Why you need fiber from your food

➤ The different kinds of fiber

➤ Foods that are high in fiber

➤ How fiber lowers your cholesterol

➤ Helping bowel problems with fiber

➤ How fiber helps diabetes

You're giving yourself all sorts of good nutrition whenever you chomp through a juicy piece of fresh fruit or a nice crunchy vegetable. You're getting vitamins, minerals, flavonoids, and antioxidants of all sorts. You're also getting one more fabulous nutritional benefit: Lots of fiber.

What's so great about this stuff? Why do you hear about it all the time these days? It's because fiber has been shown to lower your cholesterol, cut your risk of a heart attack, and help prevent colon cancer. It's also very helpful for people with bowel problems and diabetes—it could even help you lose weight.

The best thing about fiber, though, is that it's in those same fresh fruits and vegetables we've been telling you about all through this book. It's just one more really good reason to eat them.

# Why Fiber Is Fabulous

Back in the 1970s, two British doctors, Denis Burkitt and Hugh Trowell, were studying disease in Uganda. They realized that their patients got very few of the digestive problems the doctors often saw in their patients back in England. Their African patients hardly ever had constipation, diverticulitis, colon cancer, or hemorrhoids. They also hardly ever got fat or had diabetes. Their cholesterol levels were low and they hardly ever had heart disease or high blood pressure. Why not? These patients ate mostly unprocessed foods that were very high in dietary fiber. Because of that, they had large and frequent bowel movements. The doctors drew the logical conclusion: A high-fiber diet can help prevent certain diseases, especially the digestive problems that people who eat a typical low-fiber, high-fat Western diet often get. Ever since then, we've been learning more and more about the importance of fiber in keeping you healthy.

# How Much Fiber Is Enough?

There's still no RDA for dietary fiber, but today there are strong recommendations from some concerned sources: the American Heart Association, the National Institutes of Health, and the American Cancer Association. All three say that you should aim for 20 to 30 grams of dietary fiber a day. To get more specific, the FDA has set the Daily Reference Value for fiber at 25 grams. That's based on getting 11.5 grams of fiber for every 1,000 calories you eat, assuming you eat 2,000 calories a day. Even if you don't eat that much, we suggest aiming for 25 or 30 grams of fiber a day. Most of us get far less than that—the average American eats only 12 grams of fiber a day.

# Insoluble and Soluble Fiber

Dietary fiber is a general term for the indigestible parts—mostly cell walls—of plant foods. There are basically two kinds of dietary fiber: insoluble and soluble.

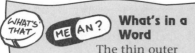

**What's in a Word**

The thin outer husks of whole grains such as rice, wheat, and oats are called *bran*. They're a rich source of insoluble fiber—and also valuable B vitamins and minerals. The bran is often removed in processing. Brown rice, for example, still has its bran, while the bran has been processed away in white rice.

## Insoluble Fiber

Insoluble fiber is cellulose, the main fiber in the cell walls of all plant foods. Insoluble fiber absorbs water, but it doesn't dissolve in it. As we'll discuss a little further on, the ability to absorb water makes insoluble fiber very helpful for your colon and bowel problems. Bran of any sort is an excellent source of insoluble fiber.

## Soluble Fiber

Most of the fiber in plant foods is soluble fiber of one sort or another. Soluble fibers dissolve in water to form a soft gel in your intestines. As the gel moves through your intestines, it can help a lot of health problems, including high cholesterol and diabetes (we'll explain how later on). Here's a breakdown of the different kinds:

➤ **Pectin.** If you've ever made jam, you know that pectin forms a gel. Pectin is found in all plant cell walls, but it's most abundant in the skins and rinds of fruits and vegetables. Apple peel, for example, is about 15 percent pectin.

➤ **Mucilage.** Sounds really gross, doesn't it? Mucilage is a general term for the gum-like soluble fiber found in seeds, beans, grains, and nuts. Guar gum is the most common mucilage. It's found in beans, and it's also widely used in processed foods as a thickener. Guar gum is used to make cream cheese, for example, and it's also used in salad dressings, ice cream, soup, and even toothpaste.

Both kinds of fiber are important for your health. Insoluble fiber helps keep your *stool* soft, bulky, and easy to pass, so you have regular bowel movements and avoid some problems of the large intestine—including colon cancer. Insoluble fiber also may help prevent heart attacks. Soluble fiber can help lower your blood cholesterol, remove wastes and toxins from your body, and help you control your blood sugar if you have diabetes. (We'll talk more about the health benefits of different kinds of fiber later on in this chapter.)

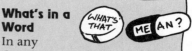

**What's in a Word**
In any discussion of fiber, your bowel movements have to be mentioned. There are a lot of words for your body's solid waste, but because this is a family book we'll use the word *stool*.

# Eating More Fiber

Imagine yourself eating six chocolate chip pecan cookies in a row. All too easy, isn't it? Now imagine yourself eating six apples in a row. Impossible. The sugar in fruit satisfies your sweet tooth, while the fiber in it fills you up quickly—with far fewer calories and none of the fat from cookies or candy. (Actually, because fiber is by definition indigestible, it doesn't really have any calories at all.) This chart gives you the fiber and calorie counts for some favorite fruits and vegetables. All plant foods—fruits, veggies, nuts, grains, and seeds—contain both soluble and insoluble fiber in varying amounts.

| **The Fiber in Fruits and Vegetables** | | | |
| --- | --- | --- | --- |
| | Serving Size | Calories | Fiber in grams |
| *Fruits* | | | |
| Apple (with skin) | 1 medium | 81 | 3.0 |
| Applesauce | 1/2 cup | 97 | 1.5 |

*continues*

## The Fiber in Fruits and Vegetables Continued

| | Serving Size | Calories | Fiber in grams |
|---|---|---|---|
| **Fruits** | | | |
| Banana | 1 medium | 105 | 1.8 |
| Blueberries | 1 cup | 82 | 3.3 |
| Cherries | 10 | 49 | 1.1 |
| Kiwi | 1 medium | 46 | 2.6 |
| Nectarine | 1 medium | 67 | 2.2 |
| Orange | 1 medium | 65 | 2.3 |
| Peach | 1 medium | 37 | 1.4 |
| Pear | 1 medium | 98 | 4.3 |
| Raisins | 2/3 cup | 296 | 5.3 |
| Strawberries | 1 cup | 45 | 3.9 |
| **Vegetables** | | | |
| Broccoli | 1/2 cup | 22 | 2.0 |
| Brussels sprouts | 1/2 cup | 30 | 3.4 |
| Carrots | 1/2 cup | 35 | 1.5 |
| Cauliflower | 1/2 cup | 12 | 1.2 |
| Chickpeas | 1 cup | 269 | 5.7 |
| Corn kernels | 1/2 cup | 89 | 3.0 |
| Green beans | 1/2 cup | 22 | 1.1 |
| Kidney beans | 1 cup | 225 | 6.4 |
| Lima beans | 1 cup | 217 | 13.5 |
| Lettuce, iceberg | 1 leaf | 3 | 0.2 |
| Lettuce, romaine | 1/2 cup | 4 | 0.5 |
| Navy beans | 1 cup | 259 | 6.6 |
| Parsnips | 1/2 cup | 63 | 2.1 |
| Peas | 1/2 cup | 67 | 2.2 |
| Potato (with skin) | 1 medium | 220 | 3.3 |
| Spinach | 1/2 cup | 21 | 2.0 |
| Sweet potato (with skin) | 1 medium | 118 | 3.4 |
| Tomato (raw) | 1 medium | 26 | 1.6 |
| Turnip | 1/2 cup | 14 | 1.6 |
| White beans | 1 cup | 253 | 7.9 |

*Note: Fiber in vegetables assumes food is lightly steamed or baked.*

It's not that hard to add 5 or 10 grams of fiber to your ordinary diet every day. Look at what you eat for lunch, for instance. One slice of ordinary white bread has well under 1 gram of fiber, while a slice of whole-wheat bread has 1.6 grams. Just switching to whole-wheat instead of white bread for your sandwich adds about 2 grams of fiber. Have an apple instead of (or along with) some cookies and you add another 3 grams—now you're up to 5 grams without even noticing! You can easily find other ways to add fiber to your diet. If you do, you may discover one of the unsung benefits of fiber. As you eat more high-fiber foods, you'll probably lose weight, gradually and painlessly, because you'll feel full sooner. You lose weight because you're eating fewer calories, but you don't feel hungry or deprived.

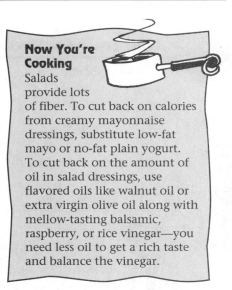

**Now You're Cooking**
Salads provide lots of fiber. To cut back on calories from creamy mayonnaise dressings, substitute low-fat mayo or no-fat plain yogurt. To cut back on the amount of oil in salad dressings, use flavored oils like walnut oil or extra virgin olive oil along with mellow-tasting balsamic, raspberry, or rice vinegar—you need less oil to get a rich taste and balance the vinegar.

As you add more fiber to your diet, you may have some problems with gas, bloating, and diarrhea. To avoid this, don't suddenly start eating a lot more fiber. Instead, add it to your diet gradually—one extra piece of fruit a day, for example. If you have any discomfort, cut back until the problem stops, then gradually begin adding more fiber again. It could take you a couple of months to get up to 30 grams a day without any unpleasant or embarrassing side effects.

# Which Type of Fiber?

Food labels today list the amount of fiber per serving, but they don't always break it down by type. The fiber in most plant foods is about 35 percent insoluble fiber and about 45 percent soluble fiber (the rest is miscellaneous other stuff). In general, you don't need to think too much about the type of fiber, because plant foods always have some of each kind. As a rough guide to the best sources of insoluble and soluble fiber, though, take a look at the chart.

| Good Sources of Fiber | |
| --- | --- |
| *Insoluble Fiber* | *Soluble Fiber* |
| Artichokes | Apples |
| Broccoli | Carrots |
| Carrots | Cauliflower |
| Cooked dried beans and peas | Citrus fruits |
| Nuts | Cooked dried beans |

*continues*

---

**Good Sources of Fiber   Continued**

| *Insoluble Fiber* | *Soluble Fiber* |
|---|---|
| Parsnips | Corn |
| Popcorn | Lentils |
| Potatoes (with skin) | Oat bran |
| Seeds | Oatmeal |
| Sweet potatoes (with skin) | Pears |
| Wheat bran | Rice bran |
| Whole grains | Sweet potatoes |

---

### Food for Thought

Not all "high-fiber" breakfast cereals, breakfast bars, and snacks are as good for you as they seem. Some of these cereals contain added oil and sugar and don't really have much in the way of whole grains—although they do have a lot of calories. Likewise, some breakfast bars and granola bars are very high in calories from fat and sugar but low in fiber. Read the labels carefully and don't be fooled by labels that say "natural." These products can be just as full of sugar and fat as the others.

Federal regulations now allow food producers to make claims for the health benefits of fiber on the labels. To claim that a food is "high fiber," it must contain at least 5 grams or more per serving. These foods must also meet the definition for low fat (3 grams or less per serving), or the level of total fat must appear next to the high-fiber claim. To claim that a food is a "good source of fiber," it must contain 2.5 to 4.9 grams per serving. To claim that a food has "more, or added fiber," it must have at least 2.5 grams more fiber per serving than that food would ordinarily have.

According to new FDA rules, food producers are allowed to make two claims for the health benefits of fiber on their labels. If a food contains a grain product, fruit, or vegetable, is a good source of fiber by itself, and is low-fat, the label can claim that the food helps prevent cancer. If a food contains a grain product, fruit, or vegetable, and is also low in saturated fat, low in cholesterol, and contains at 0.6 grams of soluble fiber per serving, the label can claim that the food helps lower your risk of heart disease.

# Fiber Supplements

It's not always easy to get enough fiber from your food. Sometimes you may want to take a fiber supplement to make sure you're getting enough. Fiber supplements are also useful if you're suffering from constipation and some colon problems.

Fiber supplements come in several different forms. The most popular is a powder (you have a choice of flavors) made from psyllium. There's about 3.4 grams of soluble fiber in one rounded teaspoon (7 grams) of psyllium powder. Psyllium also comes in capsules and in chewable wafers. Each dose has about 3 grams of fiber. You can also buy psyllium seeds in your health-food store. They're often called "flea seeds" or "natural vegetable powder."

Other fiber supplements are made from calcium polycarbophil (Equalactin®, FiberCon®), or methylcellulose (Citrucel®). They too come in a variety of forms and flavors. Of all the supplements, though, doctors recommend psyllium the most, because it's the least likely to cause gas or diarrhea.

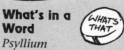

**What's in a Word**

*Psyllium powder* is actually the husks of tiny seeds from the plantago plant. Also called plantain, this is the same weed that grows on your lawn. It's available in any drugstore. Metamucil® is a popular brand; generic brands are also available.

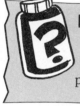

**Food for Thought**

Watching your diet and taking psyllium twice a day could lower your cholesterol level by 10 percent or more. Studies show this works best for people with the highest cholesterol levels.

To use the powder or flea seeds, stir a teaspoon or so into eight ounces of water or juice and drink it down immediately before it gets too sludgy. If you use the capsule or wafer form, you must immediately drink eight ounces of liquid. If you don't, the fiber will swell up in your stomach and could form a blockage.

Most people find they get the most predictable benefit from fiber supplements if they take them in the early evening—you should see results in about 12 to 24 hours. Don't use a larger dose or take fiber supplements more than three times a day unless your doctor recommends it. As with any fiber, taking too much could cause gas, bloating, or diarrhea. If fiber supplements cause problems for you, cut back on the dose until the problem goes away, then gradually increase the dose.

Do fiber supplements keep you from absorbing vitamins and minerals in your intestines? We're not sure. To be on the safe side, take your vitamin and mineral supplements at a different time from your fiber supplements.

**Warning!**
Do not use fiber supplements in pill form if you have any sort of problem with your esophagus!

# Water, Water Everywhere

We can't stress the importance of water enough. Every single cell in your body has water in it—in fact, half your body is nothing but water. Your kidneys and large intestine are responsible for conserving the water you take in from your food and drink, but you lose a lot of water when you breathe and in your sweat, urine, and stool. If you don't drink enough water, your large intestine will try to make up the difference by absorbing more from your stool—and that leads to constipation and other bowel problems.

Fiber in your intestines absorbs a lot of water and carries it out of your body. There's a lot of water in fresh fruits and vegetables, but you still need to be sure you're drinking enough as you increase your fiber intake. Your goal should be six to eight eight-ounce glasses of water every day. That's 48 to 64 ounces, or between 1 1/2 and 2 quarts. You can substitute juice, tea, coffee, soft drinks and the like. Plain old water is best, though. It's free, it has no calories, and it doesn't contain caffeine or anything else.

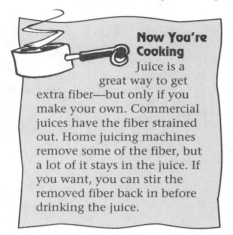

**Now You're Cooking**
Juice is a great way to get extra fiber—but only if you make your own. Commercial juices have the fiber strained out. Home juicing machines remove some of the fiber, but a lot of it stays in the juice. If you want, you can stir the removed fiber back in before drinking the juice.

# It's Official: Oatmeal Lowers Cholesterol

In 1997, the FDA decided that oatmeal makers could make this health claim on their packages: "May reduce the risk of heart disease." That's because eating oatmeal, oat bran, or foods that are high in oats helps lower your cholesterol. Most important, it lowers your LDL ("bad") cholesterol without also lowering your HDL ("good") cholesterol. How do oats accomplish this miracle? Through their unique soluble fiber. Here's why. Your liver uses cholesterol to make digestive juices called bile acids. The bile is squirted out from your gall bladder into your small intestine to help you digest your foods, especially fats. If you eat a low-fiber diet, a lot of the bile acid gets reabsorbed into your blood through your intestinal wall. Because bile acids have a lot of cholesterol in them, that can raise your blood cholesterol level. If you could keep the bile acids from being reabsorbed, your cholesterol would go down. That's exactly what oats do. Oats are full of a soluble fiber called beta glucan. When you eat oat bran, oatmeal, or oat flour, the soluble fiber forms a gel that traps the bile acids and carries them out of your body. Your liver reacts to all this by making more bile acids. To do that, it pulls cholesterol out of your blood. Because you're not reabsorbing the cholesterol from your bile acids, and because you're also using up blood cholesterol to make more of them, your cholesterol level drops.

**Now You're Cooking**
To claim that it helps lower cholesterol and prevent heart disease, an oat food must contain at least 0.75 grams of soluble fiber in a serving. You need to eat at least 3 grams a day of soluble fiber to lower your cholesterol.

If your cholesterol is on the high side, try having any sort of oat cereal for breakfast (see the chart for the fiber in some popular choices). After a few months of devoted oatmeal-eating, you could see a real drop in your cholesterol level. If you also eat a lot of beans, it could drop even further. And if your cholesterol is only borderline high (200 to 240 mg/Dl), lowering it by just 10 percent could cut your risk of a heart attack by 50 percent.

## The Fiber in Oat Cereals

| Cereal | Serving Size | Fiber in grams |
|---|---|---|
| Cheerios® | 1 1/4 cups | 2.0 |
| Honey Bunches of Oats® | 2/3 cup | 1.6 |
| Oat bran (cooked) | 1/3 cup dry | 4.2 |
| Oat bran (cold) | 1/2 cup | 3.0 |
| Oat Flakes® | 2/3 cup | 2.1 |
| Oatmeal, instant | One packet | 2.0 |
| Oatmeal, quick | 1 cup | 2.7 |
| Oatmeal, rolled | 1 cup | 3.0 |
| Oat Squares® | 1/2 cup | 2.4 |

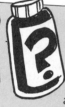

**Food for Thought**

In a major recent study of male health professionals, the men who ate the most fiber had the lowest risk of heart attack. Interestingly, it was insoluble fiber that seemed to provide the most protection against a heart attack—the amount of soluble fiber the men ate didn't seem to matter. The lesson? Eat a variety of fruits and vegetables to get both kinds of fiber.

# Oatmeal for Breakfast

Oatmeal is an inexpensive and delicious way to get more fiber into your diet. One reason oats are such a good choice is that only the inedible outer hull of the oats is removed in processing. The oat bran stays on the kernel, so you always get some bran whenever you eat oat foods. The oatmeal shelf at the supermarket can be a little confusing. Here's a rundown:

➤ **Steel-cut oats.** The most expensive kind, these are oat grains that have been cut very roughly. They take a long time to cook (20 to 30 minutes—plus you have to stir them a lot), but the extra-chewy, nutty flavor is worth it. Tip: Save some money by buying your steel-cut oats in bulk at your health food store.

➤ **Rolled oats.** Also called "old-fashioned" oats, these are the oats that come in the familiar round carton. You can also buy "table-cut" oats in bulk at health food stores. To make these oats, raw oats are steamed, rolled into flakes, and dried. Rolled oats cook in just five minutes; table-cut oats take a few minutes longer.

➤ **Quick oats.** Basically the same as old-fashioned oats, but the flakes are rolled thinner so the oats cook faster. They have slightly less fiber, but take only three minutes to cook.

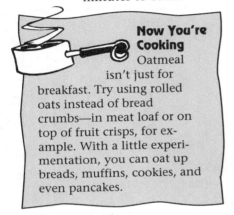

**Now You're Cooking**
Oatmeal isn't just for breakfast. Try using rolled oats instead of bread crumbs—in meat loaf or on top of fruit crisps, for example. With a little experimentation, you can oat up breads, muffins, cookies, and even pancakes.

➤ **Instant oats.** These oats are flaked into such tiny pieces that all you have to do is add boiling water and stir. The processing reduces the fiber content a little, but the real problem is that these products almost always have added sugar and artificial flavorings.

There are only 145 calories in a bowl of oatmeal, but the traditional toppings of sugar and cream add a lot of calories. Skip them and get an extra nutrition boost by topping your morning oatmeal with some sliced fresh fruit, wheat germ, raisins, dried fruits, or nuts.

# Help for Bowel Problems

In this section we're going to talk about your bowel movements. The only way to do that is to speak frankly, but if that embarrasses you, feel free to skip ahead to the next section.

Let's start with constipation. Constipation ("irregularity") happens when you have fewer bowel movements than normal for you, or when your stool is hard, dry, and difficult to pass. Too little fiber in the diet is almost always the culprit here. If you gradually increase your daily fiber intake to 30 grams a day, your constipation problems will almost certainly disappear. That's because insoluble fiber helps give bulk to your stool and keeps water in it; soluble fiber forms gels that soften the stool. In combination, they help you form a large stool that's easy to eliminate. If you eat plenty of fiber each day, you'll be able to go regularly and have a full and complete bowel movement with no trouble at all.

Straining for a bowel movement is one of the major causes of *hemorrhoids*—enlarged veins in and around your anus. By eating more fiber, you'll pass your stool easily and quickly. That helps keep hemorrhoids from getting started. If you already have them, it keeps them from getting worse. And if you're having a painful flare-up, you may need to use a fiber supplement containing psyllium—the soluble fiber will make your stool much easier to pass. If you have hemorrhoids, talk to your doctor about eating more fiber and other self-help steps you can take.

Fiber can also help diarrhea by slowing down the time it takes for food to pass through your intestines. Diarrhea is the frequent passing of loose, watery stools. It's often caused by eating something that disagrees with you, overeating, or by a "stomach bug" or "stomach flu." Fiber often helps soak up the liquid and slow things down. If you've got a stomach bug that's giving you diarrhea, go for the soluble fiber, especially pectin. Pears, bananas, blueberries, and apples (grate them with the peel) are good choices. On the other hand, the sorbitol (a type of sugar) in high-pectin fruits and juices causes diarrhea for some people, so be cautious. If your diarrhea doesn't go away in a few days, call your doctor.

A number of other serious bowel problems, including Crohn's disease, ulcerative colitis, diverticulitis, and irritable bowel syndrome, are helped a lot by fiber. If you have any of these bowel problems, discuss dietary fiber and fiber supplements with your doctor before making any changes.

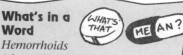

**What's in a Word**

*Hemorrhoids* (also called "piles") are a very common problem—some 25 million Americans have them. A hemorrhoid happens when a vein in your rectum (the last portion of your digestive tract) becomes swollen, itchy, and painful—in severe cases, it may bleed. Hemorrhoids are almost always a result of straining during bowel movements.

**Food for Thought**

A traditional Scandinavian remedy for diarrhea is dried blueberries (check your health food store). Soak a teaspoonful of the berries in one cup of boiling water until the berries are softened, about five minutes. Drink the liquid and then eat the berries. Repeat three to seven times daily for up to three days. Most doctors recommend a few days on the BRAT diet: bananas, rice, applesauce, and toast. Drink plenty of plain water, mild tea or herbal tea, or diluted fruit juice (the sugar in undiluted juice could make the diarrhea worse). Avoid milk and carbonated drinks.

# Beneficial Bacteria

Fiber also helps you keep a good balance of friendly bacteria in your colon. It's perfectly normal to have literally trillions of bacteria in your colon. Most of the bacteria are beneficial, but sometimes the unfriendly ones can get the upper hand, especially if you've been taking antibiotics. When that happens, you can start having problems with cramps, diarrhea, gas, and other bowel upsets. A low-fiber diet makes it easier for the unfriendly bacteria to take hold. Eating more fiber makes conditions in your colon ideal for the friendly bacteria and not so great for the unfriendly ones. The friendly bacteria multiply faster and crowd out the bad guys—and the balance tips back in your favor.

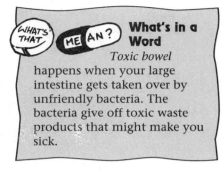

**What's in a Word**

*Toxic bowel* happens when your large intestine gets taken over by unfriendly bacteria. The bacteria give off toxic waste products that might make you sick.

**Now You're Cooking**

Beneficial bacteria supplements should be refrigerated at all times. Don't buy them if they haven't been stored properly. Look for supplements that contain ultracentrifuged bacteria from the DDS-1 acidophilus strain.

**What's in a Word**

*Fructooligo-saccharides (FOS)* are natural sugars that help feed beneficial bacteria. Small amounts of FOS are found in honey, garlic, and artichoke flour. Supplements of syrup or powder are much more concentrated—they contain 95 percent FOS.

Sometimes the bad bacteria can really take hold, though, and don't want to give up. If you have frequent gas and bloating and alternating diarrhea and constipation, along with general feelings of tiredness or depression, it could be because of an overload of unfriendly bacteria. You might have what's sometimes called *toxic bowel*—the waste products from the bad bacteria are making you sick. Just getting more fiber may not help. In mild cases, sometimes just eating live-culture yogurt, which contains beneficial acidophilus bacteria, will help. (Look for live-culture yogurt in your health food store—supermarket brands don't have live bacteria.)

In more severe cases, you may need to take supplements of beneficial bacteria to help the good guys get back in charge. Three good guys are especially helpful: acidophilus, bifidobacteria, and boulardii. If you think you have a toxic bowel, discuss the problem and how to treat it with a nutritionally oriented health care professional. He or she can arrange for a stool analysis and advise you on how to use beneficial bacteria. Clearing up the problem could take several weeks or even months.

The usual dose for a mild overgrowth of bad bacteria is one to two grams (about half a teaspoon) of acidophilus and 250 mg (about an eighth of teaspoon) of bifidobacteria, mixed with three ounces of cold water. Also swallow one or two 300-mg capsules of boulardii. Take it all on an empty stomach. For a more severe overgrowth, you may need to increase the doses to up to 10 grams of acidophilus, six of bifidobacteria, and up to six boulardii capsules, spread out over the day before meals.

To help the good bacteria get a foothold in your colon, you can also take supplements containing *fructooligosaccharides (FOS)*. These provide a sugary fuel for the good guys. FOS comes as a syrup or powder you can use as sweetener on foods or stir into drinks. Start with one gram a day and gradually work up to three or four grams daily.

# Fiber Fights Cancer

Colon cancer is one of the three leading causes of cancer deaths in the United States—some 50,000 people die from it each year. You can sharply cut your odds of getting colon cancer by eating more fiber. That's because fiber increases the bulk of your stool and makes it pass through your colon more quickly. All sorts of toxic stuff passes through your colon: your own wastes, bile acids, pesticides, food additives and preservatives, heavy metals, and chemical pollutants of all sorts. One of the jobs of your stool is to move this stuff through and out of you quickly. That way, anything that might cause cancer spends as little time as possible in contact with your colon. Because a high-fiber diet speeds the transit time for your food, it cuts the amount of time dangerous substances spend in your body, which cuts your risk of colon cancer.

Although many studies have shown that people who eat a high-fiber diet have a lower rate of colon cancer, we still don't know for sure that the fiber alone helps prevents the cancer. People who eat more fiber also tend to eat less fat, drink less alcohol, and smoke less, so the fiber connection isn't as clear-cut as you might think. Even so, the National Cancer Institute recommends a high-fiber, low-fat diet to help prevent colon cancer. Fiber in the diet may also play a role in preventing breast, cervical, and lung cancer, but here too we can't say for sure that it's the fiber alone that does the trick.

# Fiber for Diabetes

Eating a high-fiber diet can help people with diabetes better control their blood sugar. This seems to work because soluble fiber—especially the guar gum in beans—slows down your digestion of carbohydrates. If the carbos enter your bloodstream more slowly, your blood sugar doesn't jump up as sharply after you eat a meal. This helps many diabetics feel better and have fewer energy highs and lows. The National Diabetes Association now recommends a high-fiber diet for all diabetics. If you have diabetes, discuss adding soluble fiber to your diet with your doctor before you try it.

# The Least You Need to Know

➤ Dietary fiber is found in all plant foods, including fruits, vegetables, beans, whole grains, nuts, and seeds.

➤ Soluble fiber forms a soft gel in your colon. Insoluble fiber absorbs water in your colon. Plant foods contain both kinds of fiber.

➤ Most people eat too little fiber. Many doctors now recommend 30 grams of fiber a day.

➤ Eating more fiber can help lower your cholesterol and prevent heart attacks.

➤ A high-fiber diet can help prevent digestive problems and colon cancer.

➤ Eating more fiber helps people with diabetes control their blood sugar better.

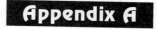
# Quick Reference Chart for Health Problems

| If you have this health problem... | see these chapters |
| --- | --- |
| Acne | 3, 19 |
| Aging | 4, 15, 17 |
| Allergies | 13 |
| Alzheimer's disease | 12, 15, 22, 23, 25 |
| Arthritis | 21, 22, 23, 24 |
| Asthma | 8, 13, 18, 24 |
| Breast cancer | 27 |
| Cancer | 3, 8, 9, 13, 15, 21, 22, 23, 25, 27 |
| Carpal tunnel syndrome | 8 |
| Cataracts | 3, 6, 13, 15 |
| Cervical dysplasia | 9 |
| Colds | 13, 19 |
| Colon cancer | 9, 14, 17, 28 |
| Constipation | 28 |
| Crohn's disease | 22, 23 |
| Dental problems | 13, 21, 25, 26 |
| Depression | 4, 8, 22 |
| Diabetes | 2, 5, 7, 8, 13, 15, 18, 19, 21, 24, 26, 28 |
| Diarrhea | 18, 20, 28 |

| If you have this health problem... | see these chapters |
| --- | --- |
| Eyesight problems | 3, 6, 13, 15, 19, 25 |
| Hair problems | 19, 23 |
| Heart disease | 3, 4, 8, 9, 15, 18, 20, 22, 23, 25, 26, 28 |
| Hemorrhoids | 28 |
| Herpes | 22 |
| High blood pressure | 2, 8, 13, 20, 17, 18, 23, 26 |
| High cholesterol | 2, 7, 13, 22, 23, 25, 26, 27, 28 |
| Immune system | 3, 4, 8, 13, 14, 15, 19, 22, 24, 26 |
| Infertility | 13, 15, 19 |
| Insomnia | 22, 27 |
| Intermittent claudication | 7, 15 |
| Jet lag | 22, 27 |
| Kidney disease | 3, 13, 18, 22 |
| Kidney stones | 8, 13, 17, 18 |
| Macular degeneration | 3, 19, 25 |
| Menopause | 17, 27 |
| Menstrual problems | 18, 21 |
| Migraines | 6, 18, 22 |
| Nail problems | 12, 19, 23 |
| Osteoporosis | 14, 16, 17, 18 |
| Pregnancy | 3, 8, 9, 13, 17, 18 |
| Premenstrual syndrome (PMS) | 7, 8, 18, 23, 27 |
| Prostate problems | 19, 25 |
| Skin problems | 12, 19, 23 |
| Stroke | 20, 25 |
| Thyroid problems | 17, 21 |
| Varicose veins | 16, 25 |
| Wound healing | 13, 19, 22 |

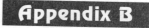 

# Resources

## Finding Nutritionally Oriented Health Care

For help finding nutritionally oriented physicians and other health care professionals near you, contact:

American Academy of Environmental Medicine
4510 West 89th Street
Prairie Village, KS 66207
(913) 642–6062

American Chiropractic Association
Council on Nutrition
1701 Clarendon Boulevard
Arlington, VA 22209
(703) 276–8800

American College for Advancement in Medicine
23121 Verdugo Drive, Suite 204
Laguna Hills, CA 92653
(800) 532–3688
(714) 583–7666

American Holistic Medical Association
4101 Lake Boone Trail, Suite 201
Raleigh, NC 27607
(919) 787–5146

Foundation for the Advancement of Innovative Medicine (FAIM)
Two Executive Boulevard, Suite 204
Suffern, NY 10901
(914) 368–9797

For more information about healthy eating or to find a qualified professional nutritionist near you, contact:

American Dietetic Association
216 West Jackson Boulevard
Chicago, IL 60606
(312) 899–0040
ADA nutrition hotline: (800) 366–1655

International and American Associations of Clinical Nutritionists
5200 Keller Springs Road, Suite 410
Dallas, TX 75248
(972) 250–2829

# Nutrition and the Elderly

The Nutrition Screening Initiative for the Elderly, a joint project of the American Academy of Family Physicians, the American Dietetic Association, and the National Council on the Aging, Inc., uses a checklist of 10 warning signs to see if an elderly person is at nutritional risk. To get the checklist and more information on the project, contact:

The Nutrition Screening Initiative
1010 Wisconsin Avenue, NW, Suite 800
Washington, DC 20007
(202) 625–1662

# Testing Labs

Not all medical testing labs can test accurately for antioxidant levels. For accurate results, ask your doctor or health-care professional to contact:

Great Smokies Diagnostic Laboratory
63 Zillicoa Street
Asheville, NC 28801
(800) 522–4762
Tests: Blood vitamin analysis

SpectraCell Laboratories, Inc.
515 Post Oak Boulevard Suite 830
Houston, TX 77027
(800) 227–5227
(713) 621–3101

Tests: Functional Intracellular Analysis (FIA™), Essential Metabolics Analysis (EMA™), Spectrabox

# Supplement Manufacturers

Choosing a quality supplement is important. These companies make a wide range of high-quality products and will be happy to provide you with details:

Enzymatic Therapy
825 Challenger Drive
Green Bay, WI 54311
(920) 469–1313
(800) 783-2286

Nature's Plus
548 Borad Hollow Road
Melville, NY 11747
(800) 645-9500

Nature's Way Products, Inc.
10 Mountain Springs Parkway
Springville, UT 84663
(801) 489-1520

Solaray
1104 Country Hills Drive
Ogden, UT 84403
(801) 621-5631

Solgar Vitamin and Herb Company, Inc.
500 Willow Tree Road
Leonia, NJ 07605
(201) 944–2311

Twinlab™
2120 Smithtown Avenue
Ronkonkoma, NY 11779
(516) 467–3140

# Supplement Information and Regulation

## General Information

For more information about nutritional supplements in general:

Council for Responsible Nutrition
1300 19th Street, NW, Suite 310
Washington, DC 20036-1609
(202) 872–1488

For more information about alternative and complementary medicine, including nutrition:

Office of Alternative Medicine
National Institutes of Health
OAM Clearinghouse
Box 8218
Silver Spring, MD 20907
(888) 644–6226

# Federal Regulations and Industry Associations

Food and Drug Administration (FDA)
5600 Fishers Lane
Rockville, MD 20857
(301) 443–3170

Several trade organizations set industry standards for integrity and good manufacturing practices:

National Nutritional Foods Association (NNFA)
3931 MacArthur Boulevard, Suite 101
Newport Beach, CA 92660
(800) 966–6632

Natural Products Quality Assurance Alliance (NPQAA)
16770 NE 79th Street, Suite 205
Redmond, WA 98052
(206) 861–8408

American Herbal Products Association (AHPA)
Box 2410
Austin, TX 87868
(512) 320–8555

# Help for Medical Problems

Many medical problems affect your nutrition and your need for vitamins and minerals. For more information about specific medical problems, talk to your doctor and contact the organizations listed here.

For more information about problems of aging:

National Institute on Aging
NIA Information Center
Box 8057
Gaithersburg, MD 20898
(800) 222-2225

For more information about Alzheimer's disease:

Alzheimer's Association
70 East Lake Street
Chicago, IL 60601
(800) 621–0379
(312) 853–3060

For more information about cholesterol, contact:

National Cholesterol Education Program
NHLBI Information Center
P.O. Box 30105
Bethesda, MD 20824–0105
(301) 951–3275

For more information about diabetes:

American Diabetes Association
1660 Duke Street
Alexandria, VA 22314
(800) 232–3472

For more information about heart disease:

American Heart Association
National Center
7272 Greenville Avenue
Dallas, TX 75231–4596
(800) 242–8721

For more information about herpes:

Herpes Resource Center
Box 13827
Research Triangle Park, NC 27709
(800) 230–6039

For more information about migraine headaches:

National Headache Foundation
5252 North Western Avenue
Chicago, IL 60625
(800) 843–2256

For more information about preventing neural tube defects (NTDs):

Spina Bifida Association of America
4590 MacArthur Boulevard, NW, Suite 250
Washington, DC 20007
(800) 621–3141

For more information about osteoporosis:

National Osteoporosis Foundation
1150 17th Street, NW, Suite 500
Washington, DC 20036
(800) 223–9994
(202) 223–2226

For more information about Parkinson's disease:

National Parkinson Foundation
1501 Northwest Ninth Avenue
Miami, FL 33136
(800) 327–4545
(800) 433–7022 (Florida)
(800) 400–8448 (California)
(305) 547–8448

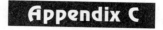

# Glossary

**Acetylcholine**   A neurotransmitter made using choline.

**Adenosine**   A flavonoid found in onions. It may be helpful for lowering cholesterol.

**Adrenal glands**   You have two adrenal glands, one on top of each kidney. Your adrenal glands produce a number of steroid hormones, including DHEA.

**Ajoene**   A flavonoid found in garlic that may help thin your blood and prevent blood clots.

**Alpha carotene**   A carotene found in red- and orange-colored foods. It is a powerful antioxidant.

**Alpha linolenic acid (LNA)**   Omega-3 fatty acids found in plant foods, especially nuts, soybeans, canola oil, and flaxseed oil.

**Alpha tocopherol**   The most active form of Vitamin E.

**Amino acids**   The building blocks of protein. Twenty-two amino acids are necessary for life. See also *Essential amino acid*; *Nonessential amino acid*

**Anemia**   A general term meaning that your red blood cells either don't have enough hemoglobin or that you have a below-normal number of them.

**Anthocyanins**   Flavonoids found in blue foods such as blueberries and grapes. They help protect your eyes against free radicals.

**Antioxidants**   Enzymes that protect your body by capturing free radicals and escorting them out of your body before they do any more damage.

**Arachidonic acid**   A type of omega-6 fatty acid.

**Arginine**   A nonessential amino acid helpful for boosting the immune system.

**Ascorbic acid**   Another name for Vitamin C.

**Atheroma**   Fatty deposit in an artery; the first stage of plaque.

**Atherosclerosis**   Fatty deposits, called plaque, build up inside your arteries, often an artery that nourishes your heart or leads to your brain.

**Aura**   Warning sign of a migraine headache, usually occurring an hour or two before the headache strikes. The aura is usually visual—many people see flashing lights or zigzag patterns.

**Benign prostatic hypertrophy** (BPH)   A condition caused by an enlarged prostate gland, which presses on the urethra and causes a need to urinate frequently.

**Beriberi**   A deficiency disease caused by a lack of thiamin.

**Beta carotene**   A carotene found in abundance in many red- and orange-colored plant foods. Your body easily converts beta carotene into Vitamin A.

**Beta-cryptoxanthin**   A carotene found in some plant foods such as oranges and peaches. It's also used to color butter.

**Biotin**   A B vitamin made in your body by friendly bacteria in your small intestine.

**Boron**   An essential trace mineral needed for bone growth.

**Bran**   The thin inner husk of grains such as wheat, rice, and oats. A good source of soluble and insoluble fiber as well as minerals and vitamins.

**B vitamins**   A group of related water-soluble vitamins. See also *Biotin*; *Choline*; *Cobalamin*; *Folic acid*; *Niacin*; *PABA*; *Pantothenic acid*; *Pyridoxine*; *Riboflavin*; *Thiamin*.

**Calciferol**   Another name for Vitamin D.

**Calcifidiol**   Another name for Vitamin $D_2$, the form of Vitamin D you get from foods or supplements.

**Calcitrol**   Yet another name for Vitamin $D_2$, the form of Vitamin D you get from foods or supplements.

**Calcium**   The most abundant mineral in your body, needed to build bones and teeth, make some hormones and enzymes, make your muscles contract, and other functions.

**Capsanthin**   A xanthophyll found in red peppers.

**Cardiac arrhythmia**   Irregular heartbeat.

**Carnitine**   An amino acid useful for people with heart disease.

**Carotenes**   Carotenoids found in many red- and orange-colored foods. Your body can convert carotenes into Vitamin A. See also *Alpha carotene*; *Beta carotene*.

**Carotenoids**   Orange- or red-colored substances found in many fruits and vegetables such as carrots. See also *Carotenes*; *Xanthophylls*.

**Cartilage**   The super-smooth, tough tissue attached to the ends of your bones. It forms joints and cushions the bones.

**Catechins**   Antioxidant flavonoids found in tea.

**Cerebral insufficiency**   Poor blood circulation to the brain, causing senility, memory loss, and depression.

**Cervix**   The neck-shaped structure leading from your vagina to your uterus.

**Cervical dysplasia**   Abnormalities in the cells of the cervix. These abnormalities can eventually lead to cervical cancer.

**Chelation**   Treating minerals to change their electrical charge, usually by binding them chemically to an amino acid or other harmless substance. This helps your body absorb the minerals better.

**Chloride**   An electrolyte mineral needed to control blood pressure and for other body functions.

**Cholecalciferol**   The form of Vitamin D you make in your body from sunshine. Also called Vitamin $D_3$.

**Cholesterol**   A waxy fat your body uses to make cell membranes, the sheaths that cover your nerves, and hormones, among other things.

**Choline**   A substance closely related to the B vitamins.

**Chromium**   A trace mineral needed to help you use glucose in your cells.

**Circadian rhythm**   Your body's 24-hour internal clock.

**Clotting factors**   Substances in your blood that help it clot and stop bleeding.

**Cobalamin**   A B vitamin, also known as Vitamin $B_{12}$.

**Cobalt**   An essential trace mineral used to make cobalamin.

**Coenzyme**   A substance, usually a vitamin or mineral, needed to complete an enzyme.

**Coenzyme $Q_{10}$**   A coenzyme your mitochondria need to produce energy. Supplements can be helpful for people with heart failure.

**Collagen**   A protein used to make the connective tissue that holds your cells together and makes up your bones, tendons, muscles, teeth, skin, blood vessels, and every other part of you.

**Constipation**   Having fewer bowel movements than normal or having stools that are hard, dry, and difficult to pass. Also called irregularity.

**Copper**   An essential trace mineral needed to make enzymes important for your blood vessels and nerves.

**Crohn's disease**   A serious inflammatory disease of the large intestine.

**Cyanocobalamin**   The form of Vitamin $B_{12}$ used in vitamin pills.

**Cysteine**   A sulfur-containing nonessential amino acid.

**Deficiency**   Serious shortage of a vitamin or mineral in your body.

**Deficiency disease**   Illness caused by a deficiency of a vitamin. Classic deficiency diseases include scurvy and beriberi.

**DHEA (dehydroepiandrosterone)**   A steroid hormone made in your adrenal glands. Your body converts DHEA into other hormones.

**Diabetes**   Inability to use glucose for fuel in your cells, sometimes because you no longer make the hormone insulin but more often because your cells have become resistant to insulin. See also *Noninsulin-dependent diabetes*.

**Diabetic neuropathy**   A complication of diabetes that causes numbness, tingling, and pain in the nerves of the feet and legs; it sometimes spreads to the nerves of the arms and trunk.

**Diarrhea**   Frequent passing of loose, watery stools.

**Diastolic pressure**   Your blood pressure when your heart is at rest between beats—the lower number in your blood pressure reading.

**Dietary fiber**   The indigestible parts—mostly cell walls—of plant foods. See also *Insoluble fiber; Soluble fiber*.

**Diosgenin**   A phytoestrogen found in Mexican wild yam root. It resembles the female hormone progesterone and was used to make the first birth control pills.

**Diuretic**   A drug or herb that makes your kidneys produce more urine. Diuretics remove water—and also some minerals and vitamins—from your body.

**Docosahexenoic acid** (DHA)   Omega-3 fatty acids found in cold-water fish.

**Eicosapentenoic acid** (EPA)   Omega-3 fatty acids found in cold-water fish.

**Electrolytes**   Minerals that dissolve in water and carry electrical charges. In your body, potassium, sodium, and chloride are the electrolyte minerals.

**Elemental calcium**   The actual amount of usable calcium in a supplement. It's usually given on the label as a percentage of the total calcium in the supplement.

**Endocrine gland**   A gland, such as your thyroid or testes, that makes hormones.

**Enzyme**   A chemical compound your body makes from various combinations of proteins, vitamins, and minerals. Enzymes speed up chemical reactions in your body.

**Epithelial tissue**   The tissue that covers the internal and external surfaces of your body. Your skin, the linings of your eyes and nose, your entire digestive tract, your lungs, your urinary tract, and your reproductive tract are all epithelial tissue.

**Ergocalciferol**   The form of Vitamin D you get from foods or supplements. Also called Vitamin $D_2$.

**Essential amino acid**   One of the nine amino acids you must get from your food.

**Essential fatty acid**   A fat you must get from your food. See also *Linoleic acid*; *Linolenic acid*.

**Estrogen**   The main female hormone, made by the ovaries and uterus.

**Fat-soluble vitamin**   A vitamin that dissolves in fat and can be stored in your body's fatty tissues. Vitamin A, Vitamin D, Vitamin E, and Vitamin K are fat-soluble.

**Fiber**   See *Dietary fiber*.

**Flavin adenine dinucleotide (FAD)**   A riboflavin-containing enzyme needed by your mitochondria to release energy.

**Flavin mononucleotide (FMN)**   A riboflavin-containing enzyme needed by your mitochondria to release energy.

**Flavonoids**   Substances found in fruits and vegetables. Flavonoids give these foods their color and taste. Flavonoids are also powerful antioxidants. See also *Anthocyanins*; *Carotenoids*; *Catechins*; *Quercetin*.

**Flea seeds**   See *Psyllium powder*.

**Fluoride**   A trace mineral that helps prevent tooth decay.

**Folacin**   An old-fashioned name for folic acid.

**Folate**   The natural form of folic acid found in foods.

**Folic acid**   The synthetic form of one of the B vitamins.

**Fortified milk**   Milk that has Vitamin D and (sometimes) Vitamin A added to it.

**FOS**   See *Fructooligosaccharides*.

**Free form amino acids**   Amino acid supplements in their pure form, sold as a powder.

**Fructooligosaccharides (FOS)**   Natural sugars found in honey, garlic, and artichoke flour that help nourish desirable bacteria in your large intestine.

**Functional medicine**   Another term for orthomolecular medicine. Functional medicine works to restore your body to its proper functioning with vitamins, minerals, and other supplements.

**Free radicals**   Unstable, destructive oxygen atoms created by your body's natural processes and also by the effects of toxins such as cigarette smoke.

**Gamma linoleic acid (GLA)**   Omega-6 fatty acid found in evening primrose and borage seed oil.

**Ginkgo biloba**   An herbal extract containing many flavonoids. It can be helpful in cases of cerebral insufficiency.

**Glucosamine**   An amino acid sugar found in the shells of shrimp and lobsters. Glucosamine supplements can be helpful for arthritis.

**Glutamine**   A nonessential amino acid useful for intestinal problems.

**Glutathione**   Your body's most abundant natural antioxidant enzyme.

**Goiter**   A swollen thyroid gland forming a lump in your neck. It's caused by a shortage of iodine.

**Guar gum**   A type of soluble fiber found in beans and also in grains, seeds, and nuts.

**Heart failure**   A condition occurring when your heart is damaged or weak and can't pump blood efficiently.

**Heme iron**   The iron found in hemoglobin.

**Hemoglobin**   The oxygen-carrying protein that gives your red blood cells their color. Every molecule of hemoglobin has four atoms of iron in it.

**Hemorrhoids**   Itchy, enlarged or swollen veins in the rectum. Also called piles.

**Herpes**   A group of viruses. Herpes simplex type 1 causes cold sores. Herpes simplex type 2 causes genital herpes. Herpes zoster causes chicken pox and shingles.

**Hesperidin**   A flavonoid found in citrus fruits. It's helpful for improving circulation in small blood vessels.

**High-density lipoprotein (HDL)**   One form of cholesterol. It's often called "good" cholesterol because it can help remove LDL cholesterol from your blood.

**High blood pressure**   Blood pressure—the pressure of your blood against your arteries as your heart beats and contracts—that is too high. Also called hypertension. If your blood pressure is 140/90 or more, you have hypertension. See also *Diastolic pressure; Systolic pressure*.

**Homocysteine**   An amino acid formed when other amino acids in your blood are broken down by normal body processes. Too much homocysteine in your blood can cause heart disease. Folic acid breaks down the homocysteine and prevents a toxic buildup.

**Hyperhomocysteinemia**   The medical term for too much homocysteine in the blood.

**Hypertension**   See *High blood pressure*

**Hypothyroidism**   An underactive thyroid gland.

**Hormone**   A chemical messenger your body makes to tell your organs what to do. Hormones regulate many activities, including your growth, blood pressure, heart rate, glucose levels, and sexual characteristics.

**Human papillomavirus (HPV)**   A sexually transmitted virus that causes venereal warts, which can cause cervical dysplasia and cancer of the cervix.

**Inositol**   A substance closely related to the B vitamins that you need to make neurotransmitters and cell membranes.

**Inositol hexaniacinate (IHN)**   A form of niacin that also contains inositol.

**Insoluble fiber**   Dietary fiber that is mostly cellulose from the cell walls of plants. Insoluble fiber absorbs water.

**Insomnia**   An inability to fall asleep or stay asleep.

**Insulin**   A hormone made by your pancreas and needed to carry glucose into your cells for fuel.

**Iodine**   An essential trace mineral needed to make thyroid hormones.

**Isoflavones**   Hormone-like substances found in soybeans.

**Jet lag**   Fatigue and insomnia caused by traveling rapidly through several time zones.

**Intrinsic factor**   A special substance secreted by your stomach to allow you to absorb cobalamin from your food.

**Iron**   An essential trace mineral needed to make hemoglobin.

**Irregularity**   See *Constipation*.

**Linoleic acid**   An essential fatty acid found in many plants and in fish, especially cold-water fish such as mackerel and cod. See also *Omega-3 fatty acids*.

**Linolenic acid**   An essential fatty acid found in many seeds, including corn. See also *Omega-6 fatty acids*.

**Lipoic acid**   A vitamin-like substance you need to make energy in your mitochondria. It's also a powerful antioxidant.

**Low-density lipoprotein (LDL)**   One form of cholesterol. It's often called "bad" cholesterol because excess amounts in your blood can lead to health problems, including heart disease.

**Lutein**   Xanthophyll that helps protect your eyes against free radicals. Lutein is found in dark-green leafy vegetables.

**Lycopene**   A carotene found in tomatoes. It's a very powerful antioxidant and may help prevent prostate cancer.

**Lysine**   An essential amino acid that may be helpful for treating herpes.

**Magnesium**   A mineral you need for many body functions, including relaxing your muscles and regulating your heartbeat.

**Manganese**   A trace mineral you need for many body functions, including blood clotting and digesting proteins.

**Marginal or subclinical deficiency**   The early stages of a vitamin or mineral deficiency.

**Megablastic or macrocytic anemia**   Anemia from cobalamin deficiency.

**Melanoma**   The most dangerous type of skin cancer. It can quickly spread to other parts of your body.

**Melatonin**   A hormone made by your pineal gland. Melatonin regulates your sleep-wake cycle.

**Menadione**   The synthetic form of Vitamin K. Also called Vitamin $K_3$.

**Menaquinone**   The form of Vitamin K made in your intestines by friendly bacteria. Also called Vitamin $K_2$.

**Metabolism**   The chemical reactions inside your cells that create energy.

**Methionine**   An essential sulfur-containing amino acid.

**Migraine**   A very severe headache usually felt on just one side of your head. Other symptoms include nausea, vomiting, sensitivity to light, and cold hands and feet.

**Mitochondria**   Tiny, rod-shaped structures found in all your cells. They function as miniaturized power plants where glucose is converted to energy, with the help of oxygen and a group of enzymes.

**Moybdenum**   An essential trace mineral important for making some enzymes and for normal growth and development.

**Mucilage**   Soluble fiber found in beans, seeds, grains, and nuts.

**NAC (N-acetyl cysteine)**   A form of the amino acid cysteine.

**Naringin**   A flavonoid found in citrus fruits.

**Neural tube defect (NTD)**   A birth defect that happens when the growing brain, spinal cord, and vertebrae (the bones of the spine) of an unborn baby don't develop properly during the first month of pregnancy.

**Neurotransmitter**   A chemical you make to transmit messages along your nerves and among your brain cells. You make a number of different neurotransmitters, including serotonin.

**Niacin**   A B vitamin also known as Vitamin $B_3$.

**Niacinamide**   Another name for niacin.

**Nicotinamide**   Another name for niacin.

**Nicotinic acid**   Another name for niacin.

**Nonessential amino acid**   One of the 11 amino acids you can get from your food or make in your body from the nine essential amino acids.

**Nonheme iron**   The iron found naturally in plant foods such as spinach and whole grains.

**Noninsulin-dependent diabetes**   The most common type of diabetes. It happens when your cells become resistant to insulin, a hormone made in your pancreas. This form of diabetes usually begins in adults over age 40, and is most common after age 55.

**Omega-3 fatty acids**   Another name for linolenic fatty acids, found in plants and cold-water fish. See also *Alpha-linolenic acid; Docosahexanoic acid; Eicosapentenoic acid.*

**Omega-6 fatty acids**   Another name for linoleic fatty acids. See also *Arachidonic acid; Gamma linoleic acid.*

**OPCs**   Oligomeric proanthocyanidins, flavonoids found in many plants and red wine. OPC supplements are usually made from grape seeds or pine bark. See also *Pycnogenol.*

**Orthomolecular medicine**   Treating the underlying causes of illness with vitamins, minerals, and other supplements. The phrase was coined by Nobel Prize-winning scientist Linus Pauling. See also *Functional medicine.*

**Osteomalacia**   Soft, weak bones in adults caused by a shortage of Vitamin D.

**Osteoporosis**   Bones that break easily because they are thin, porous, and brittle. Osteoporosis has several related causes, but too little calcium in the diet plays a big part in causing it.

**PABA**   An abbreviation for para-aminobenzoic acid. PABA makes up part of the folic acid molecule.

**Pantothenic acid**   One of the B vitamins. Pantothenic acid is found in every food.

**Pectin**   Soluble fiber found in the skins and rinds of plant foods.

**Pellagra**   A deficiency disease caused by a serious lack of niacin.

**Peptide**   A small protein made from a very short chain of amino acids—usually only two or three.

**Pernicious anemia**   Anemia caused when your stomach stops making intrinsic factor and you stop being able to absorb cobalamin from your food.

**Phenylalanine**   An essential amino acid.

**Phosphatidylcholine (PC)**   A fatty substance made from choline that you need to make the walls of your cells.

**Phosphorus**   The second most abundant mineral in your body, used to make your teeth and bones and for many metabolic processes.

**Phytoestrogens**   Hormone-like compounds found in plant foods, especially soybeans.

**Phylloquinone**   The form of Vitamin K found in plant foods. Also called Vitamin $K_1$.

**Piles**   See *Hemorrhoid*.

**Pineal gland**   A small gland found inside your brain. It produces melatonin and regulates your internal clock.

**Plaque**   Fatty deposits of cholesterol and other substances that build up inside your arteries and block them.

**Potassium**   An electrolyte mineral needed to control your blood pressure and regulate your heartbeat.

**Preformed Vitamin A**   The Vitamin A found in animal foods such as egg yolks. Your body can use preformed Vitamin A as soon as you eat it.

**Prodrome**   See *Aura*.

**Progesterone**   A female steroid hormone.

**Prostaglandins**   Hormone-like substances your body makes from fatty acids. They control many activities in your body, including swelling.

**Prostate gland**   A small male organ wrapped around the urethra. The prostate makes some of the fluids found in semen.

**Protein**   An organic substance made from hydrogen, oxygen, carbon, and nitrogen. You need protein to live; most of your body is made of it. Proteins are made from strings of amino acids.

**Prothrombin**   The most important clotting factor. You need Vitamin K to make it.

**Psyllium powder**   Soluble fiber made from the husks of plantago seeds and sold as a fiber supplement.

**Pteroylglutamic acid or pteroylmonoglutamate**   Scientific names for folic acid.

**Pycnogenol**   A type of OPC made from pine bark.

**Pyridoxal**   Another name for pyridoxine.

**Pyridoxamine**   Another name for pyridoxine

**Pyridoxine**   A B vitamin also known as Vitamin $B_6$.

**Quercetin**   An antioxidant flavonoid found in onions.

**Quinones**   Brightly colored organic substances found in all living plants and animals.

**Rectum**   The last portion of your digestive tract.

**Resveratrol**   A flavonoid found in red wine. It may help lower cholesterol and prevent blood clots.

**Retina**   The thin, light-sensitive layer of cells at the back of your eye.

**Retinoid, retinol, retinaldehyde, or retinoic acid**   Different names for the same thing: preformed Vitamin A.

**Rickets**   Crippling bone deformities in children caused by a shortage of Vitamin D.

**Rutin**   A flavonoid found in citrus fruits, buckwheat, berries, and red wine. It's helpful for improving circulation in small blood vessels.

**SAM (S-adenosylmethionine)**   A form of the amino acid methionine.

**Scurvy**   A deficiency disease caused by a prolonged lack of Vitamin C in the diet.

**Selenium**   An essential trace mineral needed to make glutathione and to help Vitamin E work more effectively.

**Serotonin**   A neurotransmitter that plays a role in your mood and emotions.

**Steroid hormones**   Hormones your body makes in your adrenal glands from cholesterol.

**Stool**   Human solid waste; feces.

**Sodium**   An electrolyte mineral needed to control your blood pressure and the amount of water in your body.

**Soluble fiber**   Dietary fiber that dissolves in water to form a soft gel. See also *Guar gum; Mucilage; Pectin.*

**Sulfur**   A mineral found in every tissue of your body. It's needed to make proteins and many vitamins, hormones, and enyzmes.

**Systolic pressure**   Your blood pressure when your heart beats to pump out blood—the higher number in your blood pressure reading.

**Taurine**   An amino acid that contains sulfur.

**Thiamin**   A B vitamin, also called Vitamin $B_1$.

**Thiamin pyrophosphate (TPP)**   An enzyme your body needs to convert carbohydrates into energy. You need thiamin to make it.

**Thioctic acid**   Another name for lipoic acid.

**Thymus gland**   A small organ found in your neck just above your breastbone. It makes some of the hormones that tell your immune system what to do.

**Thyroid gland**   A small, butterfly-shaped gland found in your neck just below your Adam's apple. It produces hormones that regulate your metabolism.

**Thyroxin**   A hormone made in your thyroid gland.

**Tocopherol**   Another name for Vitamin E. See also *Alpha tocopherol.*

**Tocotrienols**   Forms of Vitamin E found in some plant foods such as rice and barley.

**Toxic bowel**   Excess of unfriendly bacteria in the large intestine.

**Tryptophan**   An essential amino acid used in your body to make niacin, among other things.

**Tyrosine**   A nonessential amino acid.

**Ubiquinone**   See *Coenzyme Q$_{10}$.*

**Urethra**   The tube that carries urine from your kidneys to your bladder.

**Vegan**   Someone who eats no animal foods.

**Vegetarian**   Someone who doesn't eat meat. Some vegetarians limit or don't eat other animal foods as well.

**Vitamin**   An organic chemical compound essential for normal health. You must get all your vitamins from outside your body—from the foods you eat and from any supplements you take.

**Vitamin A**   A fat-soluble vitamin needed for healthy epithelial tissues, eyes, growth, bone formation, and immunity.

**Vitamin C**   A water-soluble vitamin needed to make your connective tissue and for many other functions. Vitamin C is also a powerful and abundant antioxidant.

**Vitamin D**   A fat-soluble vitamin your body makes from sunshine on your skin and also gets from some foods. It's needed to build healthy bones and to regulate the amounts of calcium in your blood.

**Vitamin E**   A fat-soluble vitamin that is a powerful antioxidant.

**Vitamin K**   A fat-soluble vitamin needed to help your blood clot.

**Water-soluble**   Vitamins that dissolve in water and can't be stored in your body. The B vitamins and Vitamin C are water-soluble.

**Wernicke-Korsakoff syndrome**   Nerve damage caused by low thiamin levels from years of alcoholism.

**Wild yam**   A tuberous plant found in the tropics. The roots contain a natural form of the female hormone progesterone. Wild yam cream or tincture can be helpful for relieving menopause symptoms.

**Xanthophylls**   Carotenoids found in dark-green leafy vegetables. See also *Lutein; Zeaxanthin.*

**Zeaxanthin**   A carotenoid found in dark-green leafy vegetables. It helps protect your eyes against free radicals.

**Zinc**   A mineral needed to make many enzymes and hormones.

# Index

## A

α-carotene, *see* alpha carotene, 31
ABC study (Alpha-tocopherol, Beta-carotene Cancer Prevention Study Group), 42
absorption blocking drugs, folic acid, 98
Accutane® (isotretinoin), Vitamin A, 42
ACE inhibitors, potassium levels, 219
acerola fruit, 134
acetylcholine (choline), 124, 325
acids
  fatty, 259-269
    cooking to preserve, 265-266
    RDA (Recommended Dietary Allowance), 265
  trans-fatty, 261
acne, vitamin therapy, 42
adenosine, 325
adrenal glands, 325
adults
  DRI (Daily Reference Intake)
    calcium, 179-180
    magnesium, 197
  DRV (Daily Recommended Values), 17
  Estimated Minimum Requirements
    chloride, 217
    potassium, 217
  RDA (Recommended Dietary Allowance)
    B vitamins, 49-50
    calcium, 180
    cobalamin, 109
    folic acid, 97
    histidine, 249
    iodine, 233
    iron, 230
    isoleucine, 249
    leucine, 249
    lysine, 249
    methionine, 249
    niacin, 75
    phenylalanine, 249

pyridoxine, 87
riboflavin, 67
selenium, 235
thiamin, 59
threonine, 249
tryptophan, 249
valine, 249
Vitamin A, 33
Vitamin C, 132
Vitamin D, 151
Vitamin E, 159
Vitamin K, 171
zinc, 208
safe dosage ranges, 19
SAI (Safe and Adequate Intake)
  biotin, 123
  copper, 236
  manganese, 238
  molybdenum, 239
  pantothenic acid, 116
toxicity symptoms, Vitamin A, 34
*see also* seniors (older adults)
age-related macular degeneration, *see* AMD
aging, resources, 322
AHA (American Heart Association)
  dietary standards, 17
  Food Certification Program, 17
ajoene, 284, 325
alanine (amino acid), 247
alcohol use, supplement guidelines
  diabetes, 198
  calcium, 182
  folic acid, 97
  magnesium, 198
  pyridoxine, 88
  thiamin deficiency, 61
  Vitamin C, 133
  zinc, 209
allergies, supplement guidelines, Vitamin C, 133, 144
allicin (flavonoid), 284-285
Allium family, antioxidant properties, 284
alpha carotene (Vitamin A), 31-32, 325
  antioxidants, 280
alpha linolenic acid (LNA), 262, 325

alpha tocopherol, 325
Alpha-tocopherol, Beta-carotene Cancer Prevention (ABC study), 42
alternative therapies for serious illness, 19
aluminum, 241
Alzheimer's disease
  choline, 125
  resources, 323
  supplement guidelines, fatty acids (essential), 268-269
AMD (age-related macular degeneration), preventing with Vitamin A, 41-44
American Heart Association, *see* AHA
amines, vital, 4
amino acids, 245-258, 325
  DNA, 247
  essential, 246
  food sources, 250-251
  homocysteine, 103, 330
  methionine, 255
  nonessential, 246, 333
  peptides, 248
  phenylketonuria (PKU), 251
  RDA (Recommended Dietary Allowances), 248-249
  supplement guidelines
    diabetes, 251
    kidney disease, 251
  taurine (amino acid), 255
  tryptophan, 75, 78
amino acid, free form, 329
amitriptyline (Elavil), riboflavin supplements, 68
Amygdalin, 55
anemia, 88, 325
  cobalamin deficiency, 110
  macrocytic, 332
  megablastic, 332
  pernicious, 333
antacids (aluminum), calcium stealing drugs, 182
anthocyanins (flavonoids), 285, 325
anti-infective agent (Vitamin A), 30
anti-stress vitamin (pantothenic acid), 118

antibiotics
    deficiencies, biotin, 123
    supplement guidelines
        calcium, 183
        Vitamin C, 133
antioxidant enzymes, 12-13
antioxidant levels, testing labs, 320-321
antioxidants, 12-13, 325
    alpha carotene, 280
    carotenes, 31
    catalase, 274
    cryptoxanthin, 280
    food sources, 279
    garlic, 284
    glutathione, 71, 250, 271
    lipoic acid, 275-276, 331
    niacin, 74
    onions, 284
    superoxide dismutase (SOD), 274
    tea, 282-283
    Vitamin C, 141
    Vitamin E, 158
arachidonic acid, 262, 326
arginine (amino acid), 246-247, 326
    boosting, immune system, 252
arsenic, 241
arthritis, treating with glucosamine (amino acid sugar), 257-258
ascorbic acid, 326
asparagine (amino acid), 247
aspartic acid (amino acid), 247
aspirin, supplement guidelines, Vitamin C, 133
asthma, 203
    preventing with magnesium, 203
    supplement guidelines
        pyridoxine, 91
        Vitamin C, 133, 144
        warning, 144
atheromas, 162, 326
atherosclerosis, 23, 162, 326
    preventing with Vitamin E, 163-164
athletic performance, boosting with coenzyme $Q_{10}$, 292
aura, 326

**B**

B vitamins, 45-55, 326
    boosting immune systems, 54-55
    brewer's yeast, 52
    deficiencies, 50-51, 54
    food sources, 51-52
    memory, 53-54

numbers, meaning of, 47
preventing heart disease, 53
RDA (Recommended Dietary Allowances), 48-50
safe dosage ranges, 20
unofficial, 47
β-carotene, *see* beta carotene, 31
bacteria supplements (beneficial), 313-315
beans, reducing gas, 101
begnign breast disease, treating with Vitamin E, 166
beneficial bacteria supplements, 313, 315
benign prostatic hypertrophy (BPH), 212, 326
beriberi, 59, 326
    thiamin deficiency, 59-60
beta carotene (Vitamin A), 31-32, 326
    dosage recommended, 33
    eyesight, 41-42
    preventing cancer, 42-43
    supplement guidelines, 34-35
Beta Carotene and Retinol Efficacy Trial, *see* CARE
beta-cryptoxanthin, 326
bioflavonoids, *see* flavonoids, 278
biotin, 46-47, 122-124, 326
    food sources, 123-124
    RDA (Recommended Dietary Allowance), 5
    safe dosage range, 20
    SAI (Safe and Adequate Intake), 123
    supplements, 124
birth control pills, supplement guidelines
    folic acid, 98
    pyridoxine, 87
    Vitamin C, 133
blood
    lead content, 141
    cholesterol levels, measuring, 23
blood clotting, Vitamin K, 170
blood pressure, 23-24
    levels, lowering (Vitamin C), 142
blood sugar, thiamin deficiency, 63
bone density test (osteoporosis), 192
bone meal supplements, calcium, 187
bones, calcium content, 178
boron, 240, 326
    RDA (Recommended Dietary Allowances), 226
bowels, toxic, 314
brain tumors (childhood), preventing with vitamin supplements, 21

bran, 304, 326
breastfeeding, 111
    supplement guidelines
        cobalamin, 111
        folic acid, 97
        pyridoxine, 87
        Vitamin C, 133
        zinc, 209
brewer's yeast, B vitamins, 52
brewing tea, 282-283

**C**

cadmium, 241
caffeine, bone loss, 182
Calcibind® (cellulose sodium phosphate) supplement, 183
calciferol, 150, 326
calcifidiol, 326
calcitrol, 326
calcium, 149, 177-194, 326
    combining with Vitamin D, 189
    deficiencies, 180-181
    DRI (Daily Reference Intake), 179-180
    effectiveness, increasing, 188-189
    food sources, 183-185
        milk, 183
    preventing
        colon cancer, 193
        heart disease, 193
        high blood pressure, 192
        kidney stones, 193
        osteoporosis, 178, 190-191
    RDA (Recommended Dietary Allowance), 7, 179-180
    safe dosage range, 20
    supplement guidelines
        alcohol use, 182
        types of, 185-188
        warning, 182-183
calcium carbonate supplements, 186
calcium citrate supplements, 186
calcium content, bones, 178
calcium glubionate supplements, 186
calcium gluconate supplements, 186
calcium lactate supplements, 186
calcium pantothenate, 118
calcium phosphate supplements, 186
calcium stealing drugs, 181-182
    high cholesterol, 182
    steroid drugs, 181
    thyroid supplements, 182
calcium-fortified foods, 180
Cambridge Heart Antioxidant Study (CHAOS), 163

cancer
   drug toxicity, pyridoxine treatment, 93
   preventing with
      beta carotene, 42-43
      fatty acids (essential), 267-268
      fiber, 315
      folic acid, 104
      molybdenum, 240
      selenium, 236
      soy foods, 297-299
      Vitamin A, 42
      Vitamin C, 145
      Vitamin E, 165
   treating, coenzyme $Q_{10}$, 293
canker sores (aphthous stomatitis), thiamin deficiency, 63
capsanthin (carotenoids), 282, 326
Captopril®, potassium levels, 219
cardiac arrhythmias, 202, 326
   magnesium deficiency, 202
CARET (Beta Carotene and Retinol Efficacy Trial), 35, 42
carnitine (amino acid), 246-247, 326
   treating
      chronic fatigue syndrome (CFS), 252
      heart disease, 252
      high cholesterol, 252-253
carotenes, 31, 280, 326
   antioxidants, 31
   cooking, 38
   importance of, 30
   lycopene, 280
carotenoids, 31-32, 279, 327
   capsanthin, 282
   lutein, 282
   xanthophylls, 281
   zeaxanthin, 282
carpal tunnel syndrome (CTS), pyridoxine treatment, 92
carrots, 39
   nutritional value, 33
cartilage, 327
catalase antioxidant, 274
cataracts, preventing with
   riboflavin, 71-72
   Vitamin A, 41
   Vitamin E, 166
   vitamin supplements, 18
catechins (flavonoid), 285, 327
cells, 8
   epithelial tissues, 30
   folic acid, manufacturing, 96
   oxidation, 12
   red blood, 108
   respiration, 70
   tumor, Vitamin K, 174

cellulose sodium phosphate (Calcibind®), supplement warning, calcium, 183
cerebral insufficiency, 287-288, 327
cervical cancer, preventing with folic acid, 104
cervical dysplasia, 327
   folic acid, 104
cervix, 327
CHAOS (Cambridge Heart Antioxidant Study), 163
chelated, 25
   minerals, 25
chelation, 327
children, dietary needs, 21-22
   DRI (Daily Reference Intake)
      calcium, 179-180
      magnesium, 197
   Estimated Minimum Requirements
      potassium, 217
      sodium, 217
   RDA (Recommended Dietary Allowance)
      B vitamins, 49-50
      calcium, 180
      cobalamin, 109
      folic acid, 97
      iodine, 233
      iron, 230
      niacin, 75
      pyridoxine, 87
      riboflavin, 67
      selenium, 235
      Thiamin, 58
      Vitamin A, 33
      Vitamin C, 132
      Vitamin D, 151
      Vitamin E, 159
      Vitamin K, 171
      zinc, 208
   SAI (Safe and Adequate Intake)
      biotin, 123
      copper, 236
      manganese, 238
      molybdenum, 239
      pantothenic acid, 116
   toxicity symptoms, Vitamin A, 34
chloride, 215-224, 327
   Estimated Minimum Requirements, 217
   RDA (Recommended Dietary Allowance), 7
chocolate, food source of magnesium, 199
cholecalciferol, 150, 327
cholesterol, 22-23, 327
   levels
      lowering (Vitamin C), 142

   measuring, 23
   resource center, 323
cholestyramine, 152
   calcium stealing drugs, 182
choline, 48, 52, 124-126, 327
   Alzheimer's disease, 125
   food sources, 125
   liver function, 125
   supplements, 125
      choosing, 126
Cholybar®, calcium stealing drugs, 182
chromium, 234-235, 327
   RDA (Recommended Dietary Allowance), 8, 226
   safe dosage range, 20
   SAI (Safe and Adequate Intakes), 234
chronic fatigue syndrome (CFS), treating with carnitine (amino acid), 252
circadian rhythm, 296, 327
citrus fruits, flavonoid content, 286
clotting (blood), Vitamin K, 170
clotting factors, 327
   Vitamin K, 174
      prothrombin, 172
coagulation (blood), Vitamin K, 170
cobalamin, 46-47, 107-114, 327
   food sources, 112-113
   deficiencies, symptoms, 109-111
   RDA (Recommended Dietary Allowance), 5, 109
   safe dosage range, 20
   supplement guidelines
      breastfeeding, 111
      omeprazole (Prilosec®), 111
      potassium, 111
      pregnancy, 111
      seniors (older adults), 110
      smoking, 111
      sublingual, 114
      vegan, 110
      vegetarian, 110, 112
cobalt, 108, 240, 327
   RDA (Recommended Dietary Allowances), 226
cod liver oil, 264
coenzyme $Q_{10}$, 289-294, 327
   boosting
      athletic performance, 292
      immune systems, 292
   food sources, 293-294
   supplement guidelines
      heart disease, 290-291
      high blood pressure, 291-292
      high cholesterol, 292

treating
  cancer, 293
  gingivitis, 292
coenzymes, 290, 327
collagen (protein), 130, 327
colloidal minerals, 25
colon cancer, preventing with
  calcium, 193
  folic acid, 104
  Vitamin D, 155
constipation, 312, 327
cooking to preserve
  B vitamins, 51
  carotenes, 38
  fatty acids, 265-266
  flavonoids, 278
  folic acid, 103
  lycopene, 280
  niacin, 82
  thiamin, 62
  Vitamin C, 137
copper, 236-328
  deficiencies, 237
  food sources, 237
  RDA (Recommended Dietary
    Allowance), 8, 226
  safe dosage range, 20
  SAI (Safe and Adequate Intake),
    236
cortisone, supplement guidelines,
  Vitamin C, 133
coumarin (Coumadin), warning,
  Vitamin K, 173
Crohn's disease, 328
  supplement guidelines
    fatty acids, 267
    glutamine, 254
cryptoxanthin (carotene), antioxidants, 280
cyanocobalamin (cobalamin), 108,
  328
cysteine (amino acid), 246-247, 328
  supplements guidelines,
    glutathione, 274
  toxins, eliminating, 253

**D**

daidzein, 298
Daily Recommended Values, *see*
  DRV
Daily Reference Intake, *see* DRI
Daily Value (DV), 16
deficiencies, 328
  B vitamins, 50-51
    depression, 54
    memory, 53-54
  biotin, 123

calcium, 180-181
cobalamine, 111
colbalamin, 109
copper, 237
electrolytes, 217-218
folic acid, 97-99
glutathione (antioxidant),
  272-273
iodine, 233
magnesium, 197-198
  cardiac arrhythmias, 202
marginal, 10-11, 332
niacin, 76
pantothenic acid, 117
pyridoxine, 87
riboflavin, 67-68
subclinical, 11, 332
  testing for, 18
thiamin, 59-60, 63
trace minerals, 227
Vitamin A, 36
Vitamin C, 130, 132, 134
Vitamin D, 151-153
Vitamin E, 160
Vitamin K, 171-172
zinc, 208-209
deficiency diseases, 6, 10, 328
dehydroepiandrosterone, *see* DHEA
dementia, niacin deficiency, 76
Department of Health and Human
  Services, 16
depression
  B vitamin deficiencies, 54
  pyridoxine treatment, 93
  treatment
    phenylalanine (amino acid),
      256
    tyrosine (amino acid), 256
DHEA (dehydroepiandrosterone),
  301-302, 328
diabetes, 328
  controlling with high-fiber diet,
    315
  insulin-dependent, 82
  noninsulin-dependent diabetes,
    24-26
  resource center, 323
  supplements guidelines, 24
    amino acids, 251
    fatty acids (essential), 267
    magnesium, 203
    Vitamin C, 133, 145
    Vitamin E, 166
    zinc, 213
diabetic neuropathy, 328
  reducing with pyridoxine, 92
  supplement guidelines, lipoic
    acid, 276
diarrhea, 328
  fiber, 313
  remedy, 313

supplement guidelines
  magnesium, 198
  niacin deficiency, 76
diastolic pressure, 23-24, 328
Dietary Approaches to Stop
  Hypertension (DASH) study, 223
dietary fiber, 328
  RDA (Recommended Dietary
    Allowances), 304
dietary needs, 20-22
dietary standards, setting, 16
Dietary Supplement Health and
  Education Act (DSHA), 25
digitalis
  potassium levels, 219
  supplement warning, calcium,
    183
digoxin (Lanoxin), potassium
  levels, 219
dihomo-linoleic acid, 262
diosgenin, 328
diseases, deficiency, 6, 10
diuretic, 328
diuretic drug use
  mineral levels, 198
  supplement guidelines
    electrolytes, 218-219
    magnesium, 198
DNA
  amino acids, 247
  effects of free radicals, 13
docosahexanoic acid (DHA), 262,
  328
dolomite supplements (calcium),
  188
DRI (Daily Reference Intake), 16
  calcium, 179-180
  magnesium 197
drug warning
  grapefruit juice, 286
  calcium stealing, 181-182
DRV (Daily Recommended Values),
  16-17
DSHA (Dietary Supplement Health
  and Education Act), 25
dunaliella (beta carotene), 40
DV (Daily Value), 16

**E**

effectiveness, increasing
  calcium, 188-189
  fatty acids (essential), 263
  iron, 232
  magnesium, 200-201
  melatonin, 297
  riboflavin, 69
  trace minerals, 228
  Vitamin A, 40
  Vitamin C, 138-139
  Vitamin D, 154

Vitamin E, 161-163
    selenium, 163
Vitamin K, 173
    zinc, 211
eggs, raw, biotin deficiency, 123
eicosapaentenoic acid (EPA), 262,
    328
Elavil (amitriptyline), riboflavin
    supplements, 68
electrolyte balance, preventing
    high blood pressure, 222-223
electrolytes, 215-224, 328
    deficiencies, 217-218
    Estimated Minimum Require-
        ments, 217
    supplement guidelines, diuretic
        drugs, 218-219
elemental calcium, 328
elements trace, 7
eliminating toxins, cysteine (amino
    acid), 253
emulsifying Vitamin A, 40
endocrine glands, 296, 328
energy from riboflavin, 66
enzymes, 4, 328
    antioxidants, 12
    flavin adenine dinucleotide, 70
    flavin mononucleotide, 70
    nicotinamide adenine dinucle-
        otide, 79
    nicotinamide adenine dinucle-
        otide phosphate, 79
    TPP (thiamin pyrophosphate),
        58
    use with vitamins, 4
    xanthine oxidase, 239
epithelial tissues, 30, 329
ergocalciferol, 150, 329
essential amino acids, 246, 329
essential fatty acids, 259-269, 329
    effectiveness, increasing, 263
    food sources, 263-265
esterized Vitamin C, 140
Estimated Minimum Requirements
    chloride, 217
    electrolytes, 217
    potassium, 217
    sodium, 217
estrogen, 298, 329
estrogen replacement therapy, 299
eyesight, Vitamin A, 41-42

**F**

fat-soluble vitamins, 4, 329
fats, 260
    monounsaturated, 260
    polyunsaturated, 260
    saturated, 260

fatty acids, 259-269
    cooking to preserve, 265-266
    essential, 261
        effectiveness, increasing, 263
        food sources, 263-265
    omega-3, 333
    omega-6, 333
    preventing
        cancer, 267-268
        heart disease, 265
        high cholesterol, 266
    RDA (Recommended Dietary
        Allowance), 265
    supplement guidelines
        Alzheimer's disease, 268-269
        Crohn's disease, 267
        diabetes, 267
        high blood pressure, 267
        PMS symptoms, 268
        rheumatoid arthritis, 267
FDA (Food and Drug Administra-
    tion), 16-17
felodipine (Plendil®), flavonoid
    warning, 286
fiber, 303-315, 329
    content, oat cereal, 311
    food sources, 305-308
    insoluble, 304
    preventing cancer, 315
    soluble, 304-315
    supplement guidelines psyl-
        lium, 309-315
    water use, 310
fish oil
    supplements, 263-268
        Vitamin E, 263
flavin adenine dinucleotide (FAD),
    329
flavin adenine dinucleotide
    enzyme, 70
flavin mononucleotide (FMN), 329
    enzymes, 70
flavonoids, 138, 278-288, 329
    allicin, 284-285
    anthocyanins, 285
    carotene, 280
    carotenoids, 279
    catechins, 285
    cooking to preserve, 278
    drug warning, grapefruit juice,
        286
    hesperidin, 286
    naring, 286
    oligomeric proanthocyanidins
        (OPC), 286
    quercetin, 283-284, 286
flaxseed oil, 266
flea seeds, 309, 329
fluoride, 237-238, 329
    RDA (Recommended Dietary
        Allowance), 226

folacin, 329
folate (folic acid), 96, 329
folic acid, 95-105, 329
    absorption blocking drugs, 98
    cells, manufacturing, 96
    cooking to preserve, 103
    deficiencies, 97-99
        symptoms, 98
    food sources, 99-100
    preventing
        cancer, 104
        heart disease, 103
        neural tube defects, 102
    RDA (Recommended Dietary
        Allowance), 5, 97
    safe dosage range, 20
    supplement recommended
        alcohol use, 97
        birth control pills, 98
        breastfeeding, 97
        pregnancy, 97
        smoking, 97
Follicular Hyperkeratosis, 36
Food and Drug Administration, *see*
    FDA
Food Certification Program,
    American Heart Association, 17
foods
    B vitamins, preserving during
        cooking, 51
    beta carotene content, 37-44
    high fat/low cholesterol, 23
    riboflavin content, 68
    sources
        amino acids, 250-251
        antioxidants, 279
        B vitamins, 51-52
        biotin, 123-124
        calcium, 183-185
        choline, 125
        cobalamin, 112-113
        coenzyme $Q_{10}$, 293-294
        copper, 237
        essential fatty acids, 263-265
        fiber, 305-308
        folic acid, 99-100
        glutathione (antioxidant),
            273-274
        iron, 230-232
        linolenic acid, 264-268
        lycopene (carotene), 281
        magnesium, 198-200
        manganese, 238
        niacin, 77-78
        pantothenic acid, 117
        potassium, 219-220
        pyridoxine, 88-90
        selenium, 236
        sodium (salt), 222

soy foods, 299-300
thiamin, 61
trace minerals, 227
tryptophan, 78
tyramine, 257
Vitamin C, 134-138
Vitamin D, 153-154
Vitamin E, 160-161
Vitamin K, 172-173
zinc, 209-210
soybean, 297-299
fortified milk, 153, 329
free form amino acids, 329
free radicals, 12, 329
DNA effects, 13
free-form amino acid supplements, 250
fructooligosaccharides (FOS), 314, 329
functional medicine, 19, 329
furosemide (Lasix), mineral levels, 198

**G**

g (grams), 6
gamma linoleic acid (GLA), 262, 330
garlic
antioxidants, 284
supplements, 285
genistein, 298
germanium, 241
gingivitis, treating with coenzyme $Q_{10}$, 292
ginkgo, 287
leaves (flavonoid), boosting memory, 287
ginkgo biloba, 330
glucocorticoids, calcium stealing drugs, 181
glucosamine (amino acid sugar), 257, 330
treating arthritis, 257-258
glutamic acid (amino acid), 247, 254
supplements, glutathione, boosting, 274
glutamine (amino acid), 247, 330
treating
Crohn's disease, 254
ileitis, 254
glutathione (antioxidant), 71, 250, 271-274, 330
boosting
cysteine (amino acid) supplements, 274
deficiencies, 272-273

glutamic acid (amino acid) supplements, 274
glycine (amino acid) supplements, 274
riboflavin supplements, 275
food sources, 273-274
supplements, 274
glutathione peroxidase, 235
glycine (amino acid), 247
supplements glutathione, boosting, 274
GMP (good manufacturing practices), 25
goiter, 232, 330
grapefruit juice, flavonoid drug warning, 286
green tea, antioxidant properties, 282
guar gum (soluble fiber), 305, 330
gum disease preventing with Vitamin C, 148

**H**

Harvard Medical School orthomolecular medicine, 19
HDL (high-density lipoprotein), 22-23, 330
headaches (PMS), preventing with niacin, 82
healing, improving with zinc, 213
health care, nutritionally oriented, 319-320
health problems, quick reference, 317-318
hearing loss, improving with Vitamin D, 156
heart disease
homocysteine, 53
preventing with
B vitamins, 53
calcium, 193
fatty acids (essential), 265
folic acid, 103
magnesium, 201-202
pyridoxine, 90-91
thiamin, 62
Vitamin A, 43
Vitamin C, 141-142, 163-164
resource center, 323
supplement guidelines, coenzyme $Q_{10}$, 290-291
treating with carnitine (amino acid), 252
heart failure, 291, 330
heme iron, 230, 330
hemochromatosis, 229
hemoglobin, 86, 110, 228-229, 330
hemophilia, 172

hemorrhoids, 312-313, 330
herpes
resource center, 323
treating with lysine (amino acid), 254
hesperidin (flavonoid), 286, 330
high blood pressure, 24, 330
preventing with
calcium, 192
electrolyte balance, 222-223
magnesium, 202
supplemen guidelines, coenzyme $Q_{10}$, 291-292
treating with essential fatty acids, 267
high cholesterol
preventing with
fatty acids (essential), 266
niacin, 80
soy foods, 299
supplement guidelines, coenzyme $Q_{10}$, 292
treating with
carnitine (amino acid), 252-253
oatmeal, 310-311
high cholesterol drugs, calcium stealing, 182
high-density lipoprotein, *see* HDL
high-fiber diet
controlling diabetes, 315
supplement guidelines, zinc, 209
Hippocrates, Vitamin A, 30
histidine (amino acid), 246-247
RDA (Recommended Dietary Allowance), 249
homocysteine (amino acid), 103, 330
heart disease, 53
hormone replacement therapy, 301
hormones, 4, 295-302, 331
male, zinc, 212
melatonin, 296-297
thyroid, 232
use with vitamins, 4
human papillomavirus (HPV), 331
folic acid, 104
hypercarotenodermia, 35
hyperhomocysteinemia, 103, 330
hypertension, 24, 330
hypervitaminosis A, 34
hypothyroidism, 232, 330

**I**

ileitis, treating with glutamine (amino acid), 254
immune cells, increasing, 44

immune systems
    boosting
        arginine (amino acid), 252
        B vitamins, 54-55
        coenzyme Q$_{10}$, 292
        pyridoxine, 91
        Vitamin E, 165-166
        zinc, 211-212
    enhancing, Vitamin C, 142-143
infants
    DRI (Daily Reference Intake)
        calcium, 179-180
        magnesium, 197
    Estimated Minimum Require-
        ments
        chloride, 217
        potassium, 217
        sodium, 217
    RDA (Recommended Dietary
        Allowance)
        B vitamins, 49-50
        calcium, 179-180
        cobalamin, 109
        folic acid, 97
        iodine, 233
        iron, 230
        niacin, 75
        pyridoxine, 87
        riboflavin, 66
        selenium, 235
        thiamin, 58
        Vitamin A, 33
        Vitamin C, 132
        Vitamin D, 151
        Vitamin E, 159
        Vitamin K, 170
        zinc, 208
    SAI (Safe and Adequate Intake)
        biotin, 123
        copper, 236
        manganese, 238
        molybdenum, 239
        pantothenic acid, 116
infertility, supplement guidelines
    treating with
        Vitamin C, 146-147
        Vitamin E, 158, 166
        zinc, 212
inositol, 48, 126, 331
inositol hexaniacinate (IHN),
    niacin supplements, 80, 331
insoluble fiber, 304, 331
insomnia, 331
    treating with
        melatonin (hormone),
            296-297
        tryptophan (amino acid),
            255-256
instant oats (fiber), 312
Institute of Medicine, 6, 16
insulin, 331

insulin-dependent diabetes
    mellitus, niacin, 82
intermittent claudication
    preventing with niacin, 82
    treating with Vitamin E, 167
International Units (IU), 32
intrinsic factor, 109, 331
iodine, 232, 331
    deficiencies, 233
    RDA (Recommended Dietary
        Allowance), 8, 226, 233
iron, 229, 331
    effectiveness, increasing, 232
    food sources, 230-232
    RDA (Recommended Dietary
        Allowance), 8, 226, 230
    safe dosage range, 20
irregularity, 331
isoflavones, 331
    in soybeans, 298
isoleucine (amino acid), 247
    RDA (Recommended Dietary
        Allowance), 249
IU (International Units), 32

## J-K

jet lag, 331
    treating, melatonin (hormone),
        297

kalium, chemical symbol, 216
kidney disease
    calcium supplement warning,
        188
    supplement guidelines
        amino acids, 251
        magnesium, 198
        Vitamin A, 34
kidney stones
    preventing with
        calcium, 193
        magnesium, 204
    treating with pyridoxine, 93

## L

lactose intolerance, 184
Laetrile, 55
laxatives, magnesium, 200
LDL (low-density lipoprotein),
    22-23, 331
lead, 241
lead content in blood, 141
lead poisoning, treating with
    Vitamin C, 147
lecithin, choline source, 125
leg cramps, treating with Vitamin
    E, 167
leucine (amino acid), 247

RDA (Recommended Dietary
    Allowance), 249
levodopa, vitamin supplement
    warning, pantothenic acid, 118
linoleic acid (essential fatty acid),
    261, 331
linolenic acid (essential fatty acid),
    261, 331
    food sources, 264-268
lipoic acid, 48
    antioxidants, 275-276, 331
    supplement guidelines, diabetic
        neuropathy, 276
lipoproteins, 22
liver function, choline, 125
low-density lipoprotein (LDL),
    22-23, 331
lung cancer, Vitamin A supple-
    ments, 35
lutein (carotenoids), 282, 331
lycopene (carotene), 280, 331
    cooking to preserve, 280
    food sources, 281
lysine (amino acid), 247, 331
    RDA (Recommended Dietary
        Allowance), 249
    treating herpes, 254

## M

macrocytic anemia, 110, 332
macular degeneration
    preventing with Vitamin A, 41
    supplements recommended,
        zinc, 214
magnesium, 195-205, 332
    content in tap water, 202
    deficiencies, 197-198
        cardiac arrhythmias, 202
    DRI (Daily Reference Intake),
        197
    effectiveness, increasing,
        200-201
    food sources, 198-200
        chocolate, 199
    laxatives, 200
    preventing
        asthma, 203
        heart disease, 201-202
        high blood pressure, 202
        kidney stones, 204
        osteoporosis, 203
    RDA (Recommended Dietary
        Allowance), 7
    safe dosage range, 20
    supplement guidelines, 200-201
        alcohol use, 198
        asthma, 203
        diabetes, 198
        diarrhea, 198

diuretic drug use, 198
  kidney disease, 198
  vomiting, 198
  treating PMS symptoms, 204
male hormone levels, zinc, 212
male pattern baldness, biotin
  supplements, 124
manganese, 238-239, 332
  food sources, 238
  RDA (Recommended Dietary
    Allowance), 8, 226
  safe dosage range, 20
  SAI (Safe and Adequate Intake),
    238
manufacturers, vitamin supplements, 321
marginal deficiencies, 10-11, 332
maximizing supplement effects,
  24-26
mcg (micrograms), 6
measles, Vitamin A, 43
measuring
  blood cholesterol levels, 23
  Vitamin A, 32
    RE (Retinol Equivalent), 32
  vitamins, metrics (grams), 6
meats, cooking to preserve
  thiamin, 62
medical problems, 322-324
  organizations, 322-324
medicine
  functional, 19
  orthomolecular, 19
megaloblastic anemia (cobolamine
  deficiency), 110, 332
melanoma, 93, 332
  pyridoxine treatment, 93
melatonin (hormone), 255,
  296-297, 332
  effectiveness, increasing, 297
  treating
    insomnia, 296-297
    jet lag, 297
memory
  B vitamins, 53-54
  boosting with gingko leaves
    (flavonoid), 287
  supplement guidelines, zinc,
    214
men, RDA (Recommended Dietary
  Allowance), 5
menadione (Vitamin K₃), 170, 332
menaquinone (Vitamin K₂), 170,
  332
menopause, osteoporosis, 191
mercury, 241
metabolism, 332
methionine, 332
  RDA (Recommended Dietary
    Allowance), 249

methionine (amino acid), 247, 255
methotrexate (Folex® or Mexate®)
  vitamin supplement warning,
    98
metrics (grams), measuring
  vitamins, 6
mg (milligrams), 6
micellized Vitamin A, 40
migraines, 332
  food causes, 257
  preventing with riboflavin,
    70-71
  resource center, 323
  treating with sumatriptan,
    256-257
milk
  food sources of calcium, 183
  fortified, 153
  nutritional values in, 186
mineral levels, diuretic drugs, 198
minerals, 7
  absorption, 25
  chelated, 25
  colloidal, 25
  safe dosage ranges, 19-20
  supplements, 228
  trace, 7-8, 226
mitochondria, 70, 332
molybdenum, 239
  preventing cancer, 240
  RDA (Recommended Dietary
    Allowance), 8, 226
  safe dosage range, 20
  SAI (Safe and Adequate Intake),
    239
monounsaturated fats, 260
morning sickness, pyridoxine
  treatment, 93
moybdenum, 332
mucilage (soluble fiber), 305, 332

## N

N-acetyl cysteine (NAC), 275, 332
naring (flavonoid), 286
naringin, 332
National Academy of Science, 6
National Nutritional Foods
  Association, 25
natrium chemical symbol, 216
neural tube defect (NTD), 102, 332
  resource center, 324
  preventing with folic acid, 102
neurotransmitter, 332
niacin, 46-47, 73-83, 332
  cooking to preserve, 82
  deficiencies, 76
    dementia, 76
    diarrhea, 76
    pellagra, 76

food sources, 77-78
  preventing
    high cholestrol, 80
    intermittent claudication, 82
    PMS headaches, 82
    tinnitus, 82
    vertigo, 82
  RDA (Recommended Dietary
    Allowance), 5, 75
  safe dosage range, 20
  supplements
    inositol hexaniacinate, 80
    recommendations, 79
    warnings, 79-80
  toxicity, 52
niacinamide, 74, 332
nickel, 240
  RDA (Recommended Dietary
    Allowance), 226
nicotinamide, 332
nicotinamide adenine dinucleotide
  (NAD), 79
nicotinamide adenine dinucleotide
  phosphate (NADP), 79
nicotinic acid, 74, 80, 333
  side effects, 81
nifedipine (Adalat®/Procardia®),
  flavonoid warning, 286
night blindness, preventing with
  Vitamin A, 41
nonessential amino acids, 246, 333
nonheme iron, 230, 333
noninsulin-dependent diabetes,
  24-26, 333
nursing women
  DRI (Daily Reference Intake),
    magnesium, 197
  RDA (Recommended Dietary
    Allowance), calcium, 180
nutrition screening, seniors (older
  adults), 320
nutritional needs, 20-22
nutritional values in milk, 186
nutritionally oriented health care,
  319-320

## O

oat cereal, fiber content, 311
oatmeal,
  treating high cholesterol,
    310-311
  types of, 311-312
older adults, *see* seniors
oleic acid, 268
Olestra® (fat substitute), 279
oligomeric proanthocyanidins
  (OPC) flavonoid, 286, 333
omega-3, *see* linolenic acid
omega-6, *see* linoleic acid

omega-9, *see* oleic acid
omeprazole (Prilosec®), supplement guidelines, cobalamin, 111
onions as antioxidants, 284
orthomolecular medicine, 19, 333
osteomalacia, 152, 333
osteoporosis, 178, 191-192, 333
  bone density test, 192
  preventing with
    calcium, 178, 190-191
    magnesium, 203
    Vitamin K, 174
  resource center, 324
overdosing, symptoms
    Vitamin A, 32
    Vitamin C, 138
oxidation in cells, 12-13
oyster shell, calcium supplements, 188

**P**

P-5-P (pyridoxal-5-phosphate) tablets, 91
PABA (para-aminobenzoic acid), 48, 126-127, 333
packaging, sodium levels on, 221
pangamic acid, 55
pantethine, 116
panthoderm, 118
panthothen, 116
pantothenic acid, 46-47, 115-119, 333
    deficiencies, 117
    food sources, 117
    levodopa, vitamin supplement warning, 118
    RDA (Recommended Dietary Allowance), 5
    safe dosage range, 20
    SAI (Safe and Adequate Intake), 116
Parkinson's disease
    resource center, 324
    supplement guidelines
      Vitamin C, 148
      Vitamin E, 167
pectin (soluble fiber), 305, 333
pellagra, 76, 79, 333
    niacin deficiency, 76
peptides, 248, 333
pernicious anemia, 110, 333
phenylalanine (amino acid), 247, 333
    RDA (Recommended Dietary Allowance), 249
    treating depression, 256
phenylketonuria (PKU), amino acids, 251

phenytoin (Dilantin®), vitamin supplement warning, 98, 101, 183
phosphatidylcholine (choline), 124-126, 333
phosphorus, 189-190, 333
    RDA (Recommended Dietary Allowance), 7
phylloquinone (Vitamin $K_1$), 170, 334
phytic acid, 126
phytochemicals, 278
phytoestrogens, 334
    in soybeans, 298
piles, 334
pineal gland, 296, 334
plaque, 23, 162, 334
PMS symptoms, 301
    preventing with pyridoxine, 93
    supplement guidelines
      fatty acids (essential), 268
    treating with magnesium, 204
polyunsaturated fats, 260
potassium, 111, 215-224, 334
    chemical symbol, 216
    Estimated Minimum Requirements, 217
    food sources, 219-220
    preventing strokes, 223
    RDA (Recommended Dietary Allowance), 7
    safe dosage range, 20
    supplement guidelines, 220-221
      cobalamin, 111
potassium levels, digitalis, 219
pravastatin (Pravachol®), 80
preformed Vitamin A, 31, 334
pregnancy
    DRI (Daily Reference Intake), magnesium, 197
    RDA (Recommended Dietary Allowances), calcium, 180
    supplement guidelines
      folic acid, 97
      Vitamin C, 133
      zinc, 209
primrose oil, PMS symptoms, 268
prodrome, 334
progesterone, 301, 334
proline (amino acid), 247
prostaglandins, 261-262, 334
prostate gland, 212, 334
prostate problems
    preventing with zinc, 212
    treating with zinc, 212
proteins, 246, 334
    collagen, 130
    efficient use of pyrodoxine, 86
prothrombin (clotting factor), 172, 334
    Vitamin K, 174

provitamin A, 31
psoriasis
    preventing with Vitamin D, 156
    vitamin therapy, 42
psyllium supplements (fiber), 309-315
psyllium powder, 309, 334
pteroylglutamic acid (folic acid), 96, 334
pteroylmonoglutamate (folic acid), 96, 334
Public Health Service, 16
pycnogenol, 334
pyridoxal (PL), *see* pyridoxine
pyridoxamine (PM), 334
pyridoxine, 46-47, 85-94, 334
    deficiencies, 87-88
    food sources, 88-90
    immune systems, boosting, 91
    preventing
      heart disease, 90-91
      PMS symptoms, 93
    RDA (Recommended Dietary Allowance), 5, 87
    safe dosage range, 20
    supplement warning, 89
    toxicity, 52
pyrodoxine supplement warning, 89-90

**Q-R**

quercetin (flavonoid), 283-284, 286, 334
quick oats (fiber), 312
quick reference, health problems, 317-318
quinones, 290, 334

RDA (Recommended Dietary Allowance), 5, 16
    amino acids, 248-249
    assumptions, faulty, 9-10
    B vitamins, 49-50
    biotin, 5
    boron, 226
    calcium, 7, 179-180
    chloride, 7
    chromium, 88, 226
    cobalamin, 5, 109
    cobalt, 226
    copper, 8, 226
    dietary fiber, 304
    fatty acids (essential), 265
    fluoride, 226
    folic acid, 5, 97
    for men/women, 5
    histidine, 249
    iodine, 8, 226, 233
    iron, 8, 226, 230

isoleucine, 249
leucine, 249
lysine, 249
magnesium, 7
manganese, 8, 226
methionine, 249
molybdenum, 8, 226
niacin, 5, 75
nickel, 226
pantothenic acid, 5
phenylalanine, 249
phosphorus, 7
potassium, 7
pyridoxine, 5, 87
riboflavin, 5, 66
selenium, 8, 226, 235
silicon, 226
sodium, 7
thiamin, 5, 58
threonine, 249
tin, 226
tryptophan, 249
valine, 249
vanadium, 226
Vitamin A, 5, 33
Vitamin C, 5, 130-132
Vitamin D, 5, 151
Vitamin E, 5, 159
Vitamin K, 5, 170-171
zinc, 8, 20, 226
RDI (Reference Daily Intake), 16
RE (Retinol Equivalent), measuring
Vitamin A, 32
rectum, 334
red blood cells, 108
red wine
flavonoids, 285
health benefits, 285-286
Reference Daily Intake, *see* RDI
regulations, supplements, 321-322
repetitive strain injuries, 92
respiratory infections, Vitamin A,
43
resveratrol, 334
Retin-A, (tretinoin), Vitamin A, 42
retina, 335
retinaldehyde (Vitamin A), 31, 335
retinoic acid (Vitamin A), 31, 335
retinoids, 31, 335
retinol (Vitamin A), 31, 335
Retinol Equivalent, *see* RE
rheumatoid arthritis, supplement
guidelines, fatty acids (essential),
267
riboflavin, 46-47, 65-72
deficiencies, 67-68
efficacy, increasing, 69
food content, 68-69

preventing
cataracts, 71-72
migraines, 70-71
RDA (Recommended Dietary
Allowance), 5, 66-67
safe dosage range, 20
supplements
glutathione, boosting, 275
recommendations, 67-68
toxicity, 71
rickets, 152, 335
preventing with Vitamin D, 153
rolled oats (fiber), 312
rutin (flavonoid), 286, 335

# S

S-adenosylmethionine (SAM), 255,
335
safe dosage ranges
minerals, 19-20
vitamins, 19-20
SAI (Safe and Adequate Intake), 8
biotin, 123
chromium, 234
copper, 236
manganese, 238
molybdenum, 239
pantothenic acid, 116
salt, reducing, 221-222
saturated fats, 260
scurvy, 130-132, 335
seaweed, food source of Vitamin K,
173
selenium, 235-236, 335
effectiveness, increasing,
Vitamin E, 163
food sources, 236
preventing cancer, 236
RDA (Recommended Dietary
Allowance), 8, 226, 235
safe dosage range, 20
seniors (older adults)
B vitamins, 54
dietary needs, 20
nutrition screening, 320
supplement guidelines
cobalamin, 110
pregnancy, 111
Vitamin C, 133
Vitamin D, 152
zinc, 209
serine (amino acid), 247
serotonin, 255, 335
silicon, 240
RDA (Recommended Dietary
Allowances), 226
skin, improving with zinc, 213
skin cancer, preventing with
Vitamin A, 42

smoking
supplement guidelines
cobalamin, 111
folic acid, 97
pyridoxine, 88
Vitamin C, 132-133
vitamin supplement warning,
42
sodium (salt), 215-224, 335
Estimated Minimum Requirements, 217
food sources, 222
levels on packaging, 221
RDA (Recommended Dietary
Allowance), 7
reducing, 221-222
soluble fiber, 304-315, 335
guar gum, 305
mucilage, 305
pectin, 305
sources (food)
amino acids, 250-251
antioxidants, 279
biotin, 123-124
boron, 240
calcium, 183-185
milk, 183
choline, 125
cobalamin, 112-113
cobalt, 240
coenzyme $Q_{10}$, 293-294
copper, 237
essential fatty acids, 263-265
fiber, 305-308
folic acid, 99-100
glutathione, 273
glutathione (antioxidant),
273-274
iron, 230-232
linolenic acid, 264-268
lycopene (carotene), 281
magnesium, 198-200
chocolate, 199
manganese, 238
nickel, 240
pantothenic acid, 117
potassium, 219-220
pyridoxine, 88-90
selenium, 236
silicon, 240
sodium (salt), 222
soy foods, 299-300
tin, 241
trace minerals, 227
vanadium, 241
Vitamin C, 134-138
Vitamin D, 153-154
Vitamin E, 160-161
Vitamin K, 172-173
zinc, 209-210

soy foods
food sources, 299-300
preventing
cancer, 297-299
high cholesterol, 299
soybean foods, 297-299
steel-cut oats (fiber), 311
steroid drugs, calcium stealing drugs, 181
steroid hormones, 298, 335
DHEA (dehydroepiandrosterone), 301
stool, 305, 335
storing vitamins, 26
stress, supplement guidelines, Vitamin C, 133
strokes, preventing with potassium, 223
subclinical deficiencies, 11, 332
sublingual cobalamin supplements, 114
sulfasalazine (Azulfidine®)
supplement guidelines, folic acid, 104
vitamin supplement warning, 98
sulfites, thiamin deficiency, 62
sulfur, 228-229, 335
sumatriptan, treating migraines, 256-257
superoxide dismutase (SOD) antioxidant, 274
surgery (recent), supplement guidelines, Vitamin C, 133, 143
systolic pressure, 23-24, 335

**T**

taurine (amino acid), 246-247, 255, 335
tea
antioxidant properties, 282-283
brewing, 282-283
thiamin deficiency, 61
teenagers dietary needs, 21-22
DRI (Daily Reference Intake), magnesium, 197
RDA (Recommended Dietary Allowance)
B vitamins, 49-50
iodine, 233
iron, 230
selenium, 235
Vitamin D, 151
Vitamin E, 159
Vitamin K, 171
zinc, 208
SAI (Safe and Adequate Intake)
manganese, 238
molybdenum, 239

terfenadine (Seldane®), flavonoid warning, 286
testing for vitamin deficiencies, 18
testing labs, 320-321
testosterone levels, zinc supplements, 212
theophylline, 91
therapies, alternative, 19
thiamin, 46-47, 57-63, 335
deficiencies
beriberi, 59-60
blood sugar, 63
Wernicke-Korsakoff syndrome, 60
effects of
alcohol, 61
sulfites, 62
tea (tannins), 61
function of, 58
RDA (Recommended Dietary Allowance), 5, 58
safe dosage range, 20
thiamin pyrophosphate (TPP), 58, 335
thiamin supplements, 62
thioctic acid, 335
threonine (amino acid), 247
RDA (Recommended Dietary Allowance), 249
thymus gland, 212, 335
thyroid gland, 232, 335
thyroid hormones, 232
thyroid supplements, calcium stealing drugs, 182
thyroxin, 335
tin, 241
RDA (Recommended Dietary Allowance), 226
tinnitus, preventing with niacin, 82
tocopherol, 158, 335
tocotrienols, 158, 335
toxic bowel, 314, 336
toxicity, B vitamins, 52
toxins, eliminating, cysteine (amino acid), 253
TPP (thiamin pyrophosphate), 58, 335
trace elements, 7
trace minerals, 7-8, 226
deficiencies, 227
effectiveness, increasing, 228
food sources, 227
trans-fatty acids, 261
transamination process, 86
triglycerides, 260
trimethoprim (Proloprim®/ Trimpex®), vitamin supplement warning, 98

tryptophan, 75, 336
amino acids, 78
food sources, 78
RDA (Recommended Dietary Allowance), 249
tryptophan (amino acid), 247
treating insomnia, 255-256
tumor cells, Vitamin K, 174
tyramine, foods containing, 257
tyrosine (amino acid), 247, 336
treating depression, 256

**U-V**

ubiquinone, *see* coenzyme Q₁₀
ulcerative colitis, folic acid treatment, 104
United States Pharmacopeia (USP), 25
urethra, 212, 336
USP (United States Pharmacopeia), 25
valine (amino acid), 247
RDA (Recommended Dietary Allowance), 249
vanadium, 241
RDA (Recommended Dietary Allowance), 226
vegans, 23, 336
dietary needs, 22
supplements recommended
cobalamin, 110
pyridoxine, 87
zinc, 209
vegetarians, 23, 336
dietary needs, 22
supplements recommended
cobalamin, 110-112
pyridoxine, 87
zinc, 209
vertigo, preventing with niacin, 82
viral infections, Vitamin A, 43
viruses, supplements recommended, Vitamin C, 133, 143
vitamin, 336
Vitamin A, 29-44, 336
boosting immunity, 43-44
deficiencies, 36
effectiveness, increasing, 40
emulsified, 40
excess, 34
eyesight, 41-42
measuring, 32
overdosing, 32
precursor, 31
preformed, 31
preventing heart disease, 43
RDA (Recommended Dietary Allowance), 5, 33

safe dosage range, 20
supplement guidelines, 40-41
toxicity, symptoms, 34
Vitamin B₁, *see* thiamin
Vitamin B₂, *see* riboflavin
Vitamin B₃, *see* niacin
Vitamin B₅, *see* pantothenic acid
Vitamin B₆, *see* pyridoxine
Vitamin B₇, *see* biotin
Vitamin B₈, *see* folic acid
Vitamin B₁₂, *see* cobalamin
Vitamin B₁₇, 55
Vitamin C, 129-148, 336
    antioxidants, 141
    cooking to preserve, 137
    deficiencies, 134
        scurvy, 130, 132
    effectiveness, increasing,
        138-139
    esterized, 140
    food sources, 134-138
    immune systems, enhancing,
        142-143
    overdosing, 138
    Parkinson's disease, slowing
        progress, 148
    preventing
        gum disease, 148
        heart disease, 163-164
        scurvy, 131
    RDA (Recommended Dietary
        Allowance), 5, 130-132
    safe dosage range, 20
    supplements, types of, 139-141
    supplements guidelines
        alcohol use, 133
        allergies, 133, 144
        antibiotics, 133
        aspirin, 133
        asthma, 133, 144
        birth-control pills, 133
        breastfeeding, 133
        cortisone, 133
        diabetes, 133
        pregnant, 133
        seniors (older adults), 133
        smoking, 133
        stress, 133
        surgery (recent), 133, 143
        viruses, 133, 143
    treating
        infertility, 146-147
        lead poisoning, 147
Vitamin D, 149-156, 336
    combining with calcium, 189
    deficiencies, 151-153
    effectiveness, increasing, 154
    food sources, 153-154
    hearing loss, improving, 156
    preventing

colon cancer, 155
    psoriasis, 156
    rickets, 153
    RDA (Recommended Dietary
        Allowance), 5, 151
    safe dosage range, 20
    supplements guidelines, seniors
        (older adults), 152
Vitamin E, 157-167, 336
    atherosclerosis, preventing,
        163-164
    boosting immune system,
        165-166
    deficiencies, 160
    effectiveness, increasing,
        161-163
        selenium, 163
    fish oil supplements, 263
    food sources, 160-161
    preserving, 165
    preventing
        cancer, 165
        cataracts, 166
    RDA (Recommended Dietary
        Allowance), 5, 159
    safe dosage range, 20
    treating
        benign breast disease, 166
        diabetes, 166
        infertility, 158, 166
        intermittent claudication,
            167
        leg cramps, 167
        Parkinson's disease, 167
Vitamin K, 169-174, 336
    clotting factors, prothrombin,
        174
    deficiencies, 171-172
    effectiveness, increasing, 173
    food sources, 172-173
        seaweed, 173
    preventing osteoporosis, 174
    prothrombin (clotting factor),
        174
    RDA (Recommended Dietary
        Allowance), 5, 170-171
Vitamin K₁ (phylloquinone), 170
Vitamin K₂ (menaquinone), 170
Vitamin K₃ (menadione), 170
vitamin supplement warnings
        methotrexate (Folex® or
            Mexate®), 98
        phenytoin (Dilantin®), 101
        sulfasalazine (Azulfidine®),
            98
        trimethoprim (Proloprim®/
            Trimpex®), 98
vitamins
    deficiencies, testing for, 18
    definition, 4
    effect on enzymes, 4

effect on homones, 4
fat-soluable, 4
metrics (grams), measuring, 6
safe dosage ranges, 19-20
storing, 26
water-soluable, 4
vomiting, supplements recom-
    mended for magnesium, 198

## W-Z

warfarin (Coumadin®)
    coenzyme Q₁₀, 291
    Vitamin E, 160
    Vitamin K, 173
water
    magnesium content, 202
    with fiber, 310
water-soluble vitamins, 4, 336
Wernicke-Korsakoff syndrome, 60,
    336
    thiamin deficiency, 60
wild yam, 336
    progesterone, 300
Wilson's disease, 237
women, RDA (Recommended
    Dietary Allowance), 5

xanthine oxidase enzyme, 239
xanthophylls (carotenoids), 281,
    336

yams, wild, progesterone, 300

zeaxanthin (carotenoids), 282, 336
zinc, 207-214, 336
    boosting immune systems,
        211-212
    deficiencies, 208-209
    effectiveness, increasing, 211
    food sources, 209-210
    male hormone levels, 212
    preventing, prostate problems,
        212
    RDA (Recommended Dietary
        Allowance), 8, 208, 226
    safe dosage range, 20
    supplement guidelines
        alcohol use, 209
        breastfeeding, 209
        diabetes, 213
        high-fiber diet, 209
        infertility (male), 212
        macular degeneration, 214
        memory (improving), 214
        pregnancy, 209
        prostate problems, 212
        seniors (older adults), 209
        vegans, 209
        vegetarians, 209